Rajesh Gupta • Robert Matthews
Lev Bangiyev • Dinko Franceschi
Mark Schweitzer

PET/MR Imaging

A Case-Based Approach

Springer

Rajesh Gupta
Department of Radiology
Stony Brook University Hospital
Stony Brook, NY, USA

Robert Matthews
Department of Radiology
Stony Brook University Hospital
Stony Brook, NY, USA

Lev Bangiyev
Department of Radiology
Stony Brook University Hospital
Stony Brook, NY, USA

Dinko Franceschi
Department of Radiology
Stony Brook University Hospital
Stony Brook, NY, USA

Mark Schweitzer
Department of Radiology
Stony Brook University Hospital
Stony Brook, NY, USA

ISBN 978-3-319-65105-7 ISBN 978-3-319-65106-4 (eBook)
https://doi.org/10.1007/978-3-319-65106-4

Library of Congress Control Number: 2017953439

Printed on acid-free paper

This Springer imprint is published by Springer Nature
The registered company is Springer International Publishing AG
The registered company address is: Gewerbestrasse 11, 6330 Cham, Switzerland

PET/MR Imaging

To my wonderful wife, Priya, for her sweet love and encouragement that propels me. To my family, especially my father, Vipin, and my brother, Apar, for their continual support. In loving memory of my mother, Ankan, to whom I am forever grateful. To my mentors and coauthors for their commitment to lifelong learning.

Rajesh Gupta

Dedicated to all the Matthews and Stone family.

Robert Matthews

To my wife, Elina, and my children, Sharon and Alan, who are the purpose of life. Also, my parents, Yakov and Natalya, to whom I owe my life.

Lev Bangiyev

To my loving wife, Maja, and our wonderful children, Ana, Dora, Nika, and Dinko Domagoj, for their love, encouragement, and support. In memory of my parents, without whose guidance I would not be here today.

Dinko Franceschi

For my beautiful wife, Sheryl, for her love and support. For Shira and Daniel, for teaching me the importance of furthering our understanding of disease.

Mark Schweitzer

Foreword

PET is fundamentally a functional imaging technique that achieves high sensitivity for various physiological processes through injection of radiolabeled ligands that are analogs of endogenous compounds, or that have high affinity for specific molecular targets. Although many radiotracers have been developed and employed in research for a range of applications in normal and disease conditions, only a handful are currently approved for the clinic, and of these by far the most dominant is the glucose analog F18-fluorodeoxyglucose (FDG). FDG is treated similarly to glucose by the body up to and including the first step of glycolysis with phosphorylation by hexokinase, after which it is trapped within the cell, unable to proceed down the glycolytic pathway due to its substitution of fluorine for a hydroxyl group. Because FDG and glucose compete for transport into cells based on their relative proportions in plasma, it is beneficial to lower and stabilize blood glucose concentrations at baseline by fasting before injecting FDG. In addition, insulin levels should be at baseline to prevent FDG from being driven into skeletal and cardiac muscle. Uptake into malignant tissue is enhanced not only by the increased metabolic demands of proliferation but also by a general preference of cancerous cells for anaerobic glycolysis, even in the presence of sufficient oxygen, which provides less ATP than aerobic glycolysis for the same amount of glucose consumed, known as the Warburg effect [1].

Although FDG PET is highly sensitive to a wide range of cancer types, it generally provides limited structural information, has poorer spatial resolution, and involves a modest dose of ionizing radiation (~10 mSv). Moreover abnormalities are sometimes difficult to distinguish from normal uptake patterns and their variations, or other pathological conditions such as infection and inflammation which can result in high FDG uptake [2]. Similarly, benign lesions such as benign primary parotid tumors and thyroid adenomas can present with high focal uptake.

The advent of PET/CT was intended to improve both sensitivity and specificity compared to PET alone while providing vastly improved anatomical detail for localization purposes [3]. In this approach, the PET and CT systems are adjacent to each other in a single gantry and share the same patient bed, allowing a high degree of alignment between the detailed structural images from CT and the functional data from PET without the need for software coregistration. Moreover, the CT provides a fast and accurate method for correction of gamma-ray attenuation in PET. PET/CT is now the clinical standard and it is employed for initial staging, therapy response, surveillance of recurrence, as well as for prognostic purposes. Because molecular imaging such as PET can reflect metabolic changes, which occur on a faster time scale than anatomical changes, PET has also become an invaluable tool in the development and screening of cancer drug candidates [4].

A drawback of PET/CT is that the CT adds radiation dose to the PET procedure which already involves a modest radiation dose [5]. In fact, the dose from the CT portion alone can be multiples of that from the PET tracer. Thus, low-dose CT protocols have been developed which reduce the CT exposure [6] compared to fully diagnostic CT which is not always necessary. Another limitation of CT is poor soft tissue contrast, which can hinder adequate evaluation of structures in the head and neck, musculoskeletal, and pelvic regions.

Contrary to CT, MRI provides superb contrast among different soft tissue types and structural abnormalities by exploiting a multitude of pulse sequences to enhance different tissue properties, with or without the use of an exogenous contrast agent. The types of sequences are mainly divided between those that reflect T1 and T2 relaxation properties, with a large number of variations that, for example, suppress water and fat or reflect water diffusion. MRI excels at structural imaging with high spatial resolution and sensitivity. While functional modes such as fMRI have been developed and continue to be refined, they have not yet found widespread clinical application.

Thus, it has long been realized that PET/MRI could be an even more powerful combination of imaging modalities than PET/CT, with initial prototype systems developed starting in the 1990s and continuing to the present [7]. MRI involves no ionizing radiation and therefore PET/MRI introduces less potential long-term risk to the patient than PET/CT. MRI can provide multiple image sets within a single imaging session, each with unique contrast mechanisms. Also, MRI can be implemented in a simultaneous mode with PET, further optimizing the spatial alignment of the images and generating the possibility to assess multiple functional parameters at the same time which has substantial implications for brain imaging research.

But the close integration of PET and MRI was a much more daunting technical challenge than PET/CT. This is related to the vulnerability of traditional PET components to the strong static and rapidly fluctuating electromagnetic fields associated with MRI, and of MRI to susceptibility artifacts, eddy currents, and radiofrequency emission from PET hardware located within the field of view [7]. For example, the photosensors used in conventional PET scanners (photomultiplier tubes) are highly sensitive to magnetic fields and do not function at all in the strong static fields used in MRI. Fortunately, the introduction of robust and compact solid-state photodetectors, including avalanche photodiodes (APDs) and then silicon photomultipliers (SiPMs), has provided a chance to move forward more quickly with this imaging approach. Early clinical systems were sequential imagers, much like PET/CT, except that the PET and MRI gantries were separate, located at opposite ends of the patient bed to minimize cross-interference [8]. This allowed optimal performance of both modalities, and even time-of-flight capability in the Philips Ingenuity TF [9], with a minimum investment in technology development, but did not optimize the imaging efficiency as well as the PET/CT. In order to minimize total imaging time and enable the exploration of multiple functional measures at the same time, simultaneous PET/MRI approaches were developed. Siemens introduced the first simultaneous PET/MRI, the Biograph mMR [10], which is based on APD photosensors, providing PET with typical whole-body spatial resolution and long axial field of view (25 cm) inside a 3 T MRI. Subsequently GE introduced the Signa PET/MR based on SiPM photosensors [11], which has a similar geometry and performance, except that it is able to provide improved time resolution that allows time-of-flight (TOF) acquisition and processing to improve SNR [12]. All the cases in this book are from the Siemens Biograph mMR PET/MR scanner, although the clinical scenarios and challenges are similar for all PET/MRI systems.

Technical Challenges

Attenuation

A particular challenge for PET/MRI is the robust determination of PET attenuation correction using MRI data only (MR attenuation correction or MRAC). This correction has up to an order of magnitude effect on the PET data and is critical for quantitative and semi-quantitative (standardized uptake value or SUV) PET imaging. In PET/CT, the CT component provides accurate photon attenuation coefficients ("mu" values) at CT energies (~100 keV) which can be robustly scaled to PET energy (511 keV) with a bilinear approach (known as CTAC) [13]. However, MRI operates on an entirely different principle and cannot determine photon attenuation coefficients in a direct way.

The first and still most common MRAC approach is to use a Dixon MRI sequence to segment tissue into the two classes of fat and water, and then to assign their known attenuation coefficients (0.085 and 0.095 cm^{-1}, respectively) to produce the mu map of the patient. Unfortunately, the Dixon sequence cannot define bone which is known to have the highest mu value of ~0.15 cm^{-1}. Although this is somewhat mitigated by the fact that bone usually occupies only a small fraction of the imaging volume, regions near bone will be underestimated. Moreover the Dixon segmentation algorithm can reverse the tissue classes about 10% of the time [14], necessitating additional, usually manual measures to verify accuracy of the attenuation correction.

A newer approach uses an ultrashort echo time (UTE) approach to create a third class for bone. While this has been an improvement, this sequence is so far restricted to head and neck imaging and often underestimates bone and overestimates air cavities. Recent approaches involve comparing an optimized MRI sequence of the patient to an atlas or database of patients who have received both the MRI sequence and CT. While this seems to be the best approach so far for the brain, it is not clear how effective it will be for those with anatomy that is not well represented in the database, and its extension to body remains a challenge. Developing improved methods for MRAC remains an active research area [15].

A general problem in MRAC is truncation of the arms in MR images which can cause underestimation of attenuation if not accounted for.

Algorithmic methods like MLAA (maximum likelihood activity and attenuation) [16] attempt to add arms to the mu map based on consistency between the measured PET and mu map. However, this needs to be performed for each bed position and the result is not always stable. It can result in discontinuous artifacts in coronal whole-body PET images at the intersection of bed positions with disparate MLAA estimates of the arms.

Spatial Resolution

Another issue in simultaneous PET/MRI systems is the reduction of spatial resolution near the edges of the FOV due to the so-called parallax effect which becomes prominent when the PET detectors are close to the FOV. A typical PET/CT system has a patient opening of ~60 cm while the PET detectors are located at a much larger diameter of ~80–90 cm, in part to reduce the effects of parallax. But in simultaneous PET/MRI systems, the PET system must fit inside the confined bore of an MRI which implies that the detectors cannot be placed much farther away to reduce the parallax effect. Modern iterative image reconstruction approaches can mitigate this effect by incorporating the point spread function into the algorithm—while this can restore the resolution to some degree, there is a cost in image noise. One advantage though is that the small diameter reduces the number of detectors and increases the axial acceptance angle which improves detection sensitivity as well as cost.

Conclusion

Simultaneous PET and MRI technology is still relatively new to the clinic and has not yet reached full acceptance, in part due to its high cost but also due to limited large-scale prospective validation studies. The initial phase of adoption focused on clinical feasibility and the degree to which it was equivalent to PET/CT for detecting lesions. In the following years, PET/MRI developed to a stage where it is superior to PET/CT for some malignancies [17, 18] and has evolved into non-oncologic clinical applications such as assessment of neurodegenerative diseases. However, cultural and historical obstacles remain in the routine clinical adoption of PET/MR imaging. Cancer specialists have considerable training and experience with PET/CT, but not necessarily in the complex language of MRI, its benefits, variety of imaging sequences and contrast mechanisms, and its limitations such as new types of artifacts to be interpreted. This book is an attempt to introduce the nuances of PET/MR imaging to oncologists, radiologists, and other specialized physicians who are already familiar with PET/CT. Our hope is that a deeper understanding of PET/MRI, including its advantages and disadvantages, by practicing physicians will help place this new technology in the most effective role in patient care.

Department of Radiology and Biomedical Engineering
Stony Brook University Medical School,
Stony Brook, NY, USA

Paul Vaska, PhD

References

1. Bensinger SJ, Christofk HR. New aspects of the Warburg effect in cancer cell biology. Semin Cell Dev Biol. 2012;23:352–61.
2. Metser U, Even-Sapir E. Increased (18)F-fluorodeoxyglucose uptake in benign, nonphysiologic lesions found on whole-body positron emission tomography/computed tomography (PET/CT): accumulated data from four years of experience with PET/CT. Semin Nucl Med. 2007;37:206–22.
3. Wechalekar K, Sharma B, Cook G. PET/CT in oncology—a major advance. Clin Radiol. 2005;60:1143–55.
4. Kelloff GJ, Hoffman JM, Johnson B, Scher HI, Siegel BA, Cheng EY, et al. Progress and promise of FDG-PET imaging for cancer patient management and oncologic drug development. Clin Cancer Res. 2005;11:2785–808.
5. Fahey F, Stabin M. Dose optimization in nuclear medicine. Semin Nucl Med. 2014;44:193–201.
6. Xia T, Alessio AM, De Man B, Manjeshwar R, Asma E, Kinahan PE. Ultra-low dose CT attenuation correction for PET/CT. Phys Med Biol. 2012;57:309–28.
7. Vaska P, Cao T. The state of instrumentation for combined positron emission tomography and magnetic resonance imaging. Semin Nucl Med. 2013;43:11–8.
8. Cho ZH, Son YD, Kim HK, Kim KN, Oh SH, Han JY, et al. A fusion PET-MRI system with a high-resolution research tomograph-PET and ultra-high field 7.0 T-MRI for the molecular-genetic imaging of the brain. Proteomics. 2008;8:1302–23.
9. Zaidi H, Ojha N, Morich M, Griesmer J, Hu Z, Maniawski P, et al. Design and performance evaluation of a whole-body ingenuity TF PET-MRI system. Phys Med Biol. 2011;56:3091–106.
10. Delso G, Fürst S, Jakoby B, Ladebeck R, Ganter C, Nekolla SG, et al. Performance measurements of the Siemens mMR integrated whole-body PET/MR scanner. J Nucl Med. 2011;52:1914–22.
11. Grant AM, Deller TW, Khalighi MM, Maramraju SH, Delso G, Levin CS. NEMA NU 2–2012 performance studies for the SiPM-based ToF-PET component of the GE SIGNA PET/MR system. Med Phys. 2016;43:10.
12. Surti S. Update on time-of-flight PET imaging. J Nucl Med. 2015;56:98–105.
13. Kinahan PE, Hasegawa BH, Beyer T. X-ray-based attenuation correction for positron emission tomography/computed tomography scanners. Semin Nucl Med. 2003;33:166–79.
14. Ladefoged CN, Hansen AE, Keller SH, Holm S, Law I, Beyer T, et al. Impact of incorrect tissue classification in Dixon-based MR-AC: fat-water tissue inversion. EJNMMI Phys. 2014;1:101.
15. Ladefoged CN, Law I, Anazodo U, St. Lawrence K, Izquierdo-Garcia D, Catana C, et al. A multi-centre evaluation of eleven clinically feasible brain PET/MRI attenuation correction techniques using a large cohort of patients. Neuroimage. 2016;147:346–59.
16. Rezaei A, Defrise M, Bal G, Michel C, Conti M, Watson C, et al. Simultaneous reconstruction of activity and attenuation in time-of-flight PET. IEEE Trans Med Imaging. 2012;31:2224–33.
17. Heusch P, Nensa F, Schaarschmidt B, Sivanesapillai R, Beiderwellen K, Gomez B, et al. Diagnostic accuracy of whole-body PET/MRI and whole-body PET/CT for TNM staging in oncology. Eur J Nucl Med Mol Imaging. 2015;42:42–8.
18. Sher AC, Seghers V, Paldino MJ, Dodge C, Krishnamurthy R, Krishnamurthy R, et al. Assessment of sequential PET/MRI in comparison with PET/CT of pediatric lymphoma: a prospective study. AJR. Am J Roentgenol. 2016;206:623–31.

Preface

Clinical applications of PET/MR imaging have been rapidly emerging over the last several years, and the use of this modality is bound to gain momentum in the diagnosis and treatment of various diseases. As this is a relatively new endeavor in the clinical realm, there is a paucity of resources that compile a collection of high-quality PET/MRI cases. Starting a new undertaking frequently brings a level of uncertainty and anxiety. In such instances, we rely on references that can help us gain confidence and expertise. We created this book to provide a case-based overview of PET/MR imaging for the novice.

Interpretation of PET/MRI requires understanding of both PET and MRI findings. In comparison to the CT component of PET imaging, MRI is more complex to master and requires comprehension of various MR sequences that can be acquired.

This collection of PET/MRI cases includes both benign and malignant pathologies organized by organ systems. Each case starts with a brief clinical history that is followed by images. The diagnosis is then revealed with detailed imaging findings along with a discussion describing disease pathology, as well as PET and MRI imaging characteristics. Suggested further reading resources are provided to give readers an opportunity to delve deeper into the individual cases. The cases in this book have been gathered over several years and represent a spectrum of cases encountered in the everyday clinical setting.

This book is intended as an introduction to PET/MR imaging, especially for radiology and nuclear medicine residents, fellows, and practicing physicians, as well as clinicians across a variety of specialties. We hope that you will find this book informative and useful as the medical community continues to incorporate PET/MR imaging into clinical practice.

Stony Brook, NY, USA

Rajesh Gupta, MD
Robert Matthews, MD
Lev Bangiyev, DO
Dinko Franceschi, MD
Mark Schweitzer, MD

Acknowledgements

We express our gratitude to the physicians, technicians, nurses, and support staff within the Department of Radiology and Clinical Services at Stony Brook University Hospital for their dedication to their patients. We would also like to thank the editorial and development staff at Springer who made this book possible.

Contents

Contributors

James Bai, MD Department of Radiology, Stony Brook University Hospital, Stony Brook, NY, USA

Lev Bangiyev, DO Department of Radiology, Stony Brook University Hospital, Stony Brook, NY, USA

David Capaldi, MD, MBA Department of Radiology, Stony Brook University Hospital, Stony Brook, NY, USA

Matthew Comito, MD Department of Radiology, Stony Brook University Hospital, Stony Brook, NY, USA

Ana M. Franceschi, MD Department of Radiology, NYU Langone Medical Center, New York, NY, USA

Michael Goodman, BA Stony Brook University School of Medicine, Stony Brook University Hospital, Stony Brook, NY, USA

Amit Gupta, MD Department of Radiology, Stony Brook University Hospital, Stony Brook, NY, USA

Apar Gupta, MD, MBA Department of Radiation Oncology, Rutgers Cancer Institute of New Jersey, New Brunswick, NJ, USA

Rajesh Gupta, MD Department of Radiology, Stony Brook University Hospital, Stony Brook, NY, USA

Michael J. Hoch, MD Department of Radiology and Imaging Sciences, Emory University Hospital, Atlanta, GA, USA

Robert Matthews, MD Department of Radiology, Stony Brook University Hospital, Stony Brook, NY, USA

Frank Papik, BA Stony Brook University School of Medicine, Stony Brook University Hospital, Stony Brook, NY, USA

Anastasia Plaunova, MD Department of Radiology, Stony Brook University Hospital, Stony Brook, NY, USA

David Pouldar, MD Albany Medical Center, College of Medicine, Albany, NY, USA

Anuj Rajput, MD Department of Radiology, Stony Brook University Hospital, Stony Brook, NY, USA

Laura L. Rosenkrantz, BS, MS Stony Brook University School of Medicine, Stony Brook University Hospital, Stony Brook, NY, USA

Elham Safaie, MD Department of Radiology, Stony Brook University Hospital, Stony Brook, NY, USA

Christopher Shackles, DO Department of Radiology, Stony Brook University Hospital, Stony Brook, NY, USA

Priya Sharma, MD Department of Psychiatry, Parkwood Institute, Western University, London, ON, Canada

Timothy M. Shepherd, MD, PhD Department of Radiology, NYU Langone Medical Center, New York, NY, USA

Eric van Staalduinen, DO Department of Radiology, Stony Brook University Hospital, Stony Brook, NY, USA

Joseph R. Stein, DO Department of Radiology, Stony Brook University Hospital, Stony Brook, NY, USA

Dharmesh Tank, MD Department of Radiology, Stony Brook University Hospital, Stony Brook, NY, USA

Kelly Tisovic, MD Department of Neurology, Stony Brook University Hospital, Stony Brook, NY, USA

Jerrin Varghese, MD Department of Radiology, Stony Brook University Hospital, Stony Brook, NY, USA

Kavitha Yaddanapudi, MD Department of Radiology, Stony Brook University Hospital, Stony Brook, NY, USA

Mark K. Youssef, MD Department of Radiology, Stony Brook University Hospital, Stony Brook, NY, USA

Jingyu Zhou, MD Department of Radiology, Stony Brook University Hospital, Stony Brook, NY, USA

Abbreviations

ADC	Apparent diffusion coefficient
BLADE	Motion-insensitive multi-shot turbo spin echo sequence
CT	Computed tomography
DOTATATE	DOTA-octreotate (radiopharmaceutical)
DWI	Diffusion-weighted imaging
FDG	F-18-fluorodeoxyglucose (radiopharmaceutical)
FLAIR	Fluid-attenuated inversion recovery
FLASH	Fast low angle shot, spoiled gradient echo sequence
GRE	Gradient echo sequence
HASTE	Half-Fourier acquisition single-shot turbo spin-echo
MIP	Maximum intensity projection
MPRAGE	3D magnetization-prepared rapid acquisition GRE
MRI	Magnetic resonance imaging
PET	Positron emission tomography
SUV	Standardized uptake value
SWI	Susceptibility-weighted imaging
STIR	Short tau inversion recovery
True FISP	Fast imaging with steay-state free precession, gradient echo sequence
TSE	Turbo spin echo sequence
VIBE	Volumetric interpolated breath-hold examination

Part I

Musculoskeletal

Case 1
Recurrent High-Grade Sarcoma

Rajesh Gupta

History

A 74-year-old female with left lower leg sarcoma, treated by below-knee amputation, has a new palpable lump at the stump, concerning for recurrence (Fig. 1.1).

Diagnosis

Recurrent high-grade sarcoma

Findings

- Moderately well-circumscribed lesion at the medial aspect of the left stump which has low signal on T1-weighted images and intermediate signal on T2-weighted images (arrows).
- Post-contrast image demonstrates heterogeneously avid contrast enhancement, mostly peripheral (arrowheads).
- PET/MR fusion images show heterogeneous abnormal FDG uptake within this soft tissue lesion along the distal portion of the tibial stump consistent with recurrence.

Discussion

Sarcomas are malignant cancers that arise from mesenchymal origins. They can arise in the muscle, bone, fat, or connective tissue. Sarcomas most often present as a mass. There are various histopathological subtypes which manifest as different clinical presentations and diagnoses. It is important to assess the grade of the tumor as it impacts staging, prognostic, and treatment implications.

MR imaging is the primary modality of choice to evaluate sarcomas, especially those arising in the soft tissues. MR can reliably identify tumor depth beneath fascial planes, tumor size, growth, and internal signal characteristics. Generally, high-grade tumors show isointense signal on T1-weighted images, heterogeneously high signal on T2-weighted images, and heterogeneous enhancement on post gadolinium images. Poorly defined tumor margin and peritumoral contrast enhancement on MRI indicate a more invasive and aggressive tumor implying a higher-grade pathology.

FDG PET imaging can reliably distinguish between low-grade and high-grade sarcomas by

R. Gupta et al., *PET/MR Imaging*, https://doi.org/10.1007/978-3-319-65106-4_1

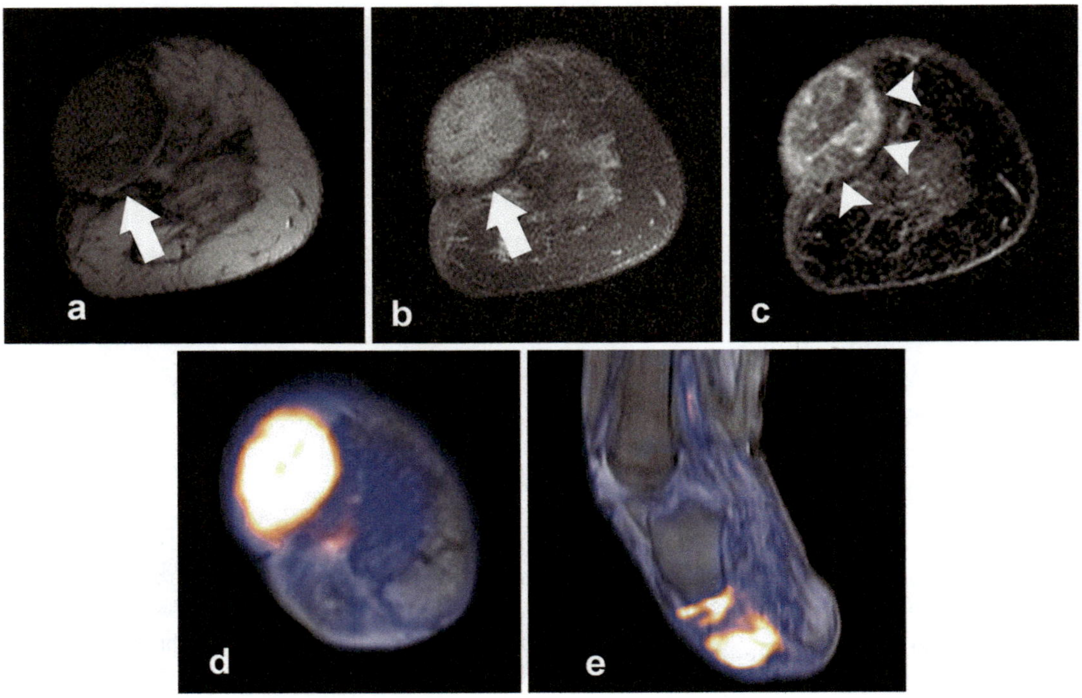

Fig. 1.1 T1 TSE axial of stump (**a**), T2 TSE with fat suppression axial of stump (**b**), T1 GRE with fat suppression post-gadolinium contrast axial of stump (**c**), PET/MR T1 VIBE axial fusion (**d**), and PET/MR T1 VIBE sagittal fusion of left knee (**e**)

the intensity of FDG uptake. FDG can detect small areas of high-grade differentiation in a large mass helping to direct biopsy targets. FDG PET is effectively used for sarcoma tumor staging and monitoring treatment response. Combined PET/MR provides excellent evaluation of the sarcoma tumor and surrounding soft tissues, as well as provides functional metabolic activity to aid in accurate tumor grading and staging. It can detect satellite lesions away from the main mass and distant metastases allowing for complete evaluation in one study.

Suggested Reading

Eary JF, Conrad EU. Imaging in sarcoma. J Nucl Med. 2011;52:1903–13.

Zhao F, Ahlawat S, Farahani SJ, Weber KL, Montgomery EA, Carrino JA, et al. Can MR imaging be used to predict tumor grade in soft-tissue sarcoma? Radiology. 2014;272:192–201.

Case 2
Bone Metastases from Lung Cancer

Rajesh Gupta

History

A 78-year-old female with lung cancer presents with bone pain (Fig. 2.1).

Diagnosis

Bone metastases from lung cancer (adenocarcinoma)

Findings

- STIR hyperintense signal at T11 vertebral body with increased signal on T1-weighted Dixon out-of-phase indicating lack of fat content.
- PET/MR image shows intense FDG uptake at T11 vertebral body (wide arrow).
- Similar hyperintense STIR signal at C7 vertebral body with increased FDG activity (curved arrow).

Discussion

Skeletal metastases arise from a variety of primary cancers, with the most prevalent being lung cancer, breast cancer, renal cell carcinoma, and prostate cancer. Metastases account for the majority of malignant bone tumors. They may be asymptomatic or cause localized bone pain. Complications include pathologic fractures, cord compression, and hyper- or hypocalcemia.

The goal of imaging in skeletal metastases is to detect metastases early, assess treatment response, and identify vertebrae with risk of fracture. It can also be useful in determining if fractures are causing spinal cord compression, which may need surgical intervention. MR imaging can detect metastatic bone marrow involvement very early on due to its high soft-tissue contrast and high spatial resolution. The T1-weighted and STIR sequences are excellent for marrow evaluation and eliminate the need for intravenous contrast in patients with poor renal function. T1-weighted images have the highest sensitivity at detecting vertebral metastases but low specificity. The addition of STIR somewhat increases the specificity. Generally, involved marrow will show low T1-weighted signal due to fatty marrow replacement by malignant cells with increased signal on STIR and T2 images. If contrast is given, these malignant lesions will demonstrate enhancement. Purely osteoblastic lesions demonstrate low signal on both T1 and T2-weighted images, as well as STIR sequences. Whole-body techniques to evaluate the skeleton in one session are gaining popularity.

The Dixon technique provides uniform fat and water separation that is resistant to inhomogeneity compared to chemical-shift fat-suppression techniques. It also has the advantage of faster scan times and maintaining image signal-to-noise ratio. Dixon MRI sequences provide an

R. Gupta et al., *PET/MR Imaging*, https://doi.org/10.1007/978-3-319-65106-4_2

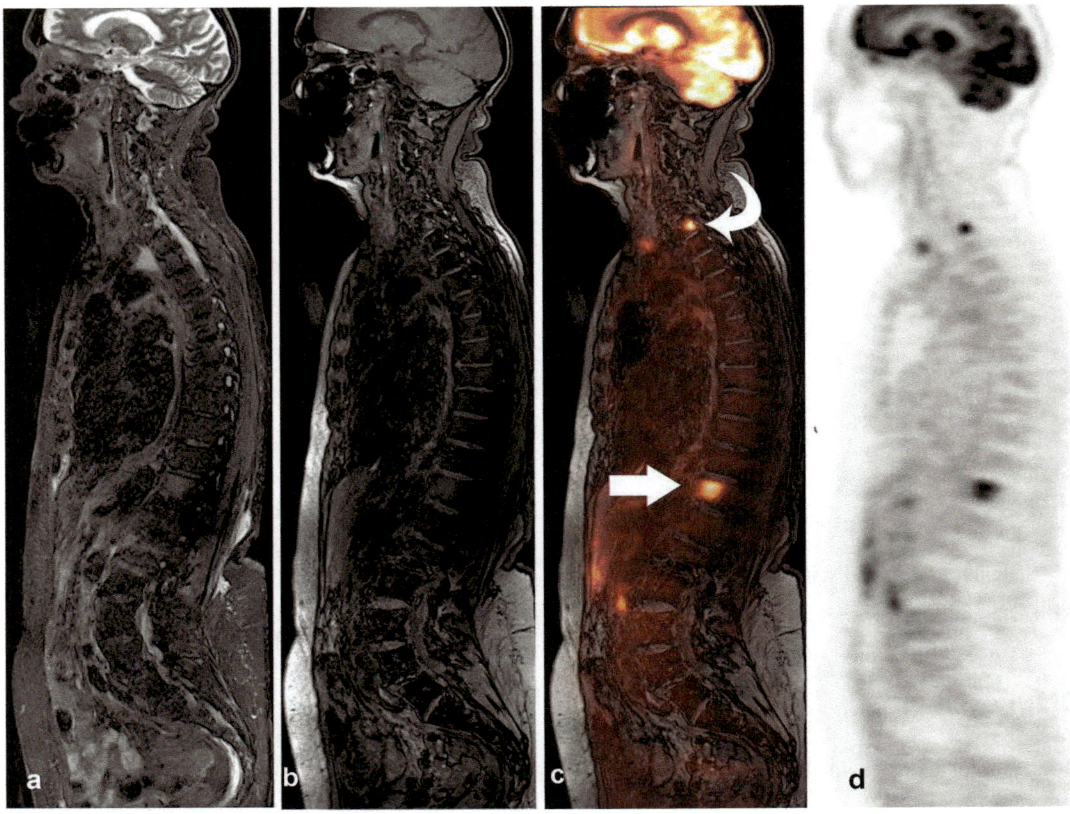

Fig. 2.1 STIR sagittal (**a**), Dixon T1-weighted out-of-phase sagittal (**b**), PET/MR Dixon T1-weighted out-of-phase sagittal fusion (**c**), and PET sagittal (**d**)

out-of-phase, in-phase image, fat-only, and water-only images. Metastatic bone lesions replace the bone marrow and do not drop on opposed-phase imaging. Dixon-based whole-body MRI has been shown to be specific and more sensitive than bone scan in detecting bone metastases, especially in breast cancer.

Overall MRI and PET imaging are roughly equal in sensitivity in detecting metastases. However, MRI has better resolution and can detect smaller lesions, while PET has the capability to effectively detect lesions on whole-body images. It can provide metabolic information related to the aggressiveness of the lesion and can determine whether the lesion is active following treatment. The use of FDG in PET/MR imaging allows for superior anatomic localization and functional assessment of malignant skeletal lesions and their response to therapy.

Suggested Reading

Costelloe CM, Kundra V, Ma J, Chasen BA, Rohren EM, Bassett RL Jr, et al. Fast Dixon whole-body MRI for detecting distant cancer metastasis: a preliminary clinical study. J Magn Reson Imaging. 2012;35(2):399–408.

Heindel W, Gübitz R, Vieth V, Weckesser M, Schober O, Schäfers M. The diagnostic imaging of bone metastases. Dtsch Arztebl Int. 2014;111(44):741–7.

O'Sullivan GJ, Carty FL, Cronin CG. Imaging of bone metastasis: an update. World J Radiol. 2015;7(8):202–11.

Case 3
Benign Notochordal Remnant

Rajesh Gupta

History

A 24-year old male with Hodgkin's lymphoma presents for restaging after treatment completion (Fig. 3.1).

Diagnosis

Benign notochordal remnant

Findings

- Well-circumscribed lesion within L3 vertebral body that is T1 hypointense and STIR hyperintense (thin arrow).
- No abnormal FDG activity associated with lesion.
- No evidence for bone expansion, destruction, or extraosseous extension.

Discussion

The notochord, in humans, is an embryonic structure that induces vertebral column formation and then disappears, leaving cellular remnants in the nucleus pulposus of the intervertebral discs. It is believed that notochord regression can arrest at any point, leaving notochordal cells along its course which can undergo hyperplasia. Notochordal remnants are occasionally found in the fetal and adult vertebrae on autopsy. Giant vertebral notochordal rest and notochordal hamartoma are terms that have been used to describe what is now collectively referred to as benign notochordal cell tumors. These tumors are intraosseous lesions of notochordal cell origin. It is important to distinguish this benign entity from chordoma, its malignant counterpart that also arises from notochordal cells.

There are several MR imaging features that can help distinguish a benign notochordal remnant from chordoma. Both arise in the midline and exhibit low to intermediate signal on T1 and high signal on T2-weighted images. However, chordomas usually enhance, are destructive and expansile, and can be associated with a soft tissue component. On the other hand, benign notochordal cell remnants are usually confined to bone without expansion and do not enhance following contrast administration.

Benign notochordal remnants will not show hypermetabolic activity on FDG-PET imaging. Chordomas most commonly arise in the sacrococcygeal region and have been described to demonstrate heterogeneously increased FDG uptake. Although benign notochordal remnants are likely to be an incidental finding, PET/MR imaging allows for thorough evaluation of these benign lesions to ensure that there is no malignant potential.

R. Gupta et al., *PET/MR Imaging*, https://doi.org/10.1007/978-3-319-65106-4_3

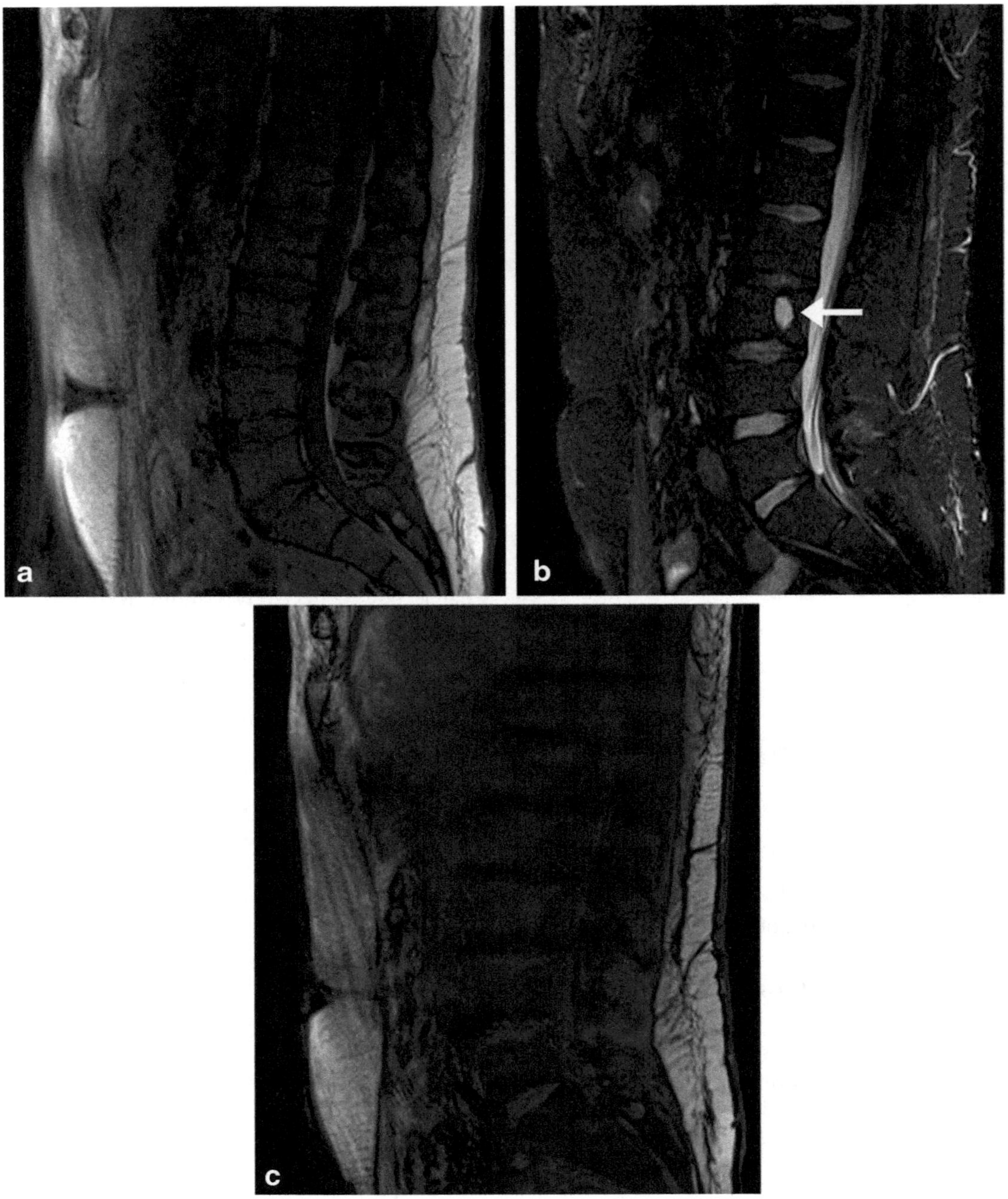

Fig. 3.1 Dixon T1-weighted fat-only sequence sagittal (**a**), STIR sagittal (**b**), and PET/MR STIR sagittal fusion image (**c**)

Suggested Reading

Kreshak J, Larousserie F, Picci P, Boriani S, Mirra J, Merlino B, et al. Difficulty distinguishing benign notochordal cell tumor from chordoma further suggests a link between them. Cancer Imaging. 2014;14:4.

Park SA, Kim HS. F-18 FDG PET/CT evaluation of sacrococcygeal chordoma. Clin Nucl Med. 2008;33(12):906–8.

Yamaguchi T, Iwata J, Sugihara S, McCarthy EF Jr, Karita M, Murakami H, et al. Distinguishing benign notochordal cell tumors from vertebral chordoma. Skelet Radiol. 2008;37(4):291–9.

Case 4
Ewing Sarcoma

Apar Gupta

History

A 13-year-old female with right knee pain radiating down the lateral side of the right lower leg (Fig. 4.1).

Diagnosis

Ewing sarcoma of the bone

Findings

- Large mass originating from the right proximal femur that is hyperintense on proton density and isointense on T1 imaging.
- Mass replaces the bone marrow of the right proximal fibula while permeating and destroying the bone cortex seen as areas of higher signal intensity within the dark cortex (arrowheads).
- Extensive infiltration of the mass into the surrounding soft tissue (curved arrows).
- Intense hypermetabolic activity on the fusion images compatible with malignancy.
- Periosteal reaction appearing as a hypointense double line at the bone cortex (thin arrow) on T2 images.
- Edematous changes are seen associated with the mass as T2 hyperintensities without FDG activity.

Discussion

Ewing sarcoma is the second most common malignant primary bone tumor of childhood, with the most common being osteosarcoma. It accounts for 3% of all pediatric cancers. Ewing sarcoma typically occurs between the ages of 4 and 25 years with a peak prevalence between the ages of 10 and 15 years. It has a slight predilection for male patients and marked predominance for Caucasians. It tends to affect the femur followed by the ilium, tibia, humerus, fibula, ribs, and sacrum. The most common presenting symptom is pain localized to the site of the tumor. Ewing sarcoma is a small round blue cell tumor with a karyotype abnormality of a translocation involving chromosomes 11 and 22. It shares this translocation and microscopic features with other Ewing sarcoma family tumors such as primitive neuroectodermal tumor and Askin tumor. Treatment involves systemic chemotherapy with either surgery, radiation, or both. Ewing sarcoma can be aggressive with up to 30% of cases demonstrating metastatic disease at presentation, most commonly to the bone, liver, or lung.

On imaging, Ewing sarcoma typically presents with a moth-eaten destructive permeative pattern and lucent bone lesions on conventional radiographs. It is often associated with a large soft tissue component. MRI reveals marrow replacement, cortical destruction, and a circum-

R. Gupta et al., *PET/MR Imaging*, https://doi.org/10.1007/978-3-319-65106-4_4

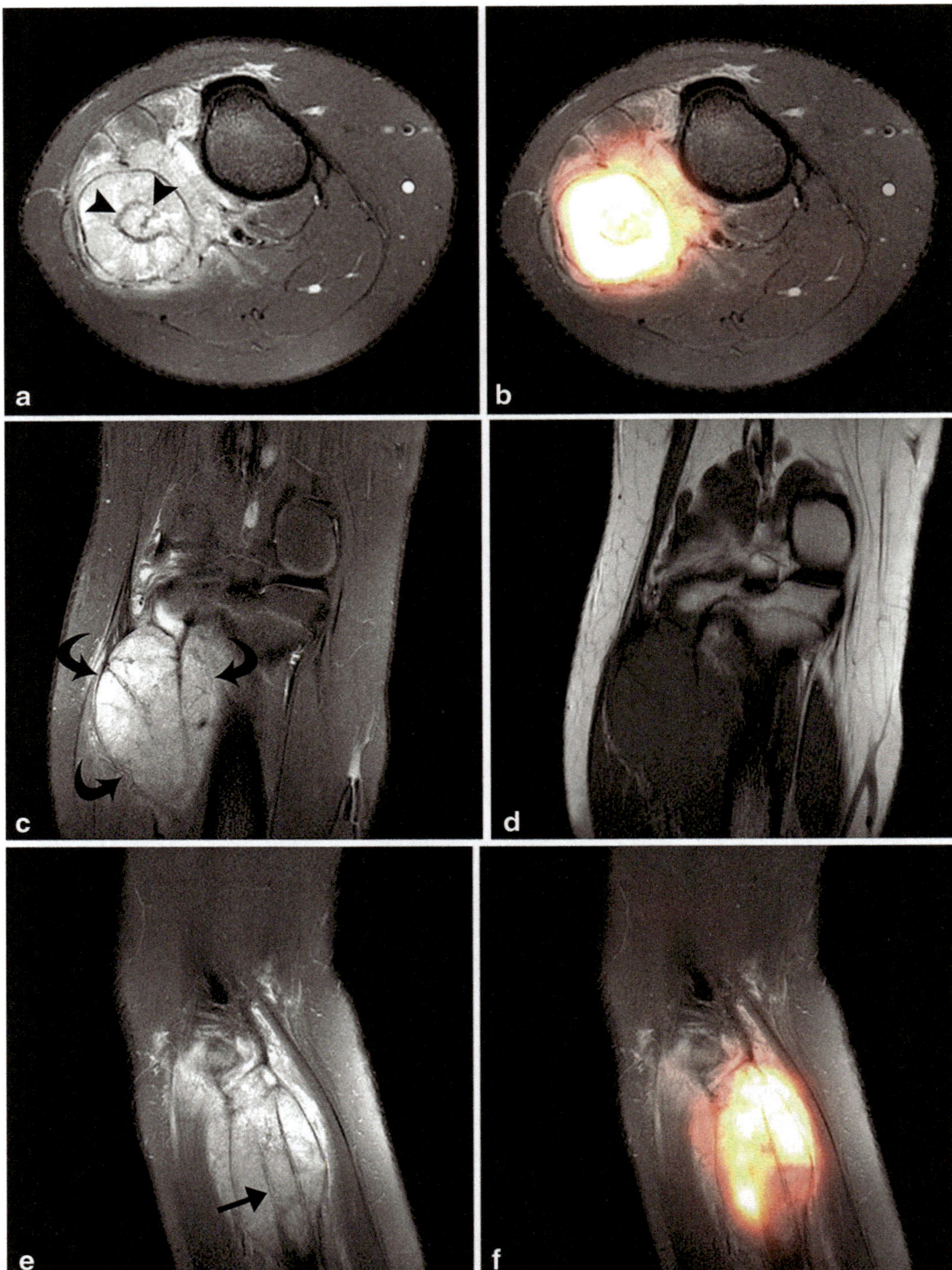

Fig. 4.1 Proton density with fat suppression axial (**a**), FDG PET/MR proton density with fat suppression axial fusion (**b**), Proton density with fat suppression coronal (**c**), T1 TSE coronal (**d**), T2 with fat suppression sagittal (**e**), and PET/MR T2 with fat suppression sagittal fusion (**f**)

ferential soft tissue mass. It is usually homogenous and low to intermediate signal intensity on T1-weighted images. On T2-weighted images, it is typically low to intermediate signal intensity due to its high degree of cellularity. High signal on T2-weighted and proton density (shared T1 and T2 weighting) images predominates in larger lesions and may represent hemorrhage or necrosis. In addition, linear low T2-weighted signal striations can be seen as the tumor extends through the Haversian canals and neurovascular channels of the cortex. The tumor enhances avidly post-contrast administration.

FDG PET provides unique information in regard to the metabolic activity of Ewing sarcomas. The functional information obtained by PET can estimate histologic tumor grade which is helpful to stage, restage, and assess treatment response in patients. FDG PET can help predict patient prognosis before and after neoadjuvant therapy. FDG PET has been shown to be superior to other modalities in detecting lymph node or osseous metastases as well as identifying tumor recurrence. Because the biochemical properties of the tumor change earlier than its morphology, functional information obtained by PET imaging can determine response to treatment. FDG PET combined with MR is useful in surgical planning as it can help delineate tumor margins. PET/MR imaging allows for superior evaluation of Ewing sarcomas as it provides important physiological information and accurate anatomical localization.

Suggested Reading

Bestic JM, Peterson JJ, Bancroft LW. Use of FDG PET in staging, restaging, and assessment of therapy response in Ewing sarcoma. Radiographics. 2009;29(5):1487–500.

Murphey MD, Senchak LT, Mambalam PK, Logie CI, Klassen-Fischer MK, Kransdorf MJ. From the radiologic pathology archives: Ewing sarcoma family of tumors: radiologic-pathologic correlation. Radiographics. 2013;33(3):803–31.

Case 5
Multiple Myeloma

Rajesh Gupta

History

A 57-year-old male presents with severe back pain (Fig. 5.1).

Diagnosis

Multiple myeloma

Findings

- Innumerable STIR hyperintense lesions throughout the spine with mild heterogenous FDG uptake.
- Mild hypermetabolic activity associated with compression fractures at T6 and T7 vertebral bodies with mild retropulsion leading to spinal canal stenosis (arrows).
- No evidence for spinal cord compression.

Discussion

Multiple myeloma is the most common primary bone malignancy. Myeloma occurs mostly in the elderly and is the second most common hematologic malignancy after non-Hodgkin lymphoma. It arises in the red marrow and involves monoclonal proliferation of mature plasma cells. Multiple myeloma is more prevalent in males and people of African descent. The common signs and symptoms include anemia, bone pain, renal insufficiency, fatigue, hypercalcemia, and weight loss. The overall 5-year survival is poor, despite current therapeutic options.

The use of MR and FDG PET in multiple myeloma has been increasing as these modalities provide information to detect early bone involvement, differentiate precursor lesions from true multiple myeloma, better define lytic lesions, detect extramedullary disease, predict prognosis, and assess response to treatment. Bone marrow involvement in multiple myeloma includes tumor replacement of fat which manifests as decreased T1-weighted signal intensity and increased T2-weighted or STIR signal. Out-of-phase imaging is particularly useful to detect early marrow involvement. MR imaging patterns of marrow involvement include normal marrow, a micronodular pattern (variegated or salt-and-pepper appearance), focal pattern, or diffuse infiltration. Lesions can also show contrast enhancement, although contrast-enhanced sequences are not generally performed as these patients are at a higher risk of having renal insufficiency.

FDG PET has been shown to have increased sensitivity in detecting bone marrow lesions which show mild to moderate increased FDG uptake. PET can also provide prognostic information as it has been shown that the presence of three or more FDG-avid osseous lesions on PET

R. Gupta et al., *PET/MR Imaging*, https://doi.org/10.1007/978-3-319-65106-4_5

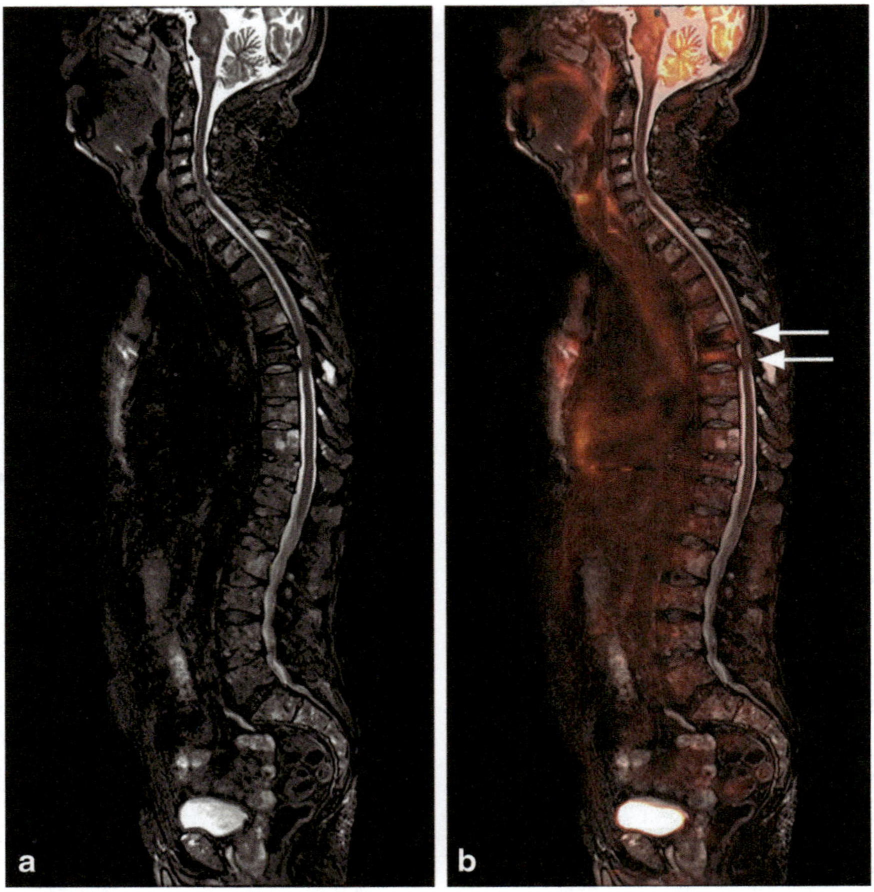

Fig. 5.1 STIR sagittal (**a**) and PET/MR STIR sagittal fusion (**b**)

imaging or maximum SUV over 4.2 in a single lesion was associated with a worse overall survival in multiple myeloma patients. Higher maximum SUV values have also been used to predict pathologic fractures in these patients. FDG PET/MR can be used to assess response to chemotherapy or stem cell therapy by showing decreasing FDG uptake. It is also useful in detecting residual or recurrent disease.

Suggested Reading

Ferraro R, Agarwal A, Martin-Macintosh EL, Peller PJ, Subramaniam RM. MR imaging and PET/CT in diagnosis and management of multiple myeloma. Radiographics. 2015;35(2):438–54.

Hanrahan CJ, Christensen CR, Crim JR. Current concepts in the evaluation of multiple myeloma with MR imaging and FDG PET/CT. Radiographics. 2010;30(1):127–42.

Case 6
Osteomyelitis

Rajesh Gupta

History

A 68-year-old diabetic female with a nonhealing left hallux valgus ulcer (Fig. 6.1).

Diagnosis

Osteomyelitis

Findings

- Hyperintense T1 signal involving the first proximal and distal phalanxes extending across the interphalangeal joint consistent with osteomyelitis (white arrow).
- Hyperintense STIR signal (asterisk) involving the first proximal and distal phalanxes compared to the normal marrow of the tarsal bones. A large plantar ulcer is also seen.
- Plantar surface ulcer with adjacent STIR hyperintensity involving the subcutaneous tissues consistent with soft tissue cellulitis (arrowheads).
- PET/MRI fusion image showing intense hypermetabolic FDG activity compatible with bone and soft tissue infection.
- PET images show area of absent of radiotracer uptake indicating necrosis (black arrow).

Discussion

Osteomyelitis is an infection of the bone typically due to a bacterial infection. Other less common pathogens include tuberculosis, syphilis, and fungal etiologies. In adults, it usually results from contiguous spread, often from a diabetic ulcer, of infection. Other routes of spread include hematogenous (more often in children and spinal infections) and postoperative.

The current modality of choice to diagnose osteomyelitis is MRI, which can determine the extent of osseous and soft tissue involvement. The simplest method of confirming osteomyelitis on MRI is to identify a deep ulcer or a sinus tract from a foot ulcer that leads to the bone surface and determine the signal characteristics of the underlying bone marrow. Findings of low T1-weighted signal, high STIR signal, and post-contrast marrow enhancement confirm the presence of osteomyelitis. MRI can also help evaluate associated soft tissue findings such as foreign bodies, abscesses, and soft tissue involvement. Chronic bone infection changes make MRI interpretation more difficult, and distinguishing diabetic foot with Charcot arthropathy from bone infection on MRI is a modest challenge.

FDG PET is emerging as an effective way to diagnose osteomyelitis providing higher-resolution tomographic images and in combination with MR

R. Gupta et al., *PET/MR Imaging*, https://doi.org/10.1007/978-3-319-65106-4_6

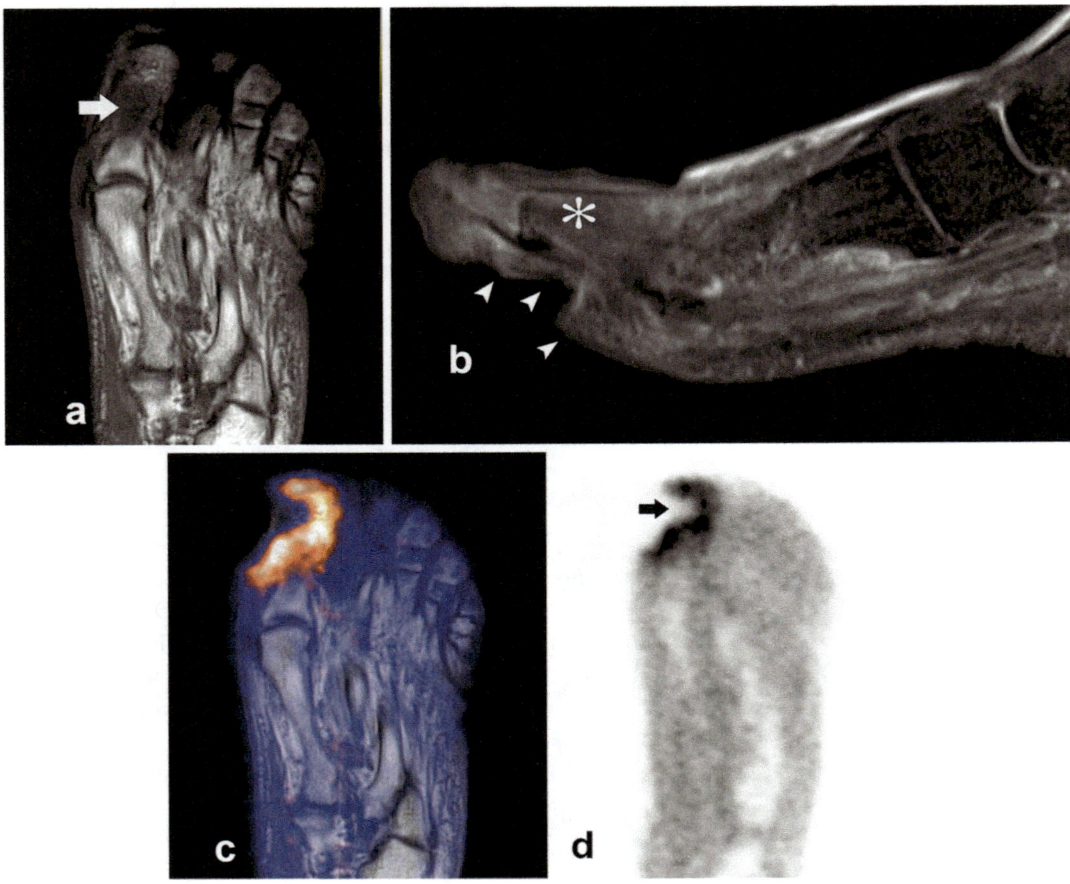

Fig. 6.1 T1-weighted axial (**a**), STIR sagittal (**b**), PET/MRI T1-weighted axial fusion (**c**), and PET axial (**d**)

anatomical location of the infection site. Multiple studies have determined high accuracy of FDG PET in the diagnosis of osteomyelitis being superior to other nuclear medicine procedures including bone scan, gallium scan, and the labeled white blood cells. FDG PET has a potential advantage over MRI in the diagnosis of osteomyelitis superimposed on Charcot arthropathy and postoperative infections. Combined use of both, FDG PET and MRI, offers benefits of obtaining high sensitivity for the presence of infection by PET and exact location of infection by MRI due to superior tissue resolution.

Suggested Reading

Donovan A, Schweitzer ME. Use of MR imaging in diagnosing diabetes-related pedal osteomyelitis. Radiographics. 2010;30:723–36.

Glaudemans AWJM, Quintero AM, Signore A. PET/MRI in infectious and inflammatory diseases: will it be a useful improvement? Eur J Nucl Med Mol Imaging. 2012;39:745–9.

Kagna O, Srour S, Melamed E, Militianu D, Keidar Z. FDG PET/CT imaging in the diagnosis of osteomyelitis in the diabetic foot. Eur J Nucl Med Mol Imaging. 2012;39:1545–50.

Case 7
Malignant Soft Tissue Myxofibrosarcoma

Rajesh Gupta

History

A 57-year-old female treated for myxofibrous sarcoma presents with suspected recurrence in the left leg (Fig. 7.1).

Diagnosis

Malignant soft tissue myxofibrosarcoma

Findings

- T1-weighted image shows a mildly hyperintense lesion in the musculature posterior to the left fibula (arrowheads).
- T2-weighted images show the lesion to be isointense to the muscle, irregular, and somewhat heterogeneous.
- PET/MR fusion shows a prominent hypermetabolic focus in the musculature posterior to the left fibula compatible with malignancy.
- After gadolinium administration, the lesion shows heterogeneous enhancement with infiltration along the fascial planes (thin arrows).

Discussion

Myxofibrosarcoma is an aggressive soft tissue neoplasm that is classified as a type of malignant fibrohistiocytic tumor. It exhibits high local recurrence and metastatic rate. It commonly presents in the sixth decade as a painless soft tissue mass within the extremities.

On MRI, the myxoid component of myxofibrosarcoma is often low in signal on T1-weighted images and high on T2-weighted and STIR sequences. On T1-weighted post-contrast imaging, the myxoid component typically does not enhance, while the surrounding tumoral and reactive tissue may enhance. T2-weighted and gadolinium-enhanced sequences are the best at evaluating the infiltrative pattern of myxofibrosarcoma.

This tumor characteristically spreads along fascial planes, often outside of the primary tumor focus. Given this type of spread, MRI alone may not be adequate in delineating the surgical margin. A subset of patients with superficial fascial infiltration will show a characteristic "tail-like" pattern on contrast-enhanced images which is associated with a poorer prognosis.

R. Gupta et al., *PET/MR Imaging*, https://doi.org/10.1007/978-3-319-65106-4_7

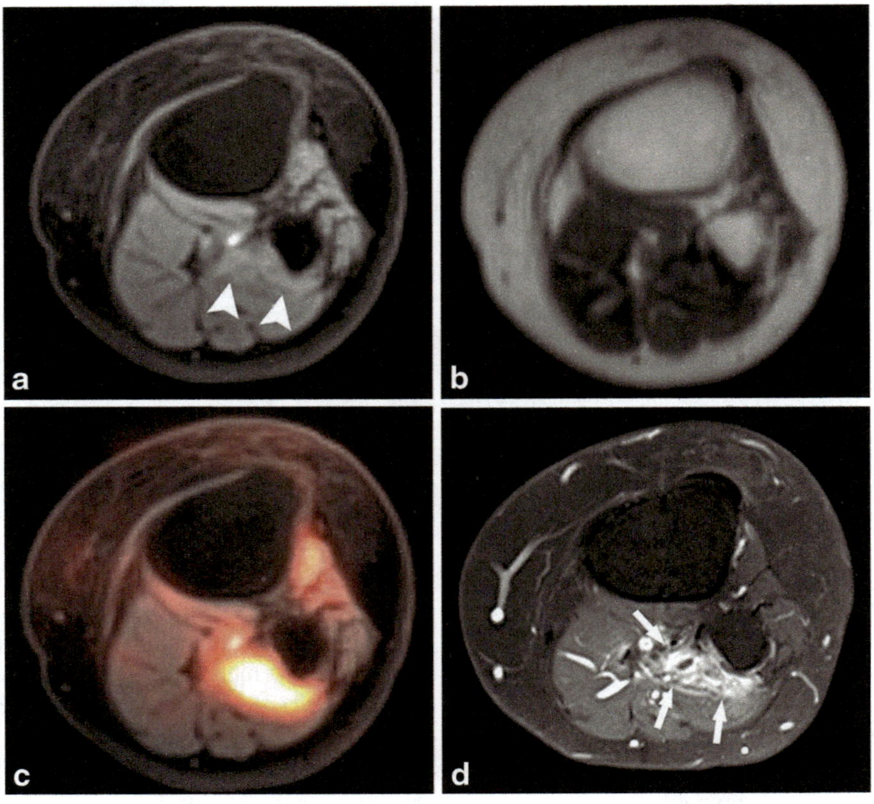

Fig. 7.1 T1 radial VIBE with fat suppression axial (**a**), T2 HASTE axial (**b**), PET/MR T1 radial VIBE with fat suppression axial fusion (**c**), and T1 TSE with fat suppression post-gadolinium contrast (**d**)

The usefulness of FDG PET in evaluation of primary and recurrent sarcomas depends on tumor grading with almost all intermediate and high-grade lesions demonstrating increased FDG activity. Low-grade tumors may have only subtle FDG uptake. This makes it difficult to differentiate low-grade myxofibrosarcomas from other benign lesions. The myxoid component of the tumor often causes a heterogeneous pattern of FDG uptake. The combination of PET/MR is helpful in determining the extent of local infiltration, define surgical margins, and detect small satellite lesions. PET/MR is also useful in monitoring response to local and systemic therapy.

Suggested Reading

Ioannidis JP, Lau J. 18F-FDG PET for the diagnosis and grading of soft-tissue sarcoma: a meta-analysis. J Nucl Med. 2003;44:717–24.

Kaya M, Wada T, Nagoya S, Sasaki M, Matsumura T, Yamaguchi T, et al. MRI and histological evaluation of the infiltrative growth pattern of myxofibrosarcoma. Skelet Radiol. 2008;37:1085–90.

Kikuta K, Kubota D, Yoshida A, Morioka H, Toyama Y, Chuuman H, et al. An analysis of factors related to the tail-like pattern of myxofibrosarcoma seen on MRI. Skelet Radiol. 2015;44:55–62.

Case 8 Vertebral Body Hemangioma

Rajesh Gupta

History

A 58-year-old male presents with mild back pain (Fig. 8.1).

Diagnosis

Vertebral body hemangioma

Findings

- STIR images show a rounded, almost popcorn-shaped region of increased signal within the L3 vertebral body lesion.
- PET images demonstrate no abnormal radiotracer uptake with the L3 lesion
- T1 radial VIBE image demonstrates low signal with fat suppression (black arrow).
- T1 VIBE post gadolinium image shows homogenous enhancement (white arrow).
- Dixon fat sequence shows the presence of fat within L3 vertebral body lesion (curved arrow).

Discussion

Hemangiomas are benign vascular tumors that can occur in a variety of soft tissues and bone. Vertebral body hemangiomas are common throughout the thoracolumbar spine with a reported incidence of 11% based on autopsy studies. They are often multiple in the spine and typically limited to the vertebral body. Rarely, they can extend into or arise from the posterior elements. Atypical and aggressive hemangiomas can behave differently and hence have more atypical imaging characteristics.

On MR imaging, vertebral body hemangiomas typically show increased T1-weighted signal due to intralesional fat. The lesions demonstrate decreased signal on fat suppression sequences. They also have increased T2-weighted and STIR signal due to their high water content. They may enhance post gadolinium as hemangiomas can be highly vascular. In- and out-of-phase imaging may be used to detect microscopic fat in atypical appearing hemangiomas. Although both hemangiomas and malignant lesions have high T2 and STIR signals, most malignant lesions are low T1 signal and replace the fat containing marrow.

On FDG PET, most vertebral body hemangiomas have normal radiotracer uptake or less commonly appear as a photopenic region within the vertebral body. Atypical hemangiomas may demonstrate mild uptake that is often heterogenous. Because hemangiomas can enhance, in a patient with cancer history, FDG PET/MR can be helpful in confirming the benign nature of a hemangioma by demonstrating that the lesion has no metabolic activity. While mild FDG uptake may be seen in both

R. Gupta et al., *PET/MR Imaging*, https://doi.org/10.1007/978-3-319-65106-4_8

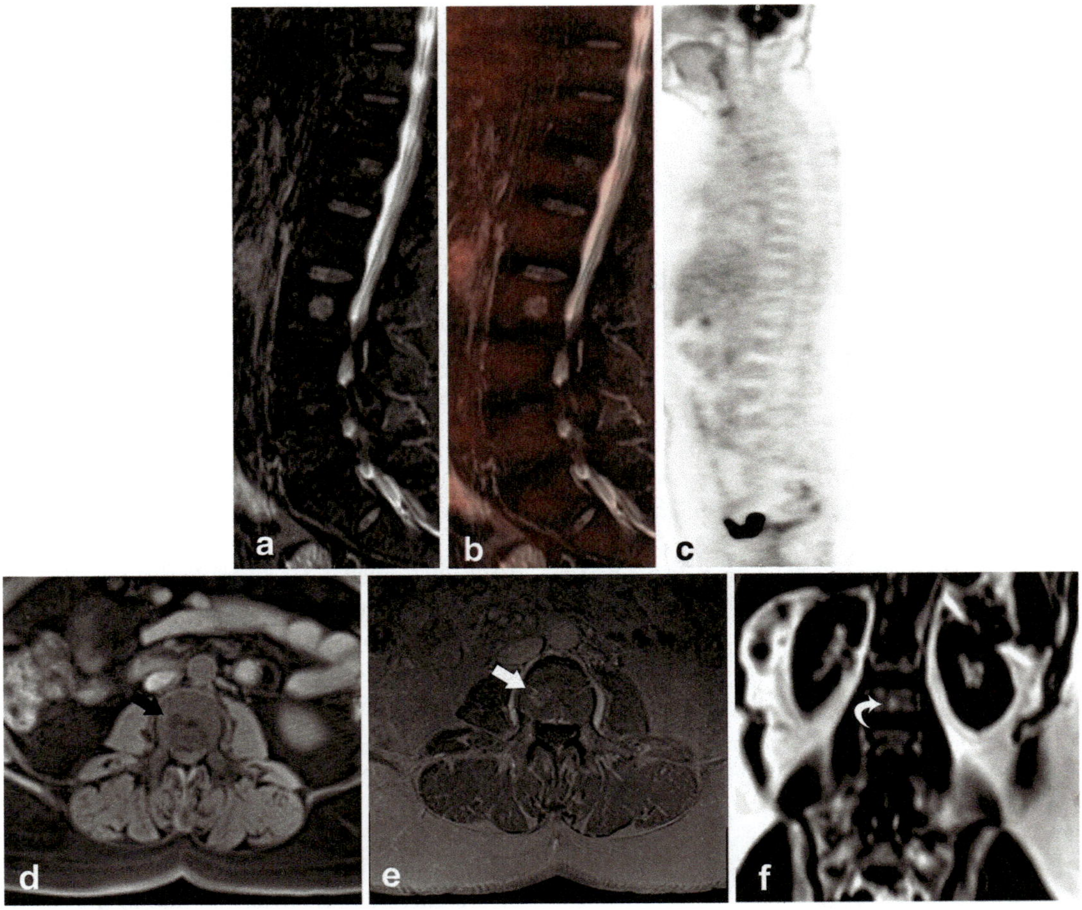

Fig. 8.1 STIR sagittal (**a**), PET/MR STIR sagittal (**b**), PET sagittal (**c**), T1 radial VIBE with fat suppression axial of L3 vertebra (**d**), T1 VIBE post-gadolinium contrast axial of L3 vertebra (**e**), and Dixon T1-weighted fat sequence coronal (**f**)

atypical hemangiomas and sclerotic metastatic bone lesions, the MRI findings are different with sclerotic lesions showing markedly low T1- and low T2-weighted signals.

Suggested Reading

Bybel B, Raja S. Vertebral hemangiomas on FDG PET scan. Clin Nucl Med. 2003;28:522–3.

Ross JS, Masaryk TJ, Modic MT, Carter JR, Mapstone T, Dengel FH. Vertebral hemangiomas: MR imaging. Radiology. 1987;165:165–9.

Case 9
Therapy-Induced Marrow Changes

Rajesh Gupta

History

A 20-year-old female with Hodgkin lymphoma, presents following chemotherapy and chest radiation (Fig. 9.1). The patient also has autoimmune hemolytic anemia treated with multiple blood tranfusions.

Diagnosis

Therapy-induced bone marrow changes

Findings

- Hypermetabolic foci involving T11, L4, and S1 vertebrae representing malignant marrow infiltration (white arrowheads). Other milder foci are seen in the cervical spine and T1 vertebra.
- Low diffuse STIR signal in multiple vertebrae including L1 through L3 due to iron deposition from blood transfusions. These vertebrae show mild FDG activity from benign red marrow stimulation.
- Heterogeneous STIR signal at L5 vertebra represents a healed neoplastic lesion which is undergoing fat conversion (thin white arrow). Other treated vertebrae are seen including T9 and T12.
- Extensive hypermetabolic retroperitoneal adenopathy consistent with malignancy (curve white arrow).
- Large volume pelvic ascites with high STIR signal no FDG uptake (black asterisk). The bladder located inferior to the ascites has intense FDG activity due to physiological urinary excretion.

Discussion

Normal bone marrow is composed of red and yellow marrow, with red marrow containing a majority of hematopoietic cells and yellow marrow consisting of a majority of fat cells. During infancy, the majority of marrow is hematopoietic, and a normal red to yellow marrow conversion takes place beginning peripherally in the phalanges and proceeding centrally to the axial skeleton (spine, pelvis, ribs, and skull). By the age of 25, most of the red marrow is limited to the axial skeleton with yellow marrow located in the appendicular skeleton. In the adult, residual appendicular red marrow can be seen in the proximal humeri and neck of femurs. During vertebral red to yellow marrow conversion, focal deposits of yellow marrow can be seen around the basivertebral vein, at the endplates, at the anterior and posterior margins, or scattered throughout the vertebral body. Yellow marrow can reconvert to red marrow as a physiological response to increased hematopoietic needs

R. Gupta et al., *PET/MR Imaging*, https://doi.org/10 1007/978-3-319-65106-4_9

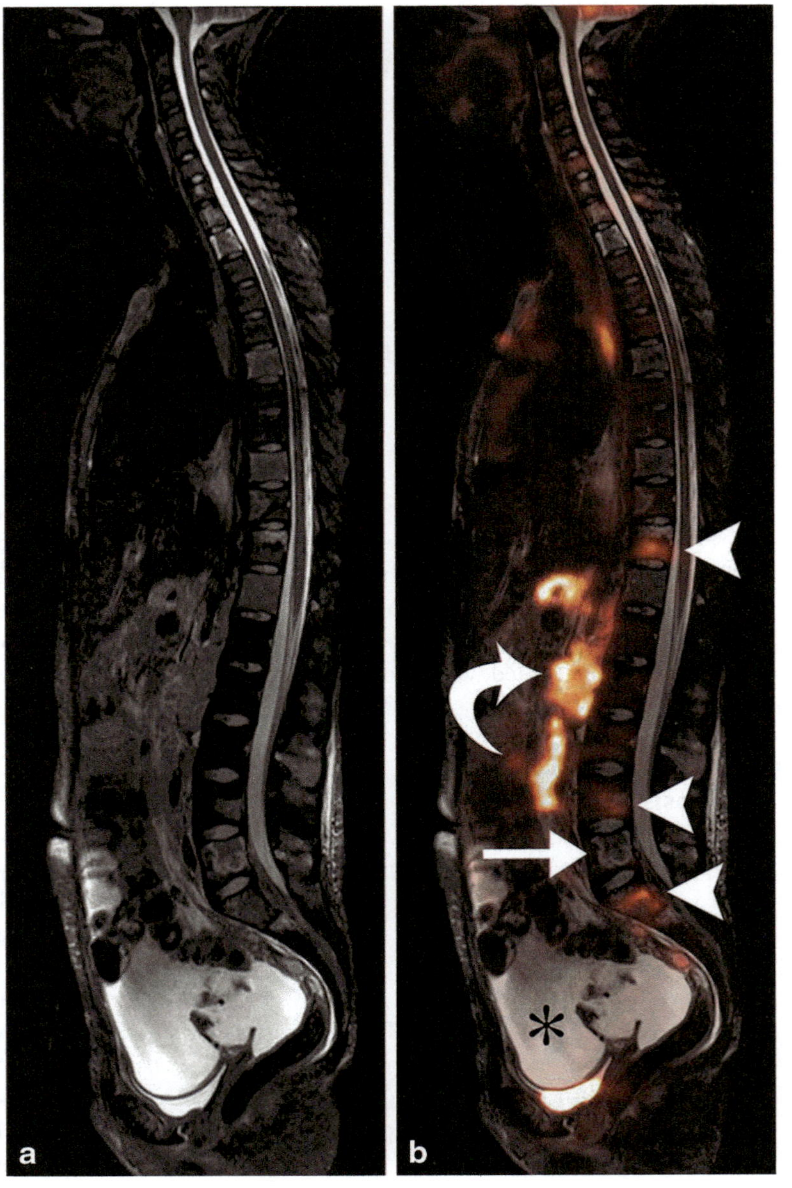

Fig. 9.1 STIR sagittal (**a**), and PET/MR STIR sagittal fusion (**b**)

and oxygen debt in the body, for example, in heavy tobacco smokers, endurance sports, obesity, chronic anemic conditions, and patients treated with hematopoietic growth factors.

The varying distribution of fat and nonfat cellular components in marrow provides for different MR imaging features. T1-weighted sequences are the most sensitive in evaluating bone marrow changes as the signal is easily influenced by fat. Bone marrow signal intensity is determined in relation to skeletal muscle or intervertebral disc signal. In adults, with predominately yellow marrow, the high fat content and low cellularity demonstrate relatively high signal on T1-weighted images and low signal on STIR and fat-suppressed T2-weighted images. Conversely, red marrow exhibits lower relative T1 and higher T2-weighted and STIR signal intensity. As red to yellow conversion occurs, gradual changes in T1 and T2-weighted signal intensity of vertebral bodies take place to reflect the change in cellular components.

Neoplastic infiltration of bone marrow results in replacement of the fatty marrow with tumor cells resulting in decreased Dixon T1-weighted in-phase and increased T2-weighted marrow signal. The distribution of neoplastic bone marrow involvement may be focal, multifocal, or diffuse. Both radiation treatment and chemotherapy have similar effects on marrow signal. In the acute period, they induce bone marrow edema leading to low T1 and high T2-weighted and STIR signal. However, the bone marrow eventually undergoes fatty replacement characterized by high T1-weighted signal close to subcutaneous fat signal and low fat-suppressed T2-weighted and STIR signals. During the post-treatment course, the bone marrow can undergo focal areas of hemorrhage. Depending on the radiation dose, the fatty conversion is often irreversible. With chemotherapy, the bone marrow can normalize with regeneration of normal hematopoietic cells in a multifocal pattern. Red blood cell transfusion therapy, administration of granulocyte colony-stimulating factor, and stem cell transplant treatment can all be accompanied by iron overload which can deposit into bone marrow and lead to diffusely decreased signal on T1, T2, and STIR sequences.

PET/MRI allows for the evaluation of benign or malignant processes within the bone marrow. It provides for precise anatomic localization, high contrast and spatial resolution, and accurate quantification of metabolic activity. Active red marrow conversion is a benign process that can have increased FDG uptake which varies based on age and level of marrow function. Likewise, malignant marrow infiltration will also usually have increased FDG uptake. Cytokine therapy can also induce increased bone marrow FDG activity. Although PET/MR imaging is a powerful tool that can help elucidate bone marrow changes, correlation with clinical history and treatment timing is essential.

Suggested Reading

Blebea JS, Houseni M, Torigian DA, Fan C Mavi A, Zhuge Y, et al. Structural and functional imaging of normal bone marrow and evaluation of its age-related changes. Semin Nucl Med. 2007;37(3):185–94.

Daldrup-Link HE, Henning T, Link TM. MR imaging of therapy-induced changes of bone marrow. Eur Radiol. 2007;17(3):743–61.

Małkiewicz A, Dziedzic M. Bone marrow reconversion - imaging of physiological changes in bone marrow. Pol J Radiol. 2012;77(4):45–50.

Case 10
Benign Spinal Cord Compression

David Pouldar and Robert Matthews

History

A 57-year-old male with pancreatic cancer treated with radiation and chemotherapy undergoes restaging (Fig. 10.1).

Diagnosis

Benign spinal cord compression

Findings

- Focal narrowing of the spinal canal consistent with spinal stenosis due to degenerative intervertebral disk disease resulting in mild compression of the spinal cord (arrow).
- Abnormal increased spinal cord signal on STIR represents either edema or myelomalacia.
- No abnormal FDG uptake within the spine to suggest malignancy. Generalized decreased FDG marrow activity within C4 through C7 and at the superior T1 vertebrae compatible with radiation therapy.

Discussion

Benign spinal cord compression is most commonly due to degenerative disk-osteophyte complexes or nucleus pulposus herniation into the epidural space, indenting the thecal sac, and resulting in spinal canal stenosis. Other causes of benign compression include posttraumatic subluxation or listhesis, infection, inflammation, variety of cysts, or benign tumors such as meningioma or nerve sheath tumor. The symptoms of benign spinal cord compression can include sudden or insidious onset of neurological deficits.

Spinal cord compression related to metastases usually denotes disseminated disease and is a common yet dreaded complication of cancer. Spine involvement occurs in 5–14% of cancer patients with more than 20,000 new patients in the USA every year. If untreated, metastatic epidural compression will inevitably progress, causing paralysis, sensory loss, and sphincter incontinence. Metastases to the spine are far more common than primary spinal neoplasms and can further be classified into epidural, leptomeningeal, and intramedullary. Approximately half of the cases of metastatic epidural compression, including compression of the spinal cord and cauda equina syndrome, in adults arises from such cancers as breast carcinoma, lymphoma, renal cell carcinoma, melanoma, prostate carcinoma, sarcoma, and multiple myeloma. In children, sarcoma, neuroblastoma, and lymphoma are typically seen. Compression occurs at thoracic levels in 70% of cases, at lumbar levels in 20% of cases, and at cervical levels in 10% of cases.

The single most important prognosticating factor is determining the level of neurologic function at the onset of therapy; thus diagnosing the condi-

R. Gupta et al., *PET/MR Imaging*, https://doi.org/10.1007/978-3-319-65106-4_10

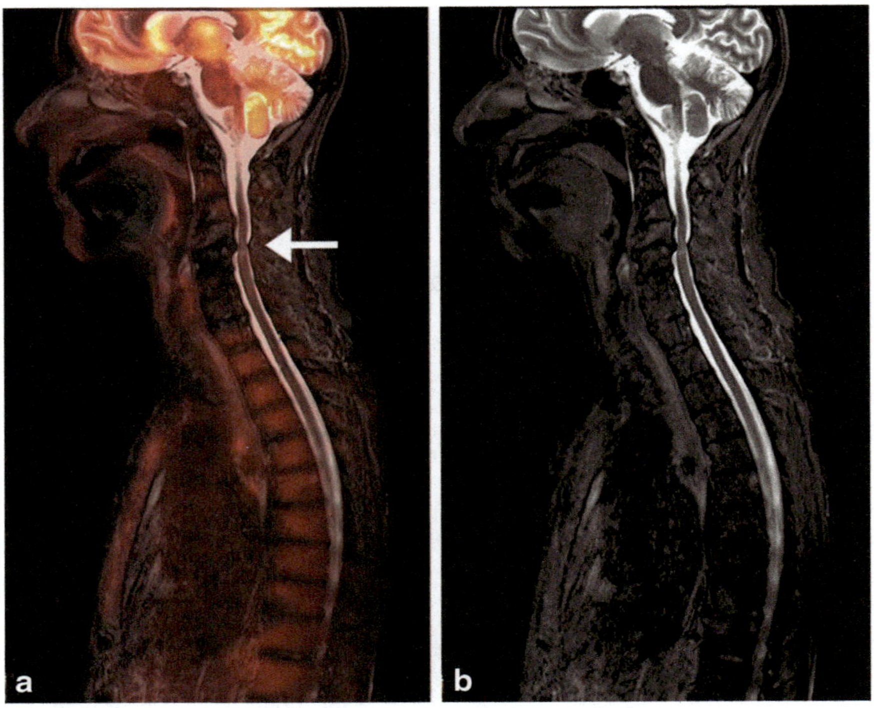

Fig. 10.1 FDG PET/MR STIR sagittal fusion (**a**) and STIR sagittal (**b**)

tion and initiating treatment before neurologic injury occurs serve as a major clinical challenge. Early diagnosis is crucial. MRI is the gold standard of diagnosis and is immediately indicated if radiculopathy or myelopathy are present with abnormal radiographs of the spine. CT myelogram is usually reserved for patients who have contraindications for MRI. In comparison to the soft tissue anatomy seen on conventional MRI and osseous integrity evaluated by CT scan, PET scanning could be advantageous in the prognostication of spinal compression, as it provides useful qualitative and quantitative estimates of impaired metabolic activity of the compromised compressed segment of spinal cord, which also closely correlates with the severity of neurologic dysfunction.

By combining the anatomical information from MRI, and the metabolic data from PET, PET/MR serves as a growing modality to further diagnose and prognosticate metastatic spinal cord compression. While the literature on PET/MRI in evaluating metastatic cord compression is limited, PET/MR could serve as a useful adjunct due to its ability to visualize cord compression, ligamentous instability, blood supply compromise, as well as quantify the metabolic effects on the cord which serve as a prognostic indicator for cord compromise.

Suggested Reading

Bozzo A, Marcoux J, Radhakrishna M, Pelletier J, Goulet B. The role of magnetic resonance imaging in the management of acute spinal cord injury. J Neurotrauma. 2011;28:1401–11.

Flowth FW, Stoffels G, Herdmann J, Eicker S, Galldiks N, Steiger HJ, et al. Prognostic value of 18F-FDG PET in monosegmental stenosis and myelopathy of the cervical spinal cord. J Nucl Med. 2011;52:1385–91.

Shah LM, Salzman KL. Imaging of spinal metastatic disease. Int J Surg Oncol. 2011;2011:769753.

Uchida K, Kobayashi S, Yayama T, Kokubo Y, Nakajima H, Kakuyama M, et al. Metabolic neuroimaging of the cervical spinal cord in patients with compressive myelopathy: a high-resolution positron emission tomography study. J Neurosurg Spine. 2004;1:72–9.

Case 11
Prostate Cancer with F-18 Sodium Fluoride

Ana M. Franceschi and Robert Matthews

History

A 65-year-old male with biopsy revealing Gleason score 4 + 4 prostate cancer (PSA 1.5) was referred for F-18 sodium fluoride PET/MR imaging (Fig. 11.1).

Diagnosis

Prostate cancer osseous metastases detected by F-18 sodium fluoride

Findings

- T12 vertebral body lesion that is hypointense on the T2-weighted image that is better visualized with fat suppression (wide white arrow).
- T12 lesion also is hypointense on T1-weighted image which is characteristic of blastic lesions. An additional lesion is seen in T11 vertebral body (curved white arrows).
- PET fusion show abnormal increased focal activity within the T11 and T12 lesions consistent with metastases.
- PET fusion of the chest reveals a left fifth rib lesion with increased FDG activity (white arrowhead).
- PET MIP demonstrates the two vertebral lesions (black thin arrows) as well as the left fifth rib lesion (black arrowhead).

Discussion

F-18 sodium fluoride (NaF) is a positron-emitting bone-specific radiotracer with uptake mechanism reflecting blood flow and osteoblastic activity. Its mechanism is similar to traditional bone scanning agents, Tc-99m labeled diphosphonates such as Tc-99m MDP. When used with PET/MRI, NaF PET provides numerous advantages over the conventional Tc-99m MDP bone scans, most importantly higher sensitivity and specificity, greater spatial resolution, and significantly shorter uptake and scan times, while maintaining a lower or similar radiation dose. NaF PET sensitivity and specificity reach 95–100% in identifying osseous metastases compared to Tc-99m MDP planar bone scintigraphy with about 70% sensitivity and 57% specificity. The most common indication for F-18 sodium fluoride bone imaging is evaluating prostate cancer metastases, but it can also be used to detect osseous metastases from breast cancer, thyroid cancer, renal cell carcinoma, and lung cancer, among others.

A lack of specificity is a limitation for both conventional bone scintigraphy with Tc-99m MDP and PET scanning with F-18 sodium fluoride, as nonmalignant skeletal diseases may also cause focal uptake of bone-specific tracers requiring further anatomic correlation with radiographs, CT, or MRI. Benign causes of abnormal focal radiotracer uptake may have the same degree of uptake leading to higher chances of false positive results when findings are inter-

R. Gupta et al., *PET/MR Imaging*, https://doi.org/10.1007/978-3-319-65106-4_11

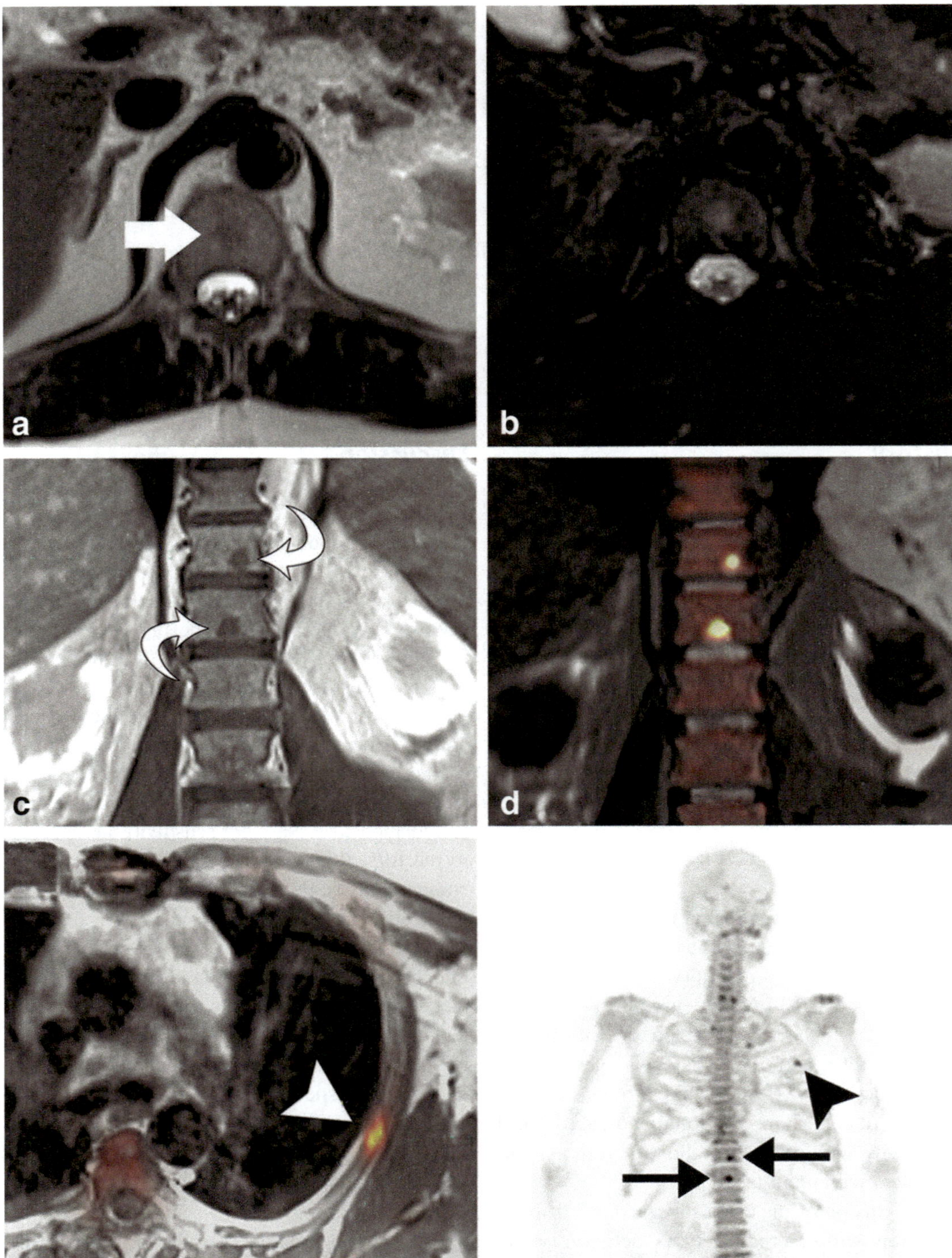

Fig. 11.1 T2 axial of T12 vertebra (**a**), T2 with fat suppression axial of T12 vertebra (**b**), T1 TSE coronal from T10 through L2 vertebra (**c**), NaF PET/MR T2 with fat suppression coronal fusion from T10 through L2 vertebra (**d**), NaF PET/MR T2 axial fusion of the chest (**e**), and NaF PET MIP (**f**)

preted with PET alone. The use of new hybrid technologies, SPECT/CT, PET/CT, and PET/MRI has greatly improved characterization of bone lesions and differentiation between benign and malignant processes markedly increasing specificity and diagnostic accuracy.

Whole-body PET/MR imaging, combining very high sensitivity of F-18 sodium fluoride PET for osteoblastic changes and the ability of MRI techniques to detect bone marrow infiltration, provides the most effective tool for early detection of bone metastasis. In particular, diffusion-weighted MRI imaging is useful to increase sensitivity. Hence for whole-body marrow imaging, a diffusion sequence is often paired with the PET. Other MRI sequences such as dynamic contrast enhanced or Dixon aid specificity to the diagnosis of osseous lesions, especially in the spine.

Suggested Reading

Bastawrous S, Bhargava P, Behnia F, Djang DS, Haseley DR. Newer PET application with an old tracer: role of 18F-NaF skeletal PET/CT in oncologic practice. Radiographics. 2014;34(5):1295–316.

Cook GJ, Azad G, Padhani AR. Bone imaging in prostate cancer: the evolving roles of nuclear medicine and radiology. Clin Transl Imaging. 2016;4(6):439–47.

Li Y, Schiepers C, Lake R, Dadparvar S. Berenji GR. Clinical utility of (18)F-fluoride PET/CT in benign and malignant bone diseases. Bone. 2012;50(1):128–39.

Mosavi F, Johansson S, Sandberg DT, Turesson I, Sörensen J, Ahlström H. Whole-body diffusion-weighted MRI compared with (18)F-NaF PET/CT for detection of bone metastases in patients with high-risk prostate carcinoma. AJR Am J Roentgenol. 2012;199(5):1114–20.

Case 12
Tarlov Cyst

Rajesh Gupta

History

A 75-year-old male with recurrent left foot sarcoma presents with lower back/hip pain (Fig. 12.1).

Diagnosis

Tarlov cyst

Findings

- T1-weighted hypointense and T2-weighted hyperintense two adjacent lesions centered in the S2-3 neuroforamen bilaterally (thin arrow).
- Lesion is hyperintense on STIR indicating that it is fluid filled (curved arrow).
- PET/MR fusion showing no FDG uptake in the lesion consistent with a Tarlov cyst.

Discussion

Tarlov cysts, which are also called sacral perineural cysts, are collections of cerebrospinal fluid between layers of the nerve root sheath near the dorsal root ganglion. They are considered type II spinal meningeal cysts as they are extradural and contain neural tissue, as opposed to type I which would be extradural without neural tissue, and type III which would be intradural. Several etiologies have been postulated, including congenital, traumatic, and inflammatory factors which cause thickening and diverticula formation of the arachnoid membrane. Since these lesions do not usually change during life, they are more likely developmental in etiology. These lesions are often incidental and asymptomatic; however potential symptoms may arise as they accumulate more fluid under high pressure through a ball valve mechanism (similar to a Baker's cyst). These rare symptoms include lower back, radiating lower extremity pain, and impaired sphincter or sexual function. Definitive treatment involves surgical resection but is rarely performed.

MRI is particularly useful in identifying the simple cystic nature of a Tarlov cyst with homogeneous high intensity on T2-weighted and lower than muscle intensity on T1-weighted images. MRI provides better soft tissue resolution compared to CT and can evaluate communication with the cyst and the subarachnoid space using flow sensitive sequences. Cysts that have free communication are usually asymptomatic as less pressure is exerted on adjacent nerve roots. Currently, it is rare to perform myelographic studies to demonstrate communication and filling characteristics of the cyst.

R. Gupta et al., *PET/MR Imaging*, https://doi.org/10.1007/978-3-319-65106-4_12

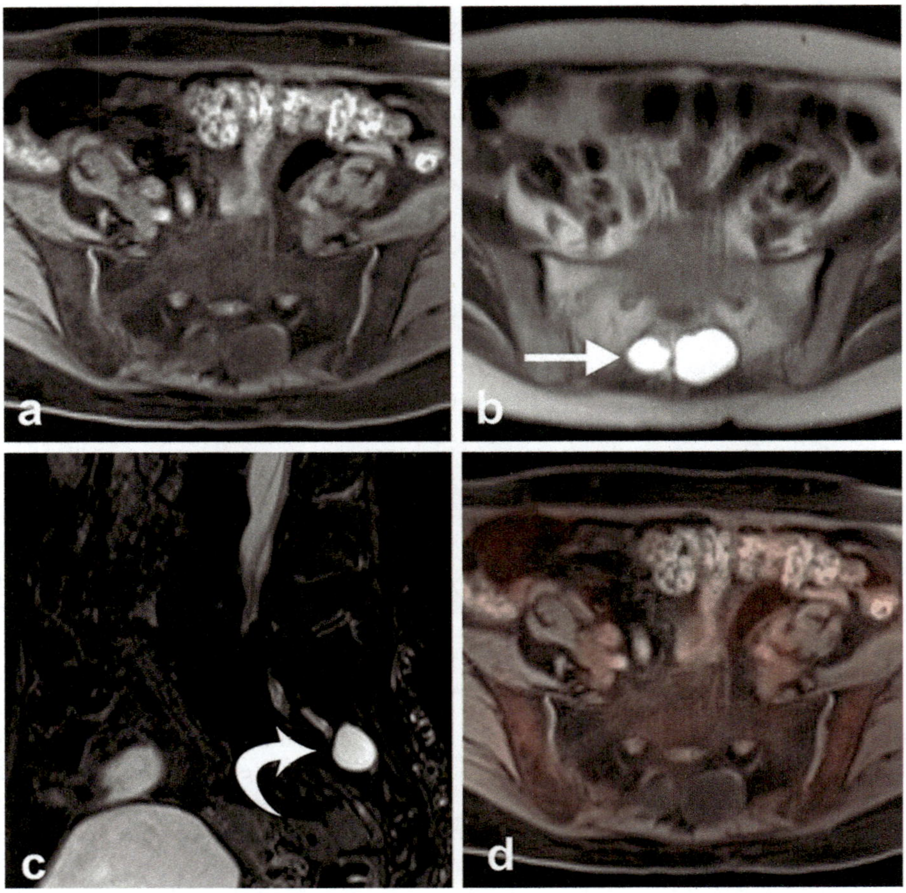

Fig. 12.1 T1 radial VIBE with fat suppression axial (**a**), T2 HASTE axial (**b**), STIR sagittal (**c**), and PET/MR T1 radial VIBE with fat suppression axial fusion (**d**)

These cysts are not metabolically active on PET imaging. Complications of the cyst such as rupture or infection might elicit increased FDG activity. Other cystic lesions of the sacrum such as chordomas and chondrosarcomas may have malignant features that could have increased activity leading to further clinical investigations.

Suggested Reading

Davis SW, Levy LM, LeBihan DJ, Rajan S, Schellinger D. Sacral meningeal cysts: evaluation with MR imaging. Radiology. 1993;187(2):445–8.

Nadler SF, Bartoli LM, Stitik TP, Chen B. Tarlov cyst as a rare cause of S1 radiculopathy: a case report. Arch Phys Med Rehabil. 2001;82(5):689–90.

Case 13
Cellulitis

Rajesh Gupta

History

A 73-year-old diabetic female with right foot soft tissue swelling and chronic ulceration over the midtarsal dorsal foot (Fig. 13.1).

Diagnosis

Cellulitis

Findings

- T1-weighted images show low signal intensity, thickened subcutaneous tissue along the dorsal aspect of the foot over the midtarsal region.
- T2-weighted images reveal intense signal along the dorsal aspect of the foot representing edema.
- PET/MR fusion demonstrates intense hypermetabolic activity within the subcutaneous tissues of the dorsal foot representing soft tissue infection (arrow).
- No evidence of marrow replacement on MRI or PET images to suggest osteomyelitis.
- T1-weighted images show a thin linear hypointense line in the medial cuneiform (arrowhead) compatible with a subchondral insufficiency fracture.
- Note the excessive fat and muscle edema in the intrinsic plantar muscles on MR, with mild FDG uptake. This is a common pattern in diabetic muscle disease.

Discussion

Cellulitis is a bacterial infection of the dermis and subcutaneous tissues that quickly spreads. Symptoms include edema, erythema, pain, and warmth. The most common causative organisms are *Staphylococcus aureus* and streptococci. Patients with peripheral vascular disease and diabetes are in particular at risk for cellulitis Proper clinical examination and imaging are important to distinguish cellulitis from more serious infections, such as osteomyelitis and most importantly necrotizing fasciitis. The latter is a rare progressive infection characterized by extensive tissue necrosis and severe systemic toxicity.

MR imaging is particularly helpful in distinguishing cellulitis from necrotizing osteomyelitis and fasciitis. Cellulitis characteristically manifests as superficial soft tissue thickening with increased signal on T2-weighted sequences and decreased signal on T1-weighted images, often in a honeycomb pattern. It often enhances following gadolinium administration. Pseudofluid collections are not infrequently seen adjacent to the deep fascia. When the patient is turned, these "collections" will move, confirm-

R. Gupta et al., *PET/MR Imaging*, https://doi.org/10.1007/978-3-319-65106-4_13

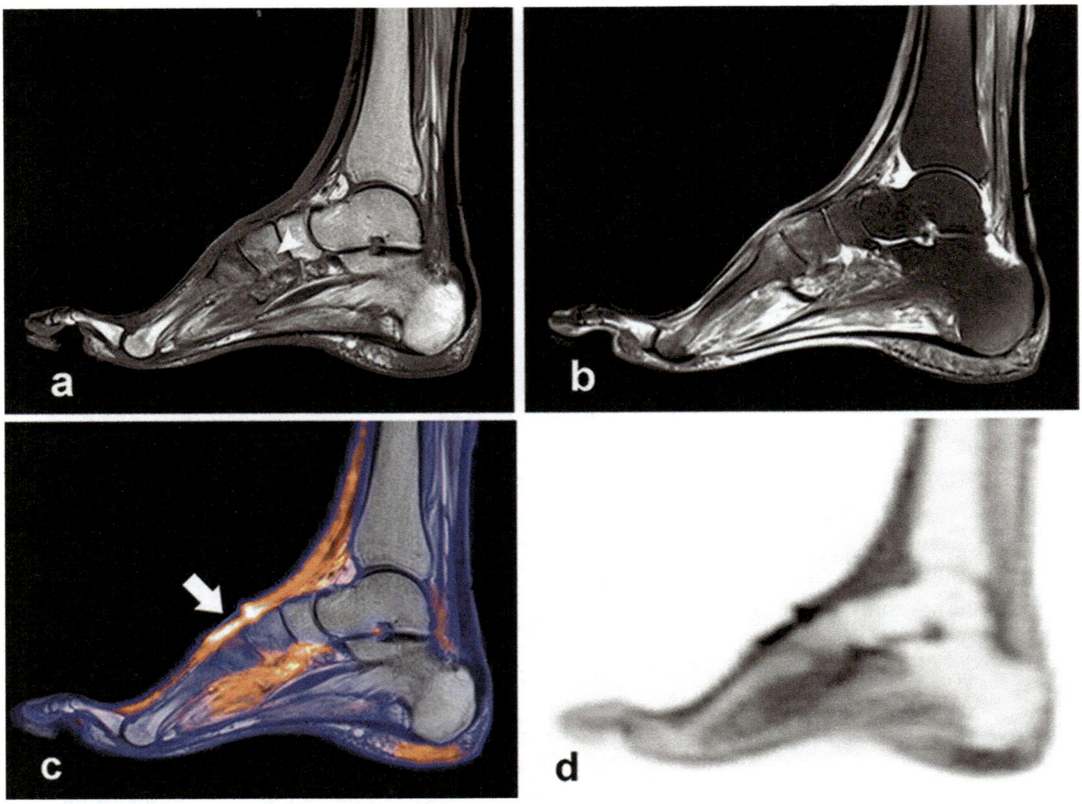

Fig. 13.1 T1 TSE sagittal (**a**), T2 TSE with fat suppression sagittal (**b**), PET/MR T1 TSE sagittal fusion (**c**), and PET sagittal (**d**)

ing that even when they rim enhance, they are not abscesses.

In necrotizing fasciitis, deeper myofascial planes are involved with high T2-weighted signal and post-contrast enhancement. Also necrotizing fasciitis shows deeper muscle edema, thickened intermuscular septae on T2-weighted images, and only subtle contrast enhancement. Osteomyelitis will have marrow replacement appearing as low signal on T1-weighted images along with high T2-weighted signal from bone marrow edema. FDG has both high sensitivity and high specificity in identifying and localizing osteomyelitis, which is often the clinical concern. PET/MR imaging can provide excellent assessment of the deeper myofascial tissues and notice secondary sites of infection.

Suggested Reading

Keidar Z, Militianu D, Melamed E, Bar-Shalom R, Israel O. The diabetic foot: initial experience with 18F-FDG PET/CT. J Nucl Med. 2005;46:444–9.

Rahmouni A, Chosidow O, Mathieu D, Gueorguieva E, Jazaerli N, Radier C, et al. MR imaging in acute infectious cellulitis. Radiology. 1994;192:493–6.

Case 14
Degenerative Spine: Modic Type I Changes

Rajesh Gupta and Robert Matthews

History

A 30-year-old male with worsening chronic back pain and suspected osteomyelitis and discitis on lumbar spine MRI without contrast was referred for PET/MRI evaluation to confirm diagnosis (Fig. 14.1).

Diagnosis

Degenerative spine: Modic type I changes

Findings

- Decreased signal on T1-weighted image and increased signal on T2-weighted image in the L5 and S1 adjacent endplates and middle vertebral bodies (wide white arrows).
- Loss of height with mild decreased T2 signal of the L5-S1 intervertebral disc (arrowhead).
- There is relative preservation of L5-S1 adjacent cortical endplates with only mild irregularity.
- Contrast enhancement of L5 inferior and S1 superior endplates (thin arrow) and adjacent vertebral bodies (curved arrows), with some peripheral enhancement of the disc.
- Overall decreased FDG uptake at the endplates of L5-S1 disc space characteristic of degenerative Modic type I changes. No significant FDG uptake to suggest osteomyelitis.

Discussion

Degenerative endplate changes in the lumbar spine are common and can have different appearances on conventional MRI. These degenerative endplate changes have been initially described by Dr. Michael Modic in 1988 and classified into three types. The classification is based on MRI appearance of marrow signal at the endplates. Modic type I changes demonstrate low signal on T1-weighted sequence, high signal on T2-weighted sequence, and can enhance after administration of contrast, which is related to bone marrow edema and inflammation. Similar imaging features are also characteristic of osteomyelitis-discitis making it difficult to differentiate between these two conditions. Modic type II endplate abnormalities are related to chronic marrow changes, with high T1 and iso to high T2 signal due to red to yellow marrow conversion. Type III degenerative changes are due to subchondral bony sclerosis and present with low T1 and T2 signal changes.

FDG PET is being increasingly used in suspected infection processes because of its high sensitivity. Inflammatory mediators, such as neutrophil granulocytes, eosinophils, and mac-

R. Gupta et al., *PET/MR Imaging*, https://doi.org/10.1007/978-3-319-65106-4_14

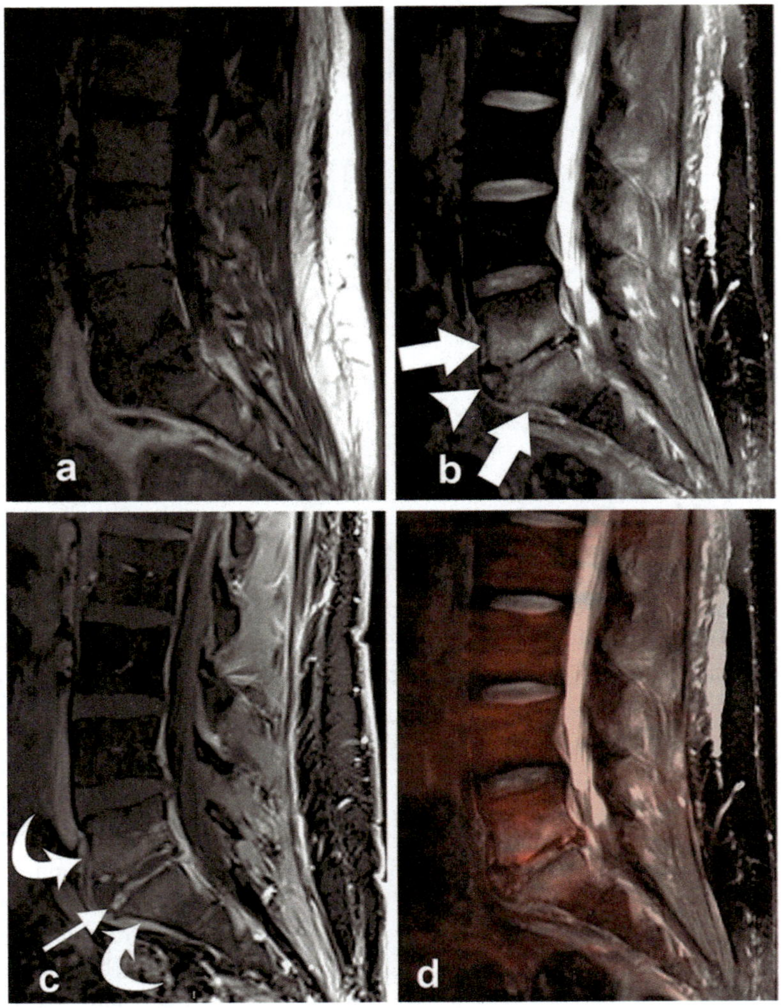

Fig. 14.1 T1 sagittal (**a**), T2 with fat suppression sagittal (**b**), T1 VIBE with fat suppression post-gadolinium contrast sagittal (**c**), and PET/MR T2 with fat suppression sagittal fusion (**d**)

rophages, are upregulated in infection with resultant increase of glucose utilization. These mediators are not present in degenerative changes. Therefore, there is little or no FDG uptake in degenerative changes of the spine unless there is presence of associated inflammatory arthropathy. FDG PET/MR imaging is an excellent tool to differentiate degenerative from infectious endplate abnormalities by determining MR signal characteristics while also demonstrating degree of metabolic FDG activity. In this case, without the PET scan disc space, infection might have been considered.

Suggested Reading

Modic MT, Steinberg PM, Ross JS, Masaryk TJ, Carter JR. Degenerative disk disease: assessment of changes in vertebral body marrow with MR imaging. Radiology. 1988;166(1 Pt 1):193–9.

Stumpe KD, Zanetti M, Weishaupt D, Hodler J, Boos N, Von Schulthess GK. FDG positron emission tomography for differentiation of degenerative and infectious endplate abnormalities in the lumbar spine detected on MR imaging. AJR Am J Roentgenol. 2002;179(5):1151–7.

Case 15 Extramedullary Multiple Myeloma

Rajesh Gupta

History

A 41-year-old male with relapsed IgG kappa multiple myeloma, initially diagnosed 2 years prior, presents with mid-back pain (Fig. 15.1).

Diagnosis

Extramedullary multiple myeloma

Findings

- Large prevertebral mass at the level of the aortic arch, which is homogenously isointense on T1-weighted image and heterogeneously hyperintense on T2.
- Mass demonstrates moderate FDG activity compatible with malignancy (arrowheads). Mild FDG activity also noted in the adjacent vertebral body due to benign bone marrow stimulation from chemotherapy.
- Mass pushes against the trachea (asterisks) and displaces the esophagus (thin arrow).

Discussion

Advances in the diagnosis, staging and treatment of multiple myeloma have increased the overall survival of patients inflicted with this disease to over 10 years from the time of initial diagnosis. This has contributed to an increase in the imaging diagnosis of extramedullary multiple myeloma that can develop at the time of relapse, especially in those patients treated with allogenic bone marrow transplant. There are two mechanisms in the development of extramedullary myeloma. The most common is through contiguous extension of osseous myelomatous masses in the spine which usually presents as large paraspinal or epidural masses. The second mechanism is through hematogenous spread of myeloma clone cells that have escaped the bone marrow and has disseminates to the skin, viscera, lymph nodes, upper airways, and brain.

MRI plays an important role in the management of extramedullary multiple myeloma as it helps in the initial diagnosis by clarifying ambiguous findings on other modalities, monitors disease activity, assesses response to treatment, and evaluates for potential complications. Extramedullary myeloma that is contiguous with the bone typically presents as large masses that are homogenous and hypo- to isointense compared to the skeletal muscle on T1-weighted images. It is hyperintense on T2-weighted images and enhances after gadolinium contrast administration. Some extramedullary myelomatous lesions that are not contiguous with bone can be hypointense on T2-weighted images, which may be explained by a biological similarity of these lesions to lymphoma. The most commonly encountered complications of extramedullary multiple myeloma are spinal cord compression

R. Gupta et al., *PET/MR Imaging*, https://doi.org/10.1007/978-3-319-65106-4_15

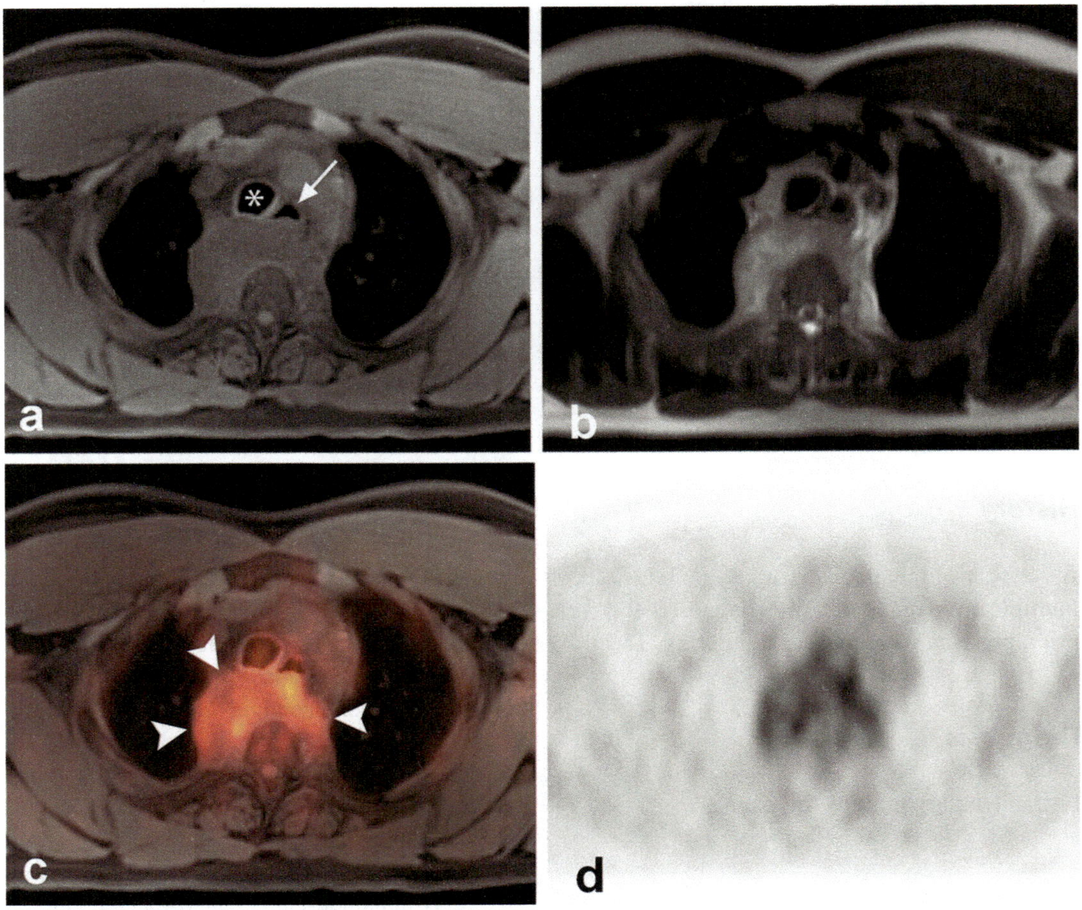

Fig. 15.1 T1 radial VIBE with fat suppression axial (**a**), T2 HASTE axial (**b**), PET/MR T1 radial VIBE with fat suppression axial fusion (**c**), and PET axial (**d**)

from epidural myelomatous masses and vertebral compression fractures which can be thoroughly evaluated with MRI.

Extramedullary myeloma is metabolically active. The advent of whole-body PET/MR imaging provides the ability for the detection of osseous multiple myeloma and extramedullary lesions in a single examination. FDG PET has been shown to be helpful in monitoring response to therapy and predicting clinical outcome based on changes in metabolic activity. It has been suggested that FDG PET should not be performed in the first 2 months following therapy to avoid false-positive results due to inflammatory postradiation or postsurgical changes.

Suggested Reading

Bredella MA, Steinbach L, Caputo G. Value of FDG PET in the assessment of patients with multiple myeloma. AJR Am J Roentgenol. 2005;184(4):1199–20.

Tirumani SH, Shinagare AB, Jagannathan JP. MRI features of extramedullary myeloma. AJR Am J Roentgenol. 2014;202(4):803–10.

Case 16
Aortitis

Rajesh Gupta

History

A 63-year-old male with back pain, fevers, and chills undergoes PET/MR imaging (Fig. 16.1).

Diagnosis

Aortitis (methicillin-resistant *Staphylococcus aureus*)

Findings

- T1-weighted image shows a complex collection surrounding the abdominal aorta.
- T2-weighted image demonstrates the low signal collection with thickening of the aortic wall (arrowhead).
- DWI shows restricted diffusion with bright signal and corresponding dark signal on ADC maps (arrows).
- PET/MR fusion reveals FDG avid semicircumferential uptake consistent with aortitis.

Discussion

Aortitis is aortic wall inflammation related to infectious or noninfectious causes. It can affect the aorta and its branches in any location along its route and with variable extent of involvement. Etiologies of noninfectious manifestations affecting larger vessels include diseases such as Takayasu arteritis, giant cell arteritis, or Behçet's disease. Collagen vascular disorders, like rheumatoid arthritis and systemic lupus erythematous, may affect the aorta in conjunction with medium and small vessels. Infectious aortitis can manifest through pyogenic infections, tuberculosis, syphilis, or salmonella involvement. Presenting symptoms vary and may include pain, fever, or vascular insufficiency.

Imaging in aortitis is useful to help differentiate infectious from noninfectious causes, assess disease progression, monitor treatment, guide biopsy, or exclude alternate diagnoses. Complications such as aneurysm, periaortic abscess, thrombus, and luminal occlusion can also be imaged. MRI provides superior assessment of the aortic wall and lumen, as well as, its branches. Multiple MRI sequences can be employed for the evaluation of aortitis. T1-weighted images show general aortic wall thickening with inflammatory mass-like extension into the surrounding fat and soft tissues. T2-weighted sequences are particularly good at showing mural edema within the vessel wall Post-gadolinium T1 images assess mural thickness and enhancement. Diffusion-weighted sequences demonstrate restricted diffusion in infection. MR angiography allows superior luminal evaluation for stenosis, thrombus, and occlusion.

FDG PET imaging demonstrates intense metabolic activity with active vascular inflammation and infection, as seen in vasculitis, atherosclero-

R. Gupta et al., *PET/MR Imaging*, https://doi.org/10.1007/978-3-319-65106-4_16

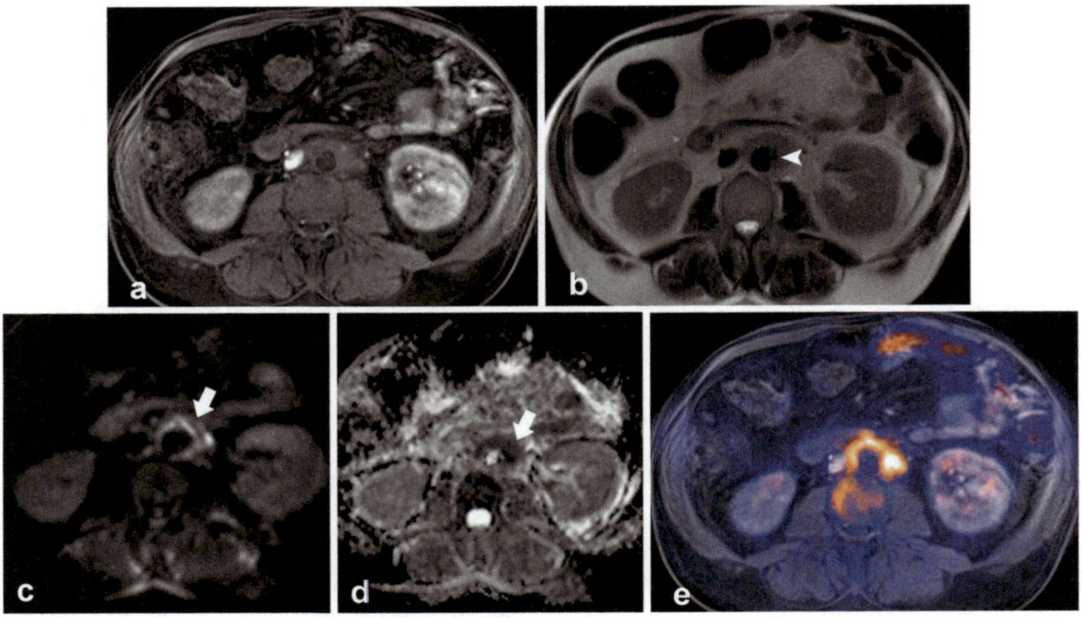

Fig. 16.1 T1 VIBE with fat suppression axial (**a**), T2 HASTE axial (**b**), Diffusion-weighted image axial (**c**), Apparent diffusion coefficient axial (**d**), and PET/MR T2 HASTE with fat suppression axial fusion (**e**)

sis, and acute dissection. However, imaging whether MR or PET, cannot reliably distinguish between infectious and noninfectious etiologies. Whole-body PET imaging can demonstrate the longitudinal extent of disease. When PET is combined with MRI, it allows for precise anatomical assessment of the aorta and other vascular structures showing increased FDG uptake characteristic of active inflammation or infection. PET/MR can also be used to monitor response to treatment by demonstrating decrease in FDG activity.

Suggested Reading

Gornik HL, Creager MA. Aortitis. Circulation. 2008;177:3039–51.

Litmanovich DE, Yıldırım A, Bankier AA. Insights into imaging of aortitis. Insights Imaging. 2012;3:545–60.

Case 17
Primary Bone Lymphoma

Rajesh Gupta

History

A 14-year-old female presents with persistent left knee pain (Fig. 17.1).

Diagnosis

Primary bone lymphoma (diffuse large B-cell lymphoma) of the distal femur

Findings

- T1-weighted images show a low signal lesion (arrow) that infiltrates the left distal femoral metaepiphysis, anteriorly. This lesion violates the physis but does not provoke a joint effusion.
- STIR sequence demonstrates high signal intensity within the mass and associated edema.
- T1-weighted images show heterogeneous post-gadolinium administration with better delineation of tumor (arrowheads).
- PET/MR fusion shows intense hypermetabolic activity confirming malignancy.

Discussion

Primary bone lymphoma (PBL) is rare manifestation of lymphoma and is defined as localized lymphomatous involvement of the bone without evidence of distant spread at the time of diagnosis. Care must be made to exclude more systemic lymphoma, most often by performing a chest, abdomen, and pelvis CT.

Diffuse large B-cell lymphoma is the most common type of PBL occurring in a wide range of ages, most commonly affecting 36- to 52-year-age group, and being rare in children under 10 years of age. The most frequent manifestation is intermittent but persistent bone pain with variable symptoms of swelling, palpable mass, and fever. Overall, the 5-year survival of patients with PBL is much better than other bone tumors.

MR imaging provides excellent bone marrow and soft tissue evaluation in PBL. On T1-weighted images, bone marrow replacement is identified with areas of low signal intensity and generally bright signal on T2-weighted sequences. This tumor appears, as in this case, more infiltrative, with less well-defined margins than other osseous neoplasms. Edema and reactive changes around the tumor may demonstrate

R. Gupta et al., *PET/MR Imaging*, https://doi.org/10.1007/978-3-319-65106-4_17

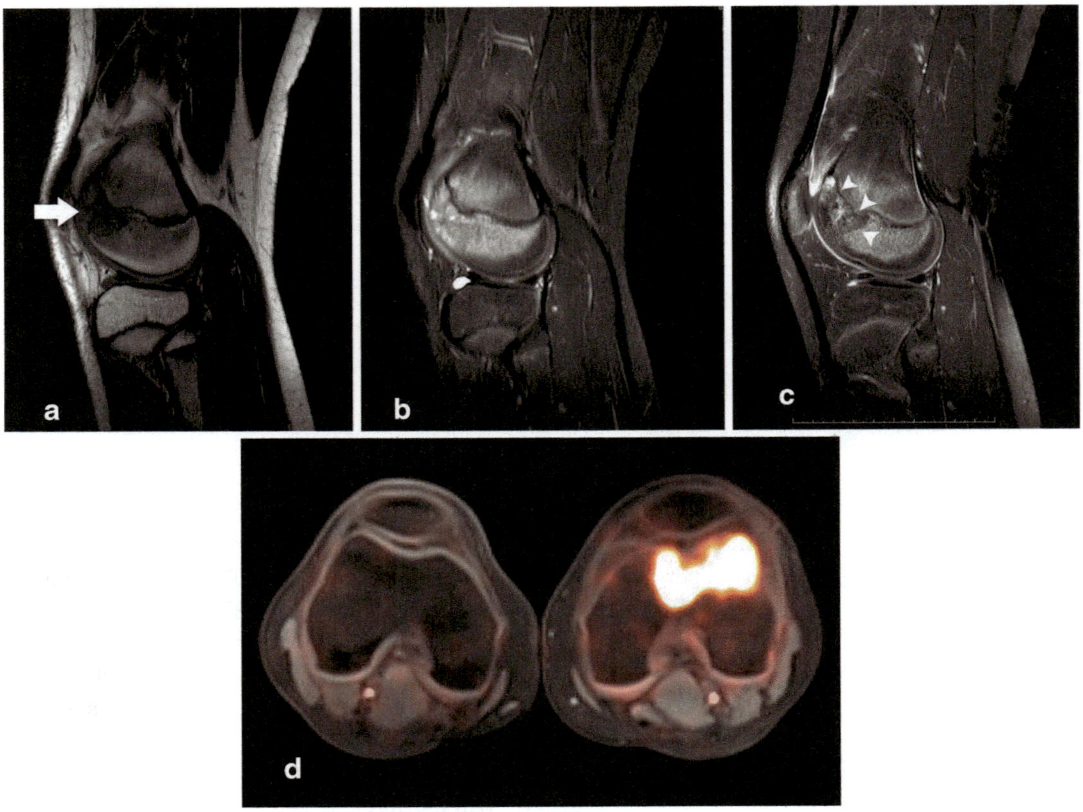

Fig. 17.1 T1-weighted sagittal of the left knee (**a**), STIR sagittal of the left knee (**b**), T1 weighted with fat suppression post-gadolinium contrast sagittal (**c**), and PET/MRI T1 radial VIBE with fat suppression axial fusion (**d**)

high T2-weighted signal. However, this pattern is less common. These tumors also show strong enhancement following administration of gadolinium contrast agents.

The use of FDG PET in lymphoma evaluation has been well studied, especially for the diffuse large B-cell histological subtype, that is >90% positive on PET. PBL and lymphomatous involvement of the bone are particularly FDG avid. FDG PET has also been shown to predict response to therapy, with negative scans after chemotherapy indicating a favorable prognosis. FDG PET has also been shown to accurately determine bone marrow involvement with concordant results when compared to bone marrow biopsy. With the superior spatial resolution of MRI and high FDG avidity on PET imaging, PET/MR is ideal in determining primary bone lymphoma and other lymphomatous involvement of bone.

Suggested Reading

Friedberg JW, Chengazi V. PET scans in the staging of lymphoma: current status. Oncologist. 2003;8:438–47.

Krishnan A, Shirkhoda A, Tehranzadeh J, Armin AR, Irwin R, Les K. Primary bone lymphoma: radiographic-MR imaging correlation. Radiographics. 2003;23:1371–83.

Case 18
Radiation Effect on Bone Marrow

David Pouldar and Robert Matthews

History

A 54-year-old female presents for restaging of cervical cancer 6 months following radiation treatment to the pelvis and chemotherapy (Fig. 18.1).

Diagnosis

Radiation effect on bone marrow

Findings

- Decreased T1 signal in L5 vertebra and the sacrum (white arrowheads) with corresponding increased T2 signal (white thin arrows) indicating increase of adipocytes in the bone marrow.
- No changes are detected on STIR images.
- PET fusion shows decreased FDG uptake in L5 vertebra and the sacrum (white curved arrow) as a result of radiation therapy.
- PET sagittal image also shows decreased FDG uptake in L5 vertebra and the sacrum (black wide arrow) with generalized increased FDG uptake in the remainder of the vertebrae as a result of chemotherapy-induced bone marrow stimulation.

Discussion

Knowledge of the evolution of bone marrow changes following radiation therapy is important in differentiating between normal postradiation changes from other marrow abnormalities. In addition, bone marrow changes may help to determine if the patient is able to undergo further antineoplastic therapy such as chemotherapy. MRI has the ability to detect the increase in adipocytes in the bone marrow which occurs as a consequence of radiation therapy. Increase in adipocytes is indicative of loss of myeloid tissue. Radiation-induced changes of bone marrow as detected by MRI are determined by both the radiation dose length of administration and the time interval following radiation treatment.

Initially, changes in the bone marrow are detected by increased signal on STIR imaging reflecting edema and necrosis. Between 3 and 6 weeks as fatty cells start to migrate, there is heterogeneous marrow signal with increased signal on T1-weighted images and the normalization of STIR hyperintensity. After 6 weeks marrow cellularity is further replaced by fatty tissue and mild increased signal on T2-weighted images. Fat sensitive T1-weighted images show increased bone marrow signal but may appear hypointense in signal. MRI changes in the marrow are most prominent 5–6 years following therapy, while

R. Gupta et al., *PET/MR Imaging*, https://doi.org/10.1007/978-3-319-65106-4_18

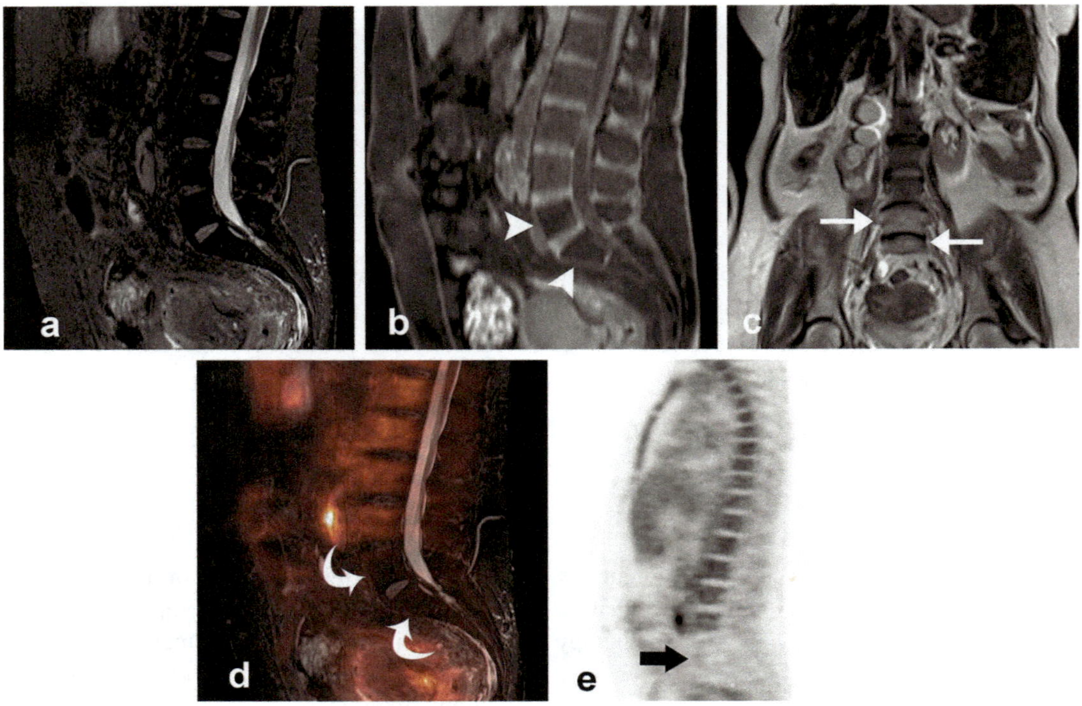

Fig. 18.1 STIR sagittal (**a**), T1 radial VIBE with fat suppression sagittal (**b**), T2 TSE coronal (**c**), PET/MR STIR sagittal fusion (**d**), and PET sagittal (**e**)

complete recovery may take up to 10–23 years after treatment with high radiation doses.

Knowing the effects of irradiated bone marrow on FDG PET/MR imaging is important in evaluating bone metastases following radiation therapy. Acute or subacute changes in FDG uptake on PET/MR following radiation can occur and make therapy response determination more difficult. Irradiated bone marrow initially has a transient rise in FDG uptake during the first 1–3 weeks reflecting inflammation. Afterward, there is a quick decline in uptake to severely decreased FDG uptake in the bone marrow reflecting replacement by adipocyte tissue. Often this decreased uptake appears more pronounced with the administration of chemotherapy agents and granulocyte-stimulating factors that dramatically increase FDG uptake in normal marrow. Return to normal FDG uptake in the irradiated bone marrow may take years. Thus, the evaluation of bone marrow in assessing treatment response using FDG PET/MR should be interpreted with caution within the first few weeks following radiation therapy. Ultimately, serial imaging may be needed to determine the significance of abnormal PET and MR findings.

Suggested Reading

Casamassima F, Caramella CR, Tinacci E, Villari N, Ruggiero M. Hematopoietic bone marrow recovery after radiation therapy: MRI evaluation. Blood. 1989;73:1677–81.

Higashi T, Fisher SJ, Brown RS, Nakada K, Walter GL, Wahl RL. Evaluation of the effect of local irradiation on normal rodent bone marrow metabolism using FDG: preclinical PET studies. J Nucl Med. 2000;41(12):2026–35.

Stevens SK, Moore SG, Kaplan D. Early and late bone-marrow changes after irradiation: MR evaluation. AJR Am J Roentgenol. 1990;154(4):754–0.

Case 19
Recurrent Myxoid Liposarcoma

Rajesh Gupta

History

A 48-year-old female with history of right upper thigh sarcoma treated by multiple resections, radiation, and chemotherapy (Fig. 19.1).

Diagnosis

Recurrent myxoid liposarcoma

Findings

- T1-weighted axial images demonstrate a low signal intensity intermuscular mass in the posterolateral upper right thigh which enhances on the post-contrast images.
- T2-weighted axial image shows slightly heterogenous, high signal intensity within the spiculated mass.
- Tissue retraction and deformity along with subcutaneous infiltration of low T1 and T2 signal overlying the recurrent tumor representing scarring from prior surgery.
- Post-contrast image shows thick irregular rim enhancement.
- PET/MR fusion images showing prominent hypermetabolic activity consistent with tumor recurrence.

Discussion

Liposarcomas are malignant tumors of fatty tissue. They are the second most common type of soft tissue sarcomas and are further classified into distinct histologic subtypes, but somewhat surprisingly are less common than the various types of fibrosarcoma that arise in the subcutaneous tissues. Myxoid liposarcoma is the second most common subtype of liposarcoma and accounts for 10% of all soft tissue sarcomas. They have no gender predilection and are most prevalent in the fourth or fifth decades of life. Myxoid liposarcoma generally affects the lower extremity arising from an intermuscular location, while muscle or subcutaneous origin is less frequent. Clinically, these lesions present as a painless, soft tissue masses. Treatment involves wide surgical excision often with adjunctive chemotherapy. Soft tissue metastases are more common than lung metastases and include the retroperitoneum, chest wall, pericardium, pleura, and pelvis.

On MR imaging, myxoid liposarcomas appear as large, intermediately defined, often lobulated masses. These lesions have high water content represented by low signal on T1-weighted images and high signal on T2-weighted images, often mimicking a cyst. However, unlike a cyst, these lesions enhance on post-contrast MRI images. Fat is usually not macroscopic and hence may not

R. Gupta et al., *PET/MR Imaging*, https://doi.org/10.1007/978-3-319-65106-4_19

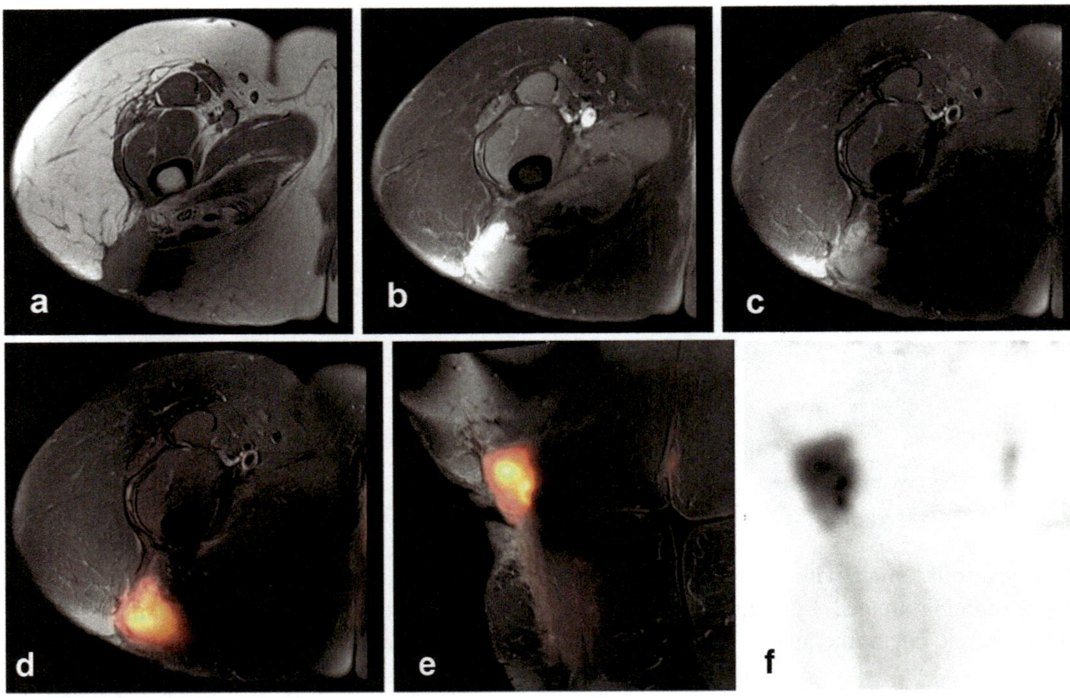

Fig. 19.1 T1 TSE axial (**a**), T1 TSE with fat suppression post-gadolinium contrast axial (**b**), T2 TSE with fat suppression axial (**c**), PET/MR T2 TSE axial fusion (**d**), PET/MR T1 TSE with fat suppression post gadolinium contrast coronal fusion (**e**), and PET coronal (**f**)

be visible on T1-weighted images. However, the identification of adipose tissue within the lesion may be seen as signal drop on in- and out-of-phase sequences.

Liposarcomas are FDG avid and PET imaging may be a useful tool for determining the more likely diagnosis in equivocal cases. In addition, the higher the SUV uptake, the more aggressive the tumor, and the worse long-term survival is associated with the diagnosis. Although PET imaging may not be useful in delineating the true extent of the primary tumor extension, PET can detect small satellite lesions and detect distant metastatic disease. PET in combination with MRI is excellent at differentiating recurrent tumor from edema, inflammation, and scarring in a patient that has undergone surgery and radiation therapy. Follow-up PET/MR imaging can provide information on changes in tumor size, metabolism, and tumor necrosis and determine response to therapy with decreasing metabolic activity being favorable.

Suggested Reading

Buchbender C, Heusner TA, Lauenstein TC, Bockisch A, Antoch G. Oncologic PET/MRI, part 2: bone tumors, soft-tissue tumors, melanoma, and lymphoma. J Nucl Med. 2012;53:1244–52.

Murphey MD, Arcara LK, Fanburg-Smith J. From the archives of the AFIP: imaging of musculoskeletal liposarcoma with radiologic-pathologic correlation. Radiographics. 2005;25:1371–95.

Partovi S, Kohan AA, Zipp L, Faulhaber P, Kosmas C, Ros PR, et al. Hybrid PET/MR imaging in two sarcoma patients – clinical benefits and implications for future trials. Int J Clin Exp Med. 2014;7:640–8.

Case 20
Osseous Sarcoidosis

Eric van Staalduinen

History

A 65-year-old male with sarcoidosis and multiple bone lesions detected on bone scan. No history of cancer (Fig. 20.1).

Diagnosis

Osseous sarcoidosis

Findings

- MRI demonstrates multiple T1 hypointense and STIR hyperintense lesions that enhance with contrast (arrowheads).
- The lesions show foci of prominent FDG uptake on PET/MR sagittal and coronal fusion images (thin arrows) suggestive of widespread metastases.
- The bone marrow also has heterogeneous FDG activity implying more extensive metastatic disease.
- Subsequent biopsy of the spine lesions showed non-necrotizing granulomas consistent with sarcoidosis.

Discussion

Sarcoidosis is a systemic granulomatous disease of unknown origin, characterized by the presence of non-necrotizing granulomas in affected organs. Skeletal sarcoidosis is thought to occur in approximately 1–13% of patients. The clinical presentation of skeletal sarcoidosis is variable, including asymptomatic presentation, nonspecific pain, arthralgia, and incidental findings on studies performed for other indications. Bone involvement generally involves the peripheral skeleton, with the phalanges, metacarpals, and metatarsals being the most frequently affected sites. However, lesions may occur in any bone, and lesions in long bones or the axial skeleton may appear similar to metastatic disease or multiple myeloma. Clear imaging discriminators that allow confident differentiation of sarcoidosis bone lesions from osseous metastases have not been established, and biopsy may be required for definitive diagnosis. Treatment generally consists of corticosteroids and is typically initiated for relief of symptoms.

MRI findings for skeletal sarcoidosis are nonspecific. Sarcoidosis lesions appear as multiple round or irregularly shaped intramedullary lesions that may contain fatty foci and are hypointense and

R. Gupta et al., *PET/MR Imaging*, https://doi.org/10.1007/978-3-319-65106-4_20

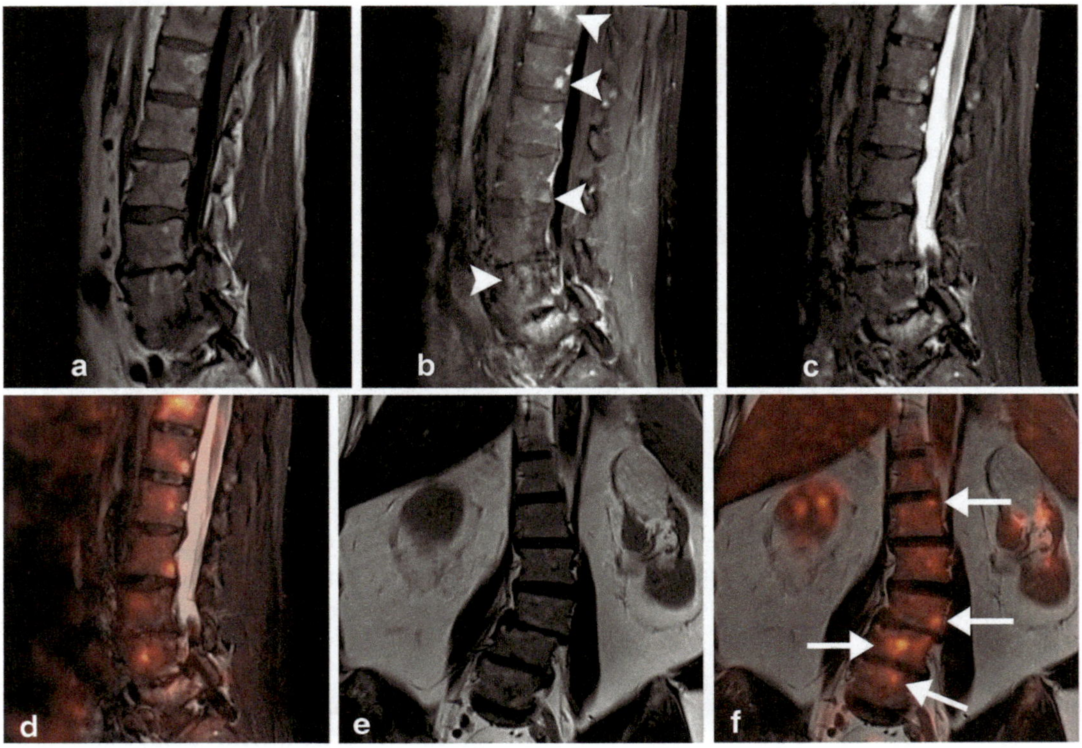

Fig. 20.1 T1 sagittal (**a**), T1 sagittal post-gadolinium contrast (**b**), STIR sagittal (**c**), PET/MR STIR sagittal fusion (**d**), T2 coronal (**e**) and PET/MR T2 coronal fusion (**f**)

homogeneous on T1-weighted imaging. On fluid-sensitive T2 and STIR sequences, these lesions are homogeneous and of high signal intensity. These lesions also show nonspecific enhancement after the intravenous administration of gadolinium chelate. The presence of fat within or replacing lesions suggests an involuting granuloma. In patients with known sarcoidosis, this strongly suggests the diagnosis of sarcoidosis rather than metastases. The use of in- and out-of-phase images can help to identify subtle areas of fat.

FDG PET can play a major role in the diagnosis of patients with suspected inflammation and infection as FDG uptake increases with disease activity. In sarcoidosis, activated macrophages are intimately involved in the formation of granulomas; this may explain why the granulomatous lesions in sarcoidosis show strong FDG uptake. It may also explain why the degree of FDG uptake correlates with activity of disease and treatment response. Although increased FDG activity is not specific for sarcoidosis, when whole-body FDG PET is performed, the distribution of FDG uptake in the chest typically reveals extensive mediastinal and bilateral hilar involvement in the characteristic pattern of sarcoidosis. Therefore, the use of whole-body FDG PET and the recognition of the patterns typical of sarcoidosis help to differentiate sarcoidosis from malignant conditions when MRI findings are nonspecific.

Suggested Reading

Aberg C, Ponzo F, Raphael B, Amorosi E, Moran V, Kramer E. FDG positron emission tomography of bone involvement in sarcoidosis. AJR Am J Roentgenol. 2004;182(4):975–7.

Moore SL, Kransdorf MJ, Schweitzer ME, Murphey MD, Babb JS. Can sarcoidosis and metastatic bone lesions be reliably differentiated on routine MRI? AJR Am J Roentgenol. 2012;198(6):1387–93.

Simpfendorfer CS, Ilaslan H, Davies AM, James SL, Obuchowski NA, Sundaram M. Does the presence of focal normal marrow fat signal within a tumor on MRI exclude malignancy? An analysis of 184 histologically proven tumors of the pelvic and appendicular skeleton. Skelet Radiol. 2008;37(9):797–804.

Talmi D, Smith S, Mulligan ME. Central skeletal sarcoidosis mimicking metastatic disease. Skelet Radiol. 2008;37(8):757–61.

Case 21 Osteoblastic Metastasis from Breast Cancer

Rajesh Gupta

History

A 47-year-old female with metastatic breast cancer presents for restaging (Fig. 21.1).

Diagnosis

Osteoblastic metastasis from breast cancer

Findings

- Left femoral head lesion demonstrates hypointense signal on T1 and T2-weighted sequences (thin arrow).
- PET fusion image shows mild FDG uptake consistent with an osteoblastic metastasis.

Discussion

Osteoblastic, also known as sclerotic, bone metastases can arise from a variety of different primary malignancies, with prostate and breast cancer being the most common causes. Prostate cancer tends to exhibit purely sclerotic metastases, whereas bone lesions in breast cancer are often mixed, lytic, or sclerotic. Less common primary tumors presenting with osteoblastic bone metastases include carcinoid, medulloblastoma, neuroblastoma, lymphoma, colon carcinoma, and transitional cell carcinoma. Various molecular mechanisms responsible for the deposition of new bone with upregulation of osteoblasts, growth factors, and adhesion molecules have been postulated.

While osteolytic metastases are usually aggressive, osteoblastic lesions tend to show a somewhat slower progression. Both lytic and sclerotic bone metastases favor areas with high red marrow content, such as the pelvis, vertebrae, ribs, and ends of long bones. MRI is excellent at assessing spread of metastatic disease in the marrow cavity as well as extension out of the marrow cavity to involve surrounding structures. Normal bone marrow contains a high fat percentage with high signal on T1-weighted images. Osseous metastatic involvement replaces the fat and leads to foci of low T1-weighted signal. On T2-weighted sequences, osteoblastic disease tends to show low to intermediate signal. This is in contrast to osteolytic metastases, which have a higher water content and therefore demonstrate high T2-weighted signal. Both types of medullary metastases show a higher signal rim on T2 images representing the reactive interface.

FDG PET provides images reflecting metabolic activity of osseous metastases. It is particularly helpful in detecting osteolytic disease, which is usually highly metabolically active when compared to osteoblastic disease. Because of the relatively low metabolic activity

R. Gupta et al., *PET/MR Imaging*, https://doi.org/10.1007/978-3-319-65106-4_21

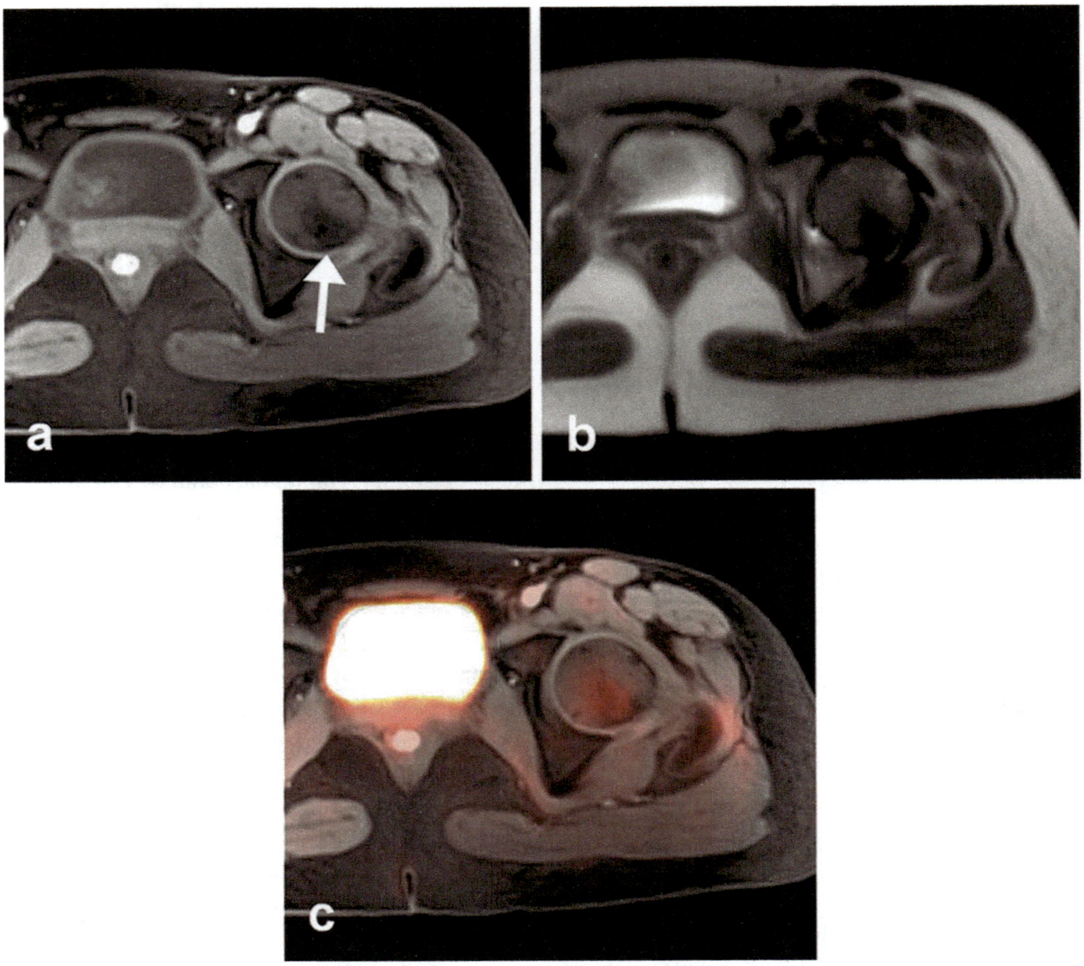

Fig. 21.1 T1 radial VIBE with fat suppression axial (**a**), T2 HASTE axial (**b**), and FDG PET/MR T1 radial VIBE with fat suppression axial fusion (**c**)

in osteoblastic metastases, lesions may show minimal to mild FDG uptake, while smaller sclerotic lesions may go undetected. Combining PET and MRI can help to improve detection of osteoblastic bone metastasis as the MR component provides excellent marrow evaluation and can demonstrate malignant marrow infiltration even when metabolic activity may be low. Future applications of PET/MR imaging include not only accurate detection of bone metastases but also evaluation of treatment response, particularly in breast cancer patients, who typically have mixed sclerotic and lytic bone metastases. In these cases MR should include in- and out-of-phase images to exclude the presence of small foci of fat.

Suggested Reading

Cook GJ, Houston S, Rubens R, Maisey MN, Fogelman I. Detection of bone metastases in breast cancer by 18FDG PET: differing metabolic activity in osteoblastic and osteolytic lesions. J Clin Oncol. 1998;16(10):3375–9.

O'Sullivan GJ, Carty FL, Cronin CG. Imaging of bone metastasis: an update. World J Radiol. 2015;7(8):202–11.

Case 22
Muscle Strain

Jingyu Zhou and Amit Gupta

History

A 36-year-old male with Hodgkin's lymphoma presents for restaging following radiation and chemotherapy (Fig. 22.1).

Diagnosis

Muscle strain

Findings

- Intense hypermetabolic activity within the bilateral temporal muscles on PET fusion imaging consistent with muscle strain (white thin arrows).
- No abnormal T1 or T2 signal within the temporal muscles.
- PET MIP image additionally shows diffuse uptake with the intercostal muscles often seen with respiratory difficulties (black arrowheads).

Discussion

Normal skeletal muscles at rest show no significant FDG uptake. However, when skeletal muscles are subjected to activity whether voluntarily or involuntarily, they may demonstrate increased FDG uptake. Chewing and exercising are examples of voluntary activities and muscle spasm is an example of involuntary activity that can result in diffuse increased muscle FDG uptake. In a patient with respiratory distress, labored breathing is manifested by increased FDG uptake in the muscles of respiration. In the resting state, diaphragm and external intercostal muscles are the main muscles for inspiration, and expiration is a relatively passive process. However, alteration in respiratory physiology, such as in pneumonia, may result in increased workload on these muscles resulting in recruitment of accessory muscles of respiration. Painful respiration from rib fractures can show recruitment of accessory muscles, such as external oblique, internal oblique, transverse abdominis, and rectus abdominis muscles. Paralysis of one group of muscles often results in increased workload of another group or contralateral muscles. For example, unilateral diaphragmatic paralysis from phrenic nerve injury leads to compensatory increase in the contralateral diaphragmatic workload and the use of accessory muscles to maintain ventilation, all showing increased FDG uptake.

It is important to be aware of these benign causes of muscular FDG uptake to differentiate them from pathological causes of FDG uptake such as neoplasms, local inflammatory processes, infections, muscle injury, myonecrosis,

R. Gupta et al., *PET/MR Imaging*, https://doi.org/10.1007/978-3-319-65106-4_22

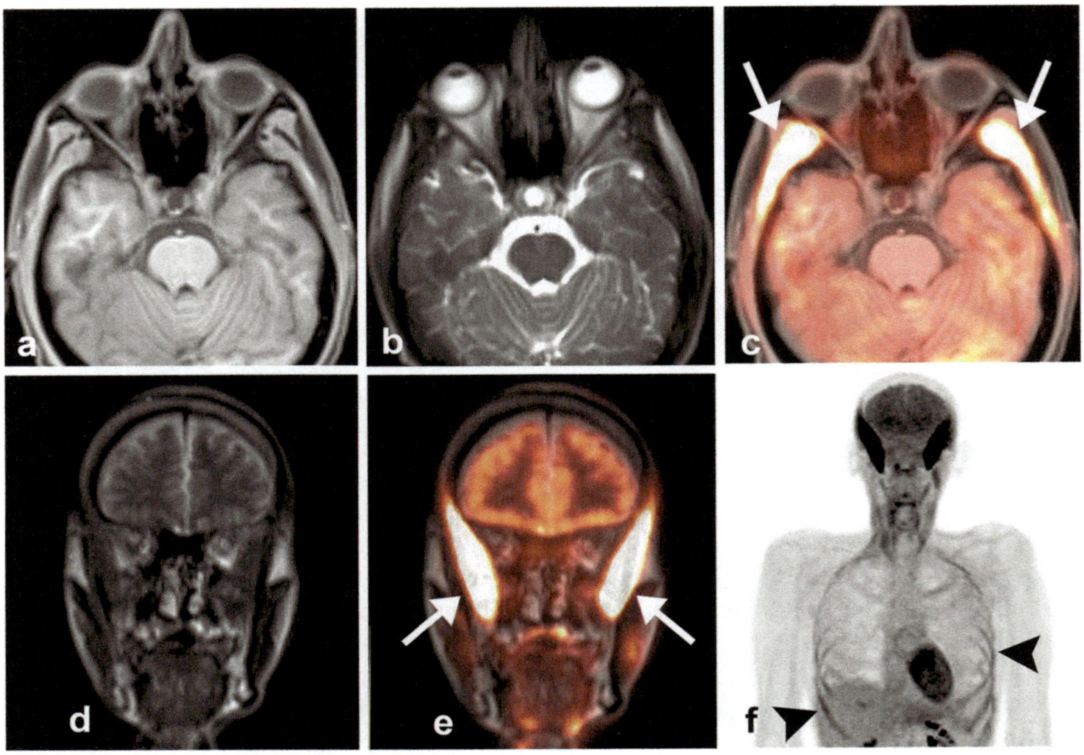

Fig. 22.1 T1 radial VIBE with fat suppression axial (**a**), T2 HASTE axial (**b**), PET/MR T1 radial VIBE with fat suppression axial fusion (**c**), T2 TSE coronal (**d**), PET/MR T2 TSE coronal fusion (**e**), and PET MIP (**f**)

and parasitic infection. Patients that have eaten recently may also have a high insulin state, driving FDG into the skeletal and cardiac muscles resulting in intense diffuse uptake. A concurrently performed MRI may help in this differentiation. A normal diaphragm and other muscles of respiration follow typical muscle MRI signal intensity and appear hypointense to fat and water on T2-weighted sequences and hypointense to fat and hyperintense to water on T1-weighted sequences. Chronic paralysis of the diaphragm will appear as decreased muscle bulk and increase in T1 and T2 signals from fatty atrophy.

Suggested Reading

Joshi P, Lele V. Left is right and right is wrong: Fluorodeoxyglucose uptake in left hemi-diaphragm due to right phrenic nerve palsy. Indian J Nucl Med. 2013;28(1):32–3.

Matthews R, Franceschi D, Cabahug C. Abdominal muscle uptake on FDG PET secondary to multiple rib fractures and use of accessory muscles of respiration. Clin Nucl Med. 2005;30(5):333–4.

Osman MM, Tran IT, Muzaffar R, Parkar N, Sachdeva A, Ruppel GL. Does ^{18}F-FDG uptake by respiratory muscles on PET/CT correlate with chronic obstructive pulmonary disease? J Nucl Med Technol. 2011;39(4):252–7.

Theodorou DJ, Theodorou SJ, Kakitsubata Y. Skeletal muscle disease: patterns of MRI appearances. Br J Radiol. 2012;85(1020):e1298–308.

Case 23
Acute Benign Vertebral Compression Fracture

Rajesh Gupta

History

A 56-year-old male with lower extremity sarcoma, presents with back pain (Fig. 23.1).

Diagnosis

Acute benign vertebral compression fracture

Findings

- Low T1-weighted signal and high STIR signal involving only the superior endplate of the L1 vertebral body are consistent with edema. Edema is seen in the adjacent disc, and there is no marrow replacement of the remainder of the vertebral body.
- Post-contrast images show intense enhancement of the superior endplate of L1 vertebral body.
- PET/MR fusion and PET images show only mild degree of FDG activity pointing toward a benign etiology (arrow).
- Minimal superior endplate depression and no evidence of middle column retropulsion or spinal canal compression.

Discussion

Acute vertebral compression fractures may occur from trauma, osteoporosis, or malignant marrow infiltration of the vertebral body. Patients will usually present with back pain and decreased mobility. It is often difficult but important to differentiate benign from malignant causes of compression fractures as spinal metastases may be the first clue to search for a primary cancer. Alternatively, osteoporotic compression fractures are common in the elderly population and can occur without a traumatic event.

MR imaging is widely used to evaluate the spine and can help diagnose and assess spinal compression fractures. Acute fractures typically show low T1-weighted signal and high T2-weighted or STIR signal representing edema. The affected bone can show mild contrast enhancement due to hyperemia. On the other hand, chronic compression fractures usually show an almost normal T1-weighted and STIR marrow signal. The use of MR to differentiate benign from malignant fractures is more difficult. Some findings that may point toward a malignant fracture include complete replacement of the normal marrow signal, indistinct fracture lines, retropulsion, posterior element involvement, and

R. Gupta et al., *PET/MR Imaging*, https://doi.org/10.1007/978-3-319-65106-4_23

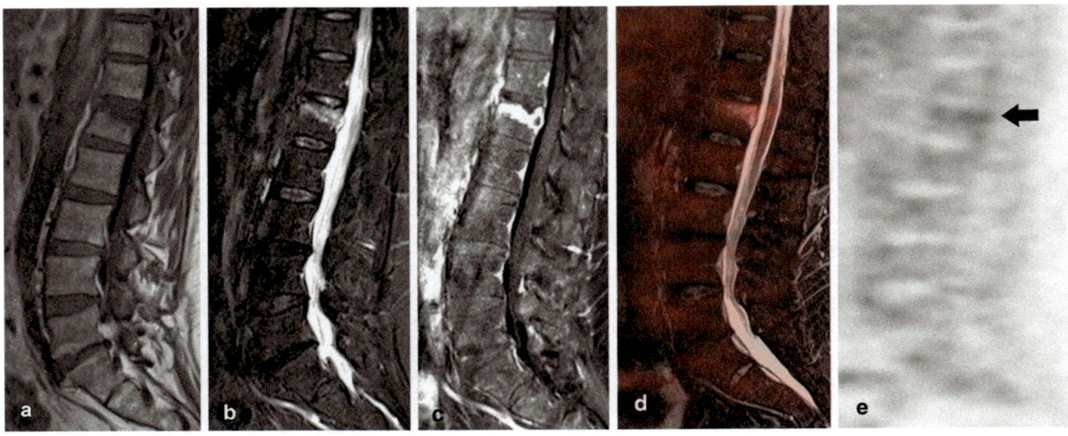

Fig. 23.1 T1-weighted sagittal (**a**), STIR sagittal (**b**), T1-weighted post-gadolinium sagittal (**c**), PET/MR STIR sagittal fusion (**d**), and PET sagittal (**e**)

presence of an epidural or foraminal soft tissue mass. Diffusion-weighted MRI has been shown to be useful in differentiating benign from malignant fractures; however, there is significant overlap between the two etiologies.

FDG PET imaging is useful in differentiating between benign and malignant compression fractures based upon its pattern of uptake as well as degree of metabolic activity. While benign fractures show mild generalized FDG uptake confined to the area of compression, malignant compression fractures demonstrate significantly higher and well-defined focal FDG uptake. PET/MR imaging allows for a more complete assessment of spinal compression fractures in its ability to characterize the type of fracture, assess for complications, determine acuity, and differentiate between benign and malignant compression fractures.

Suggested Reading

Baur A, Stäbler A, Arbogast S, Duerr HR, Bartl R, Reiser M. Acute osteoporotic and neoplastic vertebral compression fractures: fluid sign at MR imaging. Radiology. 2002;225:730–5.

Bredella MA, Essary B, Torriani M, Ouellette HA, Palmer WE. Use of FDG-PET in differentiating benign from malignant compression fractures. Skelet Radiol. 2008;37(5):405–13.

Case 24
Spinal Neuropathic Arthropathy

Anastasia Plaunova and Kelly Tisovic

History

A 72-year-old male with uncontrolled diabetes has 6-week history of lower back and hip pain. MRI of the lumbar spine showed a fracture of L5 vertebral body marrow replacing process with enhancement that was suspicious for metastases (Fig. 24.1). The adjacent L4 inferior endplate was also irregular with bright signal seen in an enlarged disc. Subsequent bone biopsy of L5 was negative for malignancy. There were no organisms seen on microscopy and cultures were negative. The QuantiFERON-TB GOLD was also negative for active or latent tuberculosis.

Diagnosis

Spinal neuropathic arthropathy

Findings

- T1 hypointense signal throughout the entire L5 vertebral body with more than 50% compression fracture (wide arrow).
- L5 vertebral body with hyperintense signal on STIR and diffuse post-contrast enhancement
- Relative cortical bone preservation, with endplate irregularity.
- Widening or ballooning of the L4-L5 and L5-S1 discs (thin arrows).
- Moderate hypermetabolic activity throughout L5 vertebral body and the inferior-posterior aspects of L4 vertebral body (curved arrows)
- T1 axial enhancing soft tissue surrounding L5 vertebral body that is also moderately hypermetabolic on PET (arrowheads)

Discussion

Spinal neuropathic arthropathy, sometimes called "Charcot spine," describes a process characterized by destructive lesions within the spine, which may also affect the adjacent disc space, surrounding vertebra, and facet joints. This process can be seen in diabetics, in patients after spinal cord injury, or in any other conditions where there is loss of the protective mechanisms of the joint, i.e., loss of deep sensation. Symptoms are often nonspecific and have significant overlap with other syndromes related to the spine including degenerative disease, infection, and malignancy. Initial symptoms often include localized deformity and pain.

The mechanism is likely related to trauma and neurovascular changes. Undetected trauma occurs due to decreased sensation and proprioception within a joint and leads to inflammation and increasing joint damage and instability. Neurovascular changes are thought to include autonomic dysregulation, leading to increased blood flow to these joints, causing increased resorption of bone and further injury to the joint

R. Gupta et al., *PET/MR Imaging*, https://doi.org/10.1007/978-3-319-65106-4_24

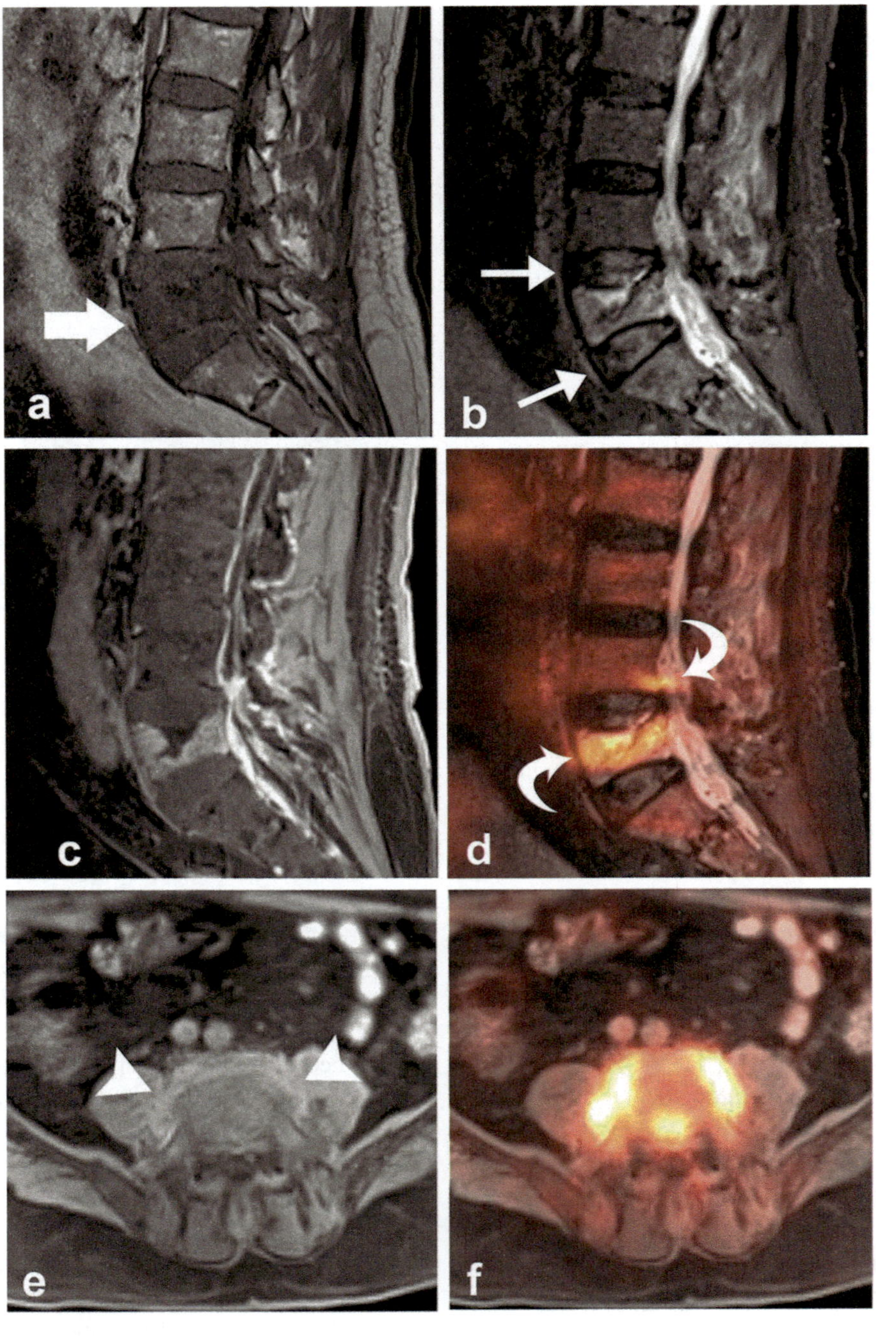

Fig. 24.1 T1 FLAIR sagittal (**a**), STIR sagittal (**b**), T1 VIBE post-gadolinium contrast sagittal (**c**), PET/MR STIR sagittal fusion (**d**), T1 radial VIBE with fat suppression post-gadolinium contrast axial (**e**), and PET/MR T1 radial VIBE with fat suppression post-gadolinium contrast axial fusion (**f**)

space. There are two main patterns of disease, atrophic and hypertrophic. The former manifests as bony resorption and can mimic septic arthritis. The latter appears as bony fragmentation, destruction of the joint space, and sclerosis and is a mimic of osteoarthritis. Importantly, spinal neuroarthropathy can mimic serious diagnoses such as osteomyelitis and metastatic disease, which require completely different treatment paths.

The radiologic findings of neuroarthropathy may overlap with those of osteomyelitis and disc space infection or even malignancy. As seen on both CT and MRI, these include productive bone formation, paraspinal soft tissue mass that may contain calcifications, endplate sclerosis or bony resorption, and endplate irregularities. On MRI, characteristics that distinguish spinal neuropathic arthropathy are debris, disorganization, spondylolisthesis, and especially vacuum disc phenomenon, with involvement of more than one spinal level, specifically facet joints. Another finding that may point to an aseptic etiology is disc bulge, although this is less sensitive than the other findings. Although disc space narrowing may be seen in both infectious and neuropathic cases, relative preservation of the disc space points toward neuropathic arthropathy. Thus, careful inspection for disc space narrowing as well as signal changes should be performed. Both infection and neuroarthropathy can appear isointense to muscle on T1 and follow fluid on T2 sequences within the bone. On gadolinium-enhanced MRI, both entities demonstrate enhancement.

Conversely, on FDG PET, spinal neuropathic arthropathy demonstrates diffuse FDG uptake in both the affected bone and paraspinal soft tissue mass indicating an inflammatory response. The SUV value is often elevated further if concurrent fracture is present. Using PET imaging alone may be difficult to distinguish spinal neuropathic arthropathy from infection or malignancy. Both infection and malignancy usually demonstrate abnormal FDG uptake within the associated disc space and more extensive soft tissue component. There may be abscess formation with intense peripheral FDG uptake and cold central defect. Malignant tumors will often spread into the spinal canal and around the nerve roots. Distant metastases may also be present. PET/MR imaging can help diagnose spinal neuropathy and its associated findings while excluding more serious entities.

Suggested Reading

Lacout A, Lebreton C, Mompoint D, Mokhtari S, Vallée CA, Carlier RY. CT and MRI of spinal neuroarthropathy. AJR Am J Roentgenol. 2009;193(6):W505–14.

Vialle R, Mary P, Tassin JL, Parker F, Guillaumat M. Charcot's disease of the spine: diagnosis and treatment. Spine. 2005;30(11):E315–22.

Wagner SC, Schweitzer ME, Morrison WB, Przybylski GJ, Parker L. Can imaging findings help differentiate spinal neuropathic arthropathy from disk space infection? Initial experience. Radiology. 2000;214(3):693–9.

Case 25 Well-Differentiated Liposarcoma

Rajesh Gupta

History

A 41-year-old female with pain radiating down her right buttock and leg (Fig. 25.1).

Diagnosis

Well-differentiated liposarcoma

Findings

- Lesion in the right gluteus muscle is high in T1-weighted signal matching the subcutaneous fat signal (wide arrow). The majority of the lesion demonstrates a dark signal with fat suppression on the T2 image.
- Lesion has thick septations that are T1 hypointense and T2 hyperintense with mild contrast enhancement (arrowheads).
- Lipomatous lesion demonstrates mild FDG uptake.

Discussion

Well-differentiated liposarcoma (WDL), also known as atypical lipomatous tumor (ALT), is a low-grade malignancy of fatty tissue that rarely metastasizes. However, they must be followed as local recurrence and dedifferentiation can occur. This is the most common histological subtype of liposarcomas. Both WDL and ALT are synonymous, as they share the same morphology and karyotype; however, they may show slight differences in behavior related to tumor location. The World Health Organization designates the term ALT for subcutaneous extremity lesions and WDL for all remaining sites. Low-grade liposarcomas typically affect adults. WDL and ALT are indolent in nature, and treatment with wide surgical excision usually has favorable outcomes. Symptoms arise based on tumor location, which can cause swelling or pain if nerve impingement occurs.

There are several imaging features that can help distinguish well-differentiated liposarcomas from their benign counterpart, lipomas. MRI findings in both show high signal intensity on both T1 and T2-weighted images due to their inherent fatty content. Larger size, deeper localization, heterogeneity, and areas of post-contrast enhancement favor WDL over lipomas. However, the most significant characteristic feature of a well-differentiated liposarcoma is the presence of thickened septa or globular areas of nonadipose tissue comprising more than 25% of the lesion. It is also important to note that high-grade liposarcomas and sarcomas differ from WDL and lipomas in that they have a higher water content and exhibit low signal intensity on T1 weighting.

R. Gupta et al., *PET/MR Imaging*, https://doi.org/10.1007/978-3-319-65106-4_25

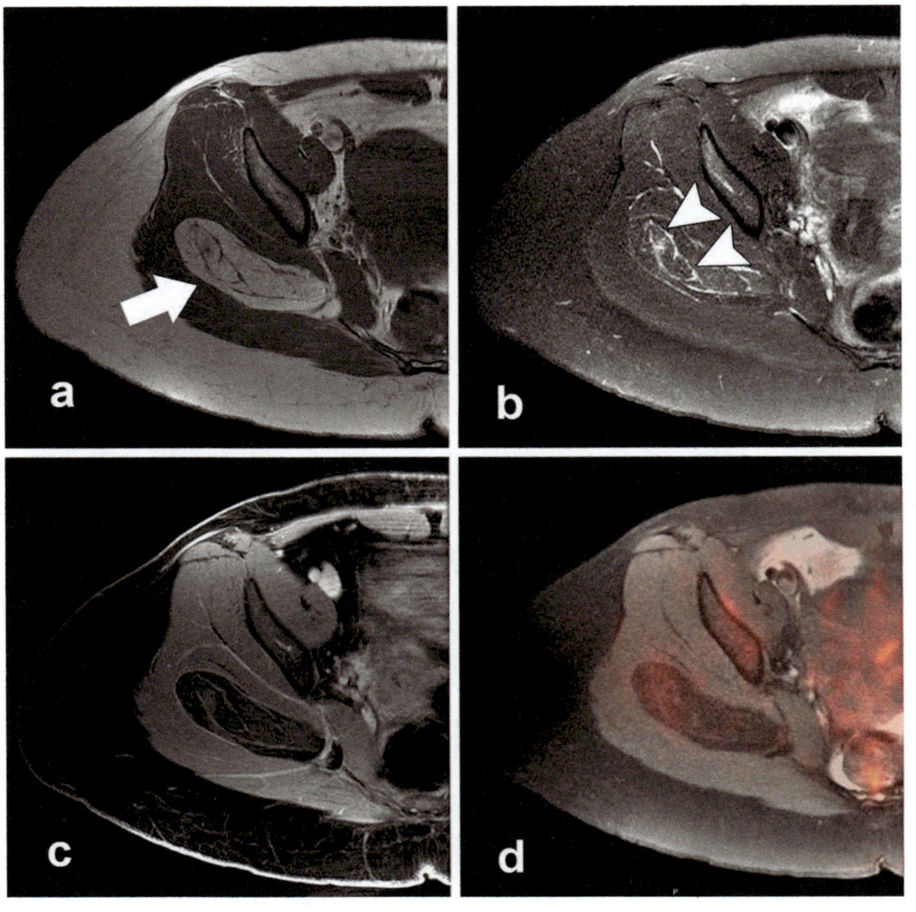

Fig. 25.1 T1 TSE axial (**a**), T2 TSE with fat suppression axial (**b**), T1 VIBE with fat suppression post-gadolinium contrast axial (**c**), and FDG PET/MR T1 VIBE with fat suppression axial fusion (**d**)

While there are several features on MRI to suggest well-differentiated liposarcoma, it is not sufficiently reliable at evaluating biological neoplastic activity in all malignant fatty lesions. It has been shown that FDG PET has a high accuracy in discerning malignant from benign adipose tissue tumors, as malignant lesions have a higher FDG uptake. Quantitative PET analysis can also differentiate between the different histological subtypes of liposarcomas, as the SUV measurements in higher-grade liposarcomas are two- to threefold higher than the well-differentiated subtype. Therefore, PET/MR imaging is helpful in the noninvasive evaluation of soft tissue adipose tumors as it provides the MR characteristics and metabolic information to discern not only between malignant and benign fatty lesions but also differentiate between different liposarcoma subtypes which can help guide initial treatment considerations.

Suggested Reading

Kransdorf MJ, Bancroft LW, Peterson JJ, Murphey MD, Foster WC, Temple HT. Imaging of fatty tumors: distinction of lipoma and well-differentiated liposarcoma. Radiology. 2002;224(1):99–104.

Nagano S, Yokouchi M, Setoguchi T, Ishidou Y, Sasaki H, Shimada H, et al. Differentiation of lipoma and atypical lipomatous tumor by a scoring system: implication of increased vascularity on pathogenesis of liposarcoma. BMC Musculoskelet Disord. 2015;16:36.

Suzuki R, Watanabe H, Yanagawa T, Sato J, Shinozaki T, Suzuki H, et al. PET evaluation of fatty tumors in the extremity: possibility of using the standardized uptake value (SUV) to differentiate benign tumors from liposarcoma. Ann Nucl Med. 2005;19(8):661–70.

Part II

Chest

Case 26 Pulmonary Sarcoidosis

Kavitha Yaddanapudi

History

A 58-year-old female with sarcoidosis referred to PET/MRI for cardiac evaluation (Fig. 26.1).

Diagnosis

Pulmonary sarcoidosis

Findings

- T1 and T2-weighted images show extensive heterogeneous opacities throughout both lungs representing multiple lung nodules and ground-glass opacities.
- PET/MR fusion image shows intense hypermetabolic activity within the lung abnormalities consistent with active pulmonary sarcoidosis (arrowheads). Some hypermetabolic lesions do not have underlying MR lung abnormalities since MR has difficulty visualizing ground-glass opacities.
- PET MIP image shows predominantly upper lobe lung involvement (black thin arrows). No FDG active lymph nodes were identified.

Discussion

Sarcoidosis is an immune-mediated multisystem disease characterized by noncaseating granulomas. Sarcoidosis mostly affects young adults, under 40 years of age with a predilection for women and people of African descent. The lungs are most commonly involved, with respiratory symptoms, night sweats, and erythema nodosum being the most common clinical presentation. However, about 50% of patients are asymptomatic and incidentally diagnosed.

Pulmonary sarcoidosis on imaging has more typical versus atypical manifestations. The typical manifestations include bilateral upper lobe and perihilar opacities, nodules, predominantly in a perilymphatic distribution, and fibrotic changes. The reversible manifestations on imaging include nodules, ground-glass opacities, and consolidations, while the irreversible changes include cysts, traction bronchiectasis, and volume loss. Mediastinal and bilateral hilar lymphadenopathy is another classic manifestation of the disease, with or without pulmonary abnormalities. Although MRI is not routinely used in the diagnosis of pulmonary sarcoidosis as its counterpart CT, studies have shown a very good

R. Gupta et al., *PET/MR Imaging*, https://doi.org/10.1007/978-3-319-65106-4_26

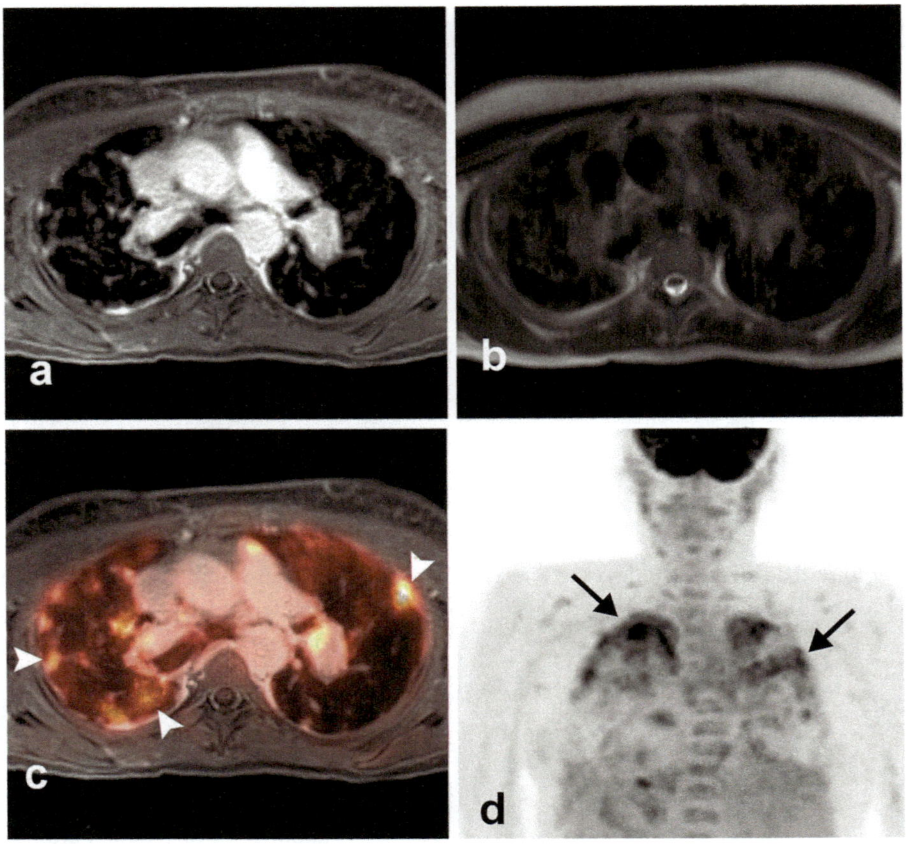

Fig. 26.1 T1 radial VIBE axial with fat suppression (**a**), T2 axial (**b**), PET/MR T1 radial VIBE axial with fat suppression fusion (**c**), and PET MIP (**d**)

correlation between CT and MRI for parenchymal abnormalities in sarcoid, including consolidation and reticular opacities, especially with upper lobe involvement. The most common MRI sequences to evaluate parenchymal disease include HASTE, VIBE, and True FISP.

FDG PET plays an important role in estimating the disease burden, identifying the active inflammatory lesions, guiding biopsy, and assessing treatment response. FDG PET is also useful in assessing for the presence of cardiac involvement and neurosarcoidosis. FDG PET is particularly beneficial in assessing response to treatment in patients on immunosuppressive therapy. PET/MR imaging fulfills all the above roles of PET/CT but has an added advantage of decreased radiation and better tissue characterization in the evaluation of cardiac and CNS involvement.

Suggested Reading

Chung JH, Little BP, Forssen AV, Yong J, Nambu A, Kazlouski D, et al. Proton MRI in the evaluation of pulmonary sarcoidosis: comparison to chest CT. Eur J Radiol. 2013;82(12):2378–85.

Criado E, Sánchez M, Ramírez J, Arguis P, de Caralt TM, Perea RJ, et al. Pulmonary sarcoidosis: typical and atypical manifestations at high-resolution CT with pathologic correlation. Radiographics. 2010;30(6):1567–86.

Case 27 Cardiac Metastasis from Renal Cell Carcinoma

Kavitha Yaddanapudi and Robert Matthews

History

A 69-year-old male with a history of renal cell carcinoma with a new mass seen on chest CT (Fig. 27.1).

Diagnosis

Cardiac metastasis from renal cell carcinoma

Findings

- T2 hyperintense, T1 isointense large left ventricular tumor (wide white arrows).
- Delayed enhancement of the tumor with frank myocardial invasion of the left ventricular apex (thin white arrow) as well as early extension into the right ventricular apex.
- PET/MR and PET MIP images demonstrate intense hypermetabolic activity within the left ventricular metastasis (curved black arrow).
- PET MIP additionally reveals a metastatic right lung lesion (black arrowhead).

Discussion

Metastases are the most common malignant cardiac tumors. Metastases can occur from renal cell carcinoma, melanomas, breast cancer, lung cancer, lymphoma, and a variety of sarcomas. The most common primary tumor to spread to the heart are metastases from lung cancer that can either directly invade the heart or metastasize to it. The most frequent site of metastatic involvement is the pericardium which can subsequently invade the underlying myocardium. Although cardiac metastases are most likely asymptomatic, there may be shortness of breath, chest wall pain, and peripheral edema caused from pericardial effusion and impaired right cardiac filling.

Although there are no specific MRI features of metastases, they are typically hypointense on T1-weighted images and hyperintense on T2-weighted images, except for melanoma which have increased T1-weighted signal. Pericardial effusions are typically hyperintense on T1-weighted images if they are hemorrhagic or exudative and hypointense on T1 if a benign

R. Gupta et al., *PET/MR Imaging*, https://doi.org/10.1007/978-3-319-65106-4_27

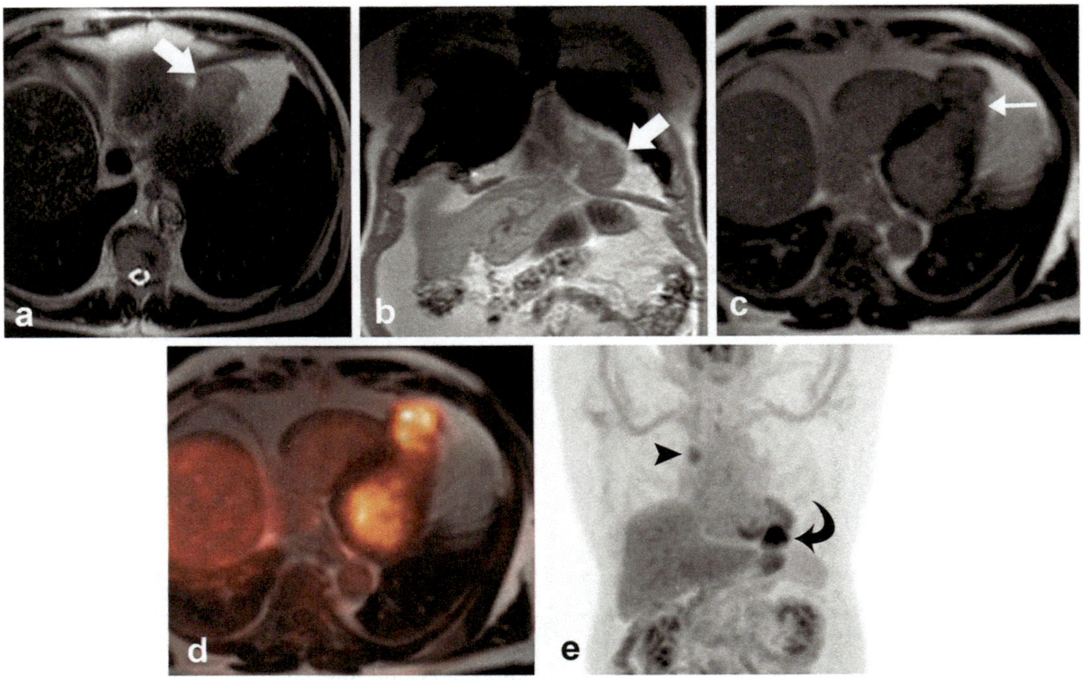

Fig. 27.1 T2 axial (**a**), T1 FLASH coronal (**b**), True FISP post-gadolinium contrast enhancement, four-chamber view (**c**), PET/MR True FISP post-gadolinium contrast enhancement, four-chamber view fusion (**d**), and PET MIP (**e**)

transudate. On MRI malignant lesions can be differentiated from benign lesions by myocardial invasion. The enhancement pattern on MR is not important, since many benign primary cardiac lesions such as myxomas and fibromas also enhance.

With PET/MR imaging, benign tumors of the heart are usually not FDG avid with the exception of tumor-like inflammatory lesions, such as thrombus. As with any cardiac tumor, biopsy is the gold standard. FDG PET/MR imaging can serve as a single-stop imaging modality for cardiac masses. MRI provides excellent anatomical detail, localization, and assessment of function and on post-contrast images determines invasion of the myocardium and associated scarring. FDG PET, with its capability for metabolic characterization, determines whether the mass is benign or malignant. FDG-negative cardiac masses with typical MRI features of a benign mass, such as a lipoma or hemangioma, can safely be followed without biopsy or surgical intervention in some cases. Imaging of malignant masses is used to assess for guidance of biopsy, presurgical evaluation of the myocardium, and postsurgical evaluation for recurrence.

Suggested Reading

Motwani M, Kidambi A, Herzog BA, Uddin A, Greenwood JP, Plein S. MR imaging of cardiac tumors and masses: a review of methods and clinical applications. Radiology. 2013;268(1):26–43.

Nensa F, Tezgah E, Poeppel TD, Jensen CJ, Schelhorn J, Köhler J, et al. Integrated 18F-FDG PET/MR imaging in the assessment of cardiac masses: a pilot study. J Nucl Med. 2015;56(2):255–60.

Yaddanapudi K, Brunken R, Tan CD, Rodriguez E, Bolen MA. PET-MR imaging in evaluation of cardiac and paracardiac masses with histopathologic correlation. J Am Coll Cardiol Img. 2016;9(1):82–5.

Case 28
Breast Cancer (Invasive Ductal Carcinoma)

Elham Safaie

History

A 60-year-old female presents for staging of primary breast cancer after the initiation of chemotherapy (Fig. 28.1).

Diagnosis

Breast cancer (invasive ductal carcinoma)

Findings

- A 5 cm mass that is isointense on T1-weighted image and mildly hyperintense on T2-weighted image (curved arrow) localized to the right breast, without chest wall invasion.
- PET images show abnormal increased FDG uptake in the right breast mass compatible with malignancy.
- No hypermetabolic lymph nodes are identified.
- Mild stimulation of the bone marrow reflecting the initiation of chemotherapy.

Discussion

Breast cancer is the most common malignancy in women, with an estimated 234,000 new cases diagnosed in 2015 and approximately 5–9% of patients presenting with metastatic disease. Patients commonly present with a palpable somewhat, immobile mass. More advanced breast cancer may present with breast pain, swelling, rash or nipple discharge, or a larger more fixed mass. Invasive ductal carcinoma is the most common type of breast cancer, accounting for up to nearly 70–80% of all breast cancer diagnoses. It is a subtype of ductal carcinoma that shows an infiltrative pattern of malignant mammary ducts.

The initial staging of breast cancer is mostly based on imaging. The role of FDG PET/MR imaging in patients with breast cancer is to stage locally advanced cancer, to evaluate for chest wall involvement, axillary or internal mammary lymph node metastases, and distant metastases. The sensitivity of FDG PET for small tumors less than 10 mm, stage T1, has been shown to range from 50 to 72%, with the sensitivity increasing to greater than 90% for tumors between 20 and 50 mm. Dedicated PET imaging of the breast using positron emission mammography attains higher resolution of 1–2 mm.

MR imaging is currently used and approved for a number of indications in patients with breast cancer including screening in high-risk women, assessment of patients with prior breast augmentation surgery, evaluation of the extent of disease in newly diagnosed cancer patients, and evaluation of response in patients who received treatment. PET/MRI with dedicated breast coil in

R. Gupta et al., *PET/MR Imaging*, https://doi.org/10.1007/978-3-319-65106-4_28

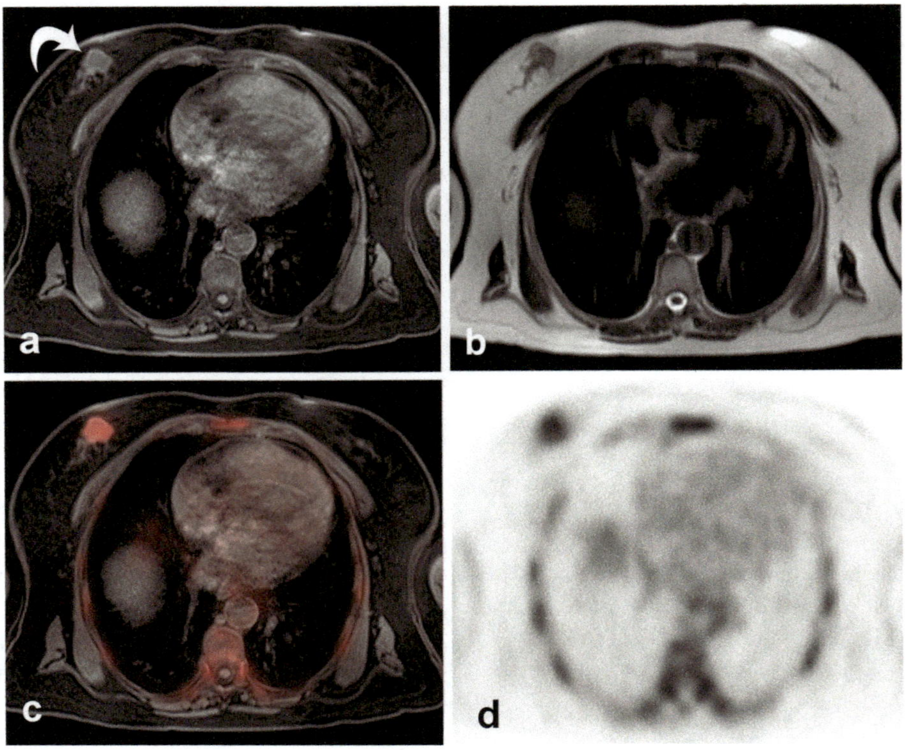

Fig. 28.1 T1 VIBE with fat suppression axial (**a**), T2 axial (**b**), PET/MR fusion with fat suppression axial fusion (**c**), and PET axial (**d**)

conjunction with administration of IV contrast with dynamic acquisition provides excellent evaluation of the breast tissue. Whole-body FDG PET/MR imaging with a body coil is less useful in evaluating primary tumors of the breast as there is volume averaging due to the small size of the lesion, but is valuable in assessing metastatic disease, especially distant metastases. In particular whole body assessment is recommended for breast cancer patients with a suspicion of metastatic disease.

Suggested Reading

Rice SL, Friedman KP. Clinical PET-MR imaging in breast cancer and lung cancer. PET Clin. 2016;11(4):387–402.

Case 29
Benign Thymic Rebound Hyperplasia

Rajesh Gupta

History

A 21-year-old male with lymphoma (Fig. 29.1).

Diagnosis

Benign thymic rebound hyperplasia

Findings

- At staging, the fusion image shows a residual thymus gland in the anterior mediastinum (curved arrow) without significant FDG activity. This would be a normal finding in an 18-year-old patient.
- Following chemotherapy, the fusion image shows hypermetabolic activity in the now significantly enlarged thymus gland.
- MR demonstrates the enlarged thymus gland, following chemotherapy, which is homogenously isointense on T1-weighted image compared to muscle and homogenously moderately hyperintense on T2-weighted image.
- PET MIP images show diffuse FDG uptake in the hyperplastic thymus gland (thin arrow).

Discussion

The thymus is a lymphoid and endocrine organ that plays a role in the development of the adaptive immune system, primarily through T-cell maturation. It is located in the superior and anterior mediastinum, behind the sternum. The thymus gland is relatively larger in infants and gradually undergoes fatty replacement and involution by adolescence or early adulthood. The thymus responds to systemic stresses such as infection, neoplasm, surgery, or chemotherapy by rapid atrophy. However it can regrow to its original size or beyond once the stressful event is over. This process is known as thymic rebound hyperplasia and although typically seen in children can occur at any age.

The size, shape, and imaging characteristics of the normal thymus change with age. Initially, it appears as a retrosternal bilobed mass with convex margins. It increases in weight through puberty to become largely fatty by 40 years of age. MR imaging characteristics change over time to reflect the microscopic fatty involution of the thymus gland with increasing T1- and T2-weighted signal as it matures. It is usually slightly hyperintense to muscle on T1-weighted

R. Gupta et al., *PET/MR Imaging*, https://doi.org/10.1007/978-3-319-65106-4_29

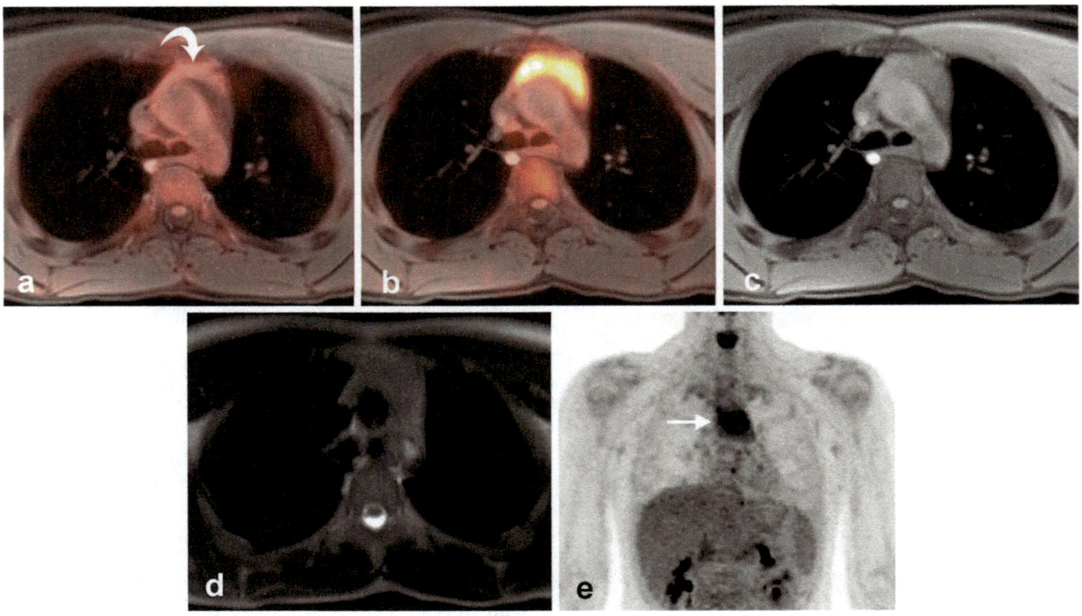

Fig. 29.1 PET/MR T1 radial VIBE with fat suppression axial fusion, at staging (**a**); PET/MR T1 radial VIBE with fat suppression axial fusion, 6 months after starting chemotherapy (**b**); T1 radial VIBE axial, 6 months after starting chemotherapy (**c**); T2 axial, 6 months after starting chemotherapy (**d**); and PET MIP, 6 months after starting chemotherapy (**e**)

images, moderately hyperintense to muscle on T2-weighted images approaching fat signal. The normal thymus should not exceed 1.8 cm in thickness under the age of 20, and thymus thickness should not exceed 1.3 cm in older patients as measured on cross-sectional imaging perpendicular to the length of a lobe. Chemical shift MR imaging has also been used to demonstrate the presence of microscopic fat in the normal thymus. In times of stress, the gland can atrophy to almost half of its original size and rebound up to double its size once the stress has resolved.

In children before puberty, the thymus gland can have mild to moderate normal physiological FDG uptake on PET imaging with SUV 2-5. In children and adults with benign thymic rebound hyperplasia, the FDG uptake is moderately increased with SUV usually in the range 3-7. Thymic rebound has been reported to occur anywhere from 1 to 10 months after the completion of chemotherapy. The fusion of FDG PET and MR provides the ability to distinguish a benign thymus from malignancy more accurately as anatomic characteristics and metabolic information can be obtained and interpreted simultaneously in conjunction with the clinical information at that time.

Suggested Reading

Ackman JB, Wu CC. MRI of the thymus. AJR Am J Roentgenol. 2011;197(1):W15–20.

Gawande RS, Khurana A, Messing S. Differentiation of normal thymus from anterior mediastinal lymphoma and lymphoma recurrence at pediatric PET/CT. Radiology. 2012;262(2):613–22.

Case 30
Pulmonary Infarct

Kavitha Yaddanapudi

History

A 23-year-old male presents with Hodgkin's lymphoma arising from posttransplant lymphoproliferative disorder following renal transplant (Fig. 30.1). He had an acute pulmonary embolism 4 months ago.

Diagnosis

Pulmonary infarct

Findings

- CT chest angiogram shows a filling defect in an enlarged right lower lobe pulmonary artery representing acute pulmonary embolism (thin arrow). A left-sided pleural effusion is also seen.
- MRI shows a wedge-shaped lesion in the right upper lobe that is hyperintense on T1-weighted image and hyperintense on T2-weighted image consistent with lung infarct from pulmonary embolism (wide arrow).
- PET/MR fusion image shows hypermetabolic activity within the lung infarct consistent with inflammation.
- Susceptibility artifact from sternotomy wires is noted.

Discussion

Pulmonary embolism has a higher incidence in cancer patients than in the general population. Pulmonary thromboembolism can lead to lung infarction in one fourth of the cases. Typically pulmonary infracts are wedge-shaped consolidations or airspace processes in the setting of pulmonary embolism. On PET/CT, pulmonary infarcts can be confused for neoplastic processes if there is uniform, intense uptake of FDG. FDG uptake in infarcts is related to increased inflammation and foamy macrophage activity. The FDG uptake of a pulmonary infarct is typically a large peripheral lung density with increased outer hypermetabolic activity and decreased central activity, referred to as a "rim sign". Increased FDG uptake related to inflammation can also be identified in central vessel emboli. In a calcifying infarct, FDG uptake is likely attributable to dystrophic calcification and associated inflammatory response.

MRI has been used to identify acute pulmonary embolism in patients who have contraindications to CT contrast and are not appropriate for nuclear lung scans. MRI can identify acute pulmonary embolism with acceptable accuracy. Infarcts on MRI are typically wedge-shaped consolidation with its base to the lung periphery. They can also appear as subpleural densities or peripheral nodules. Infarcts

R. Gupta et al., *PET/MR Imaging*, https://doi.org/10.1007/978-3-319-65106-4_30

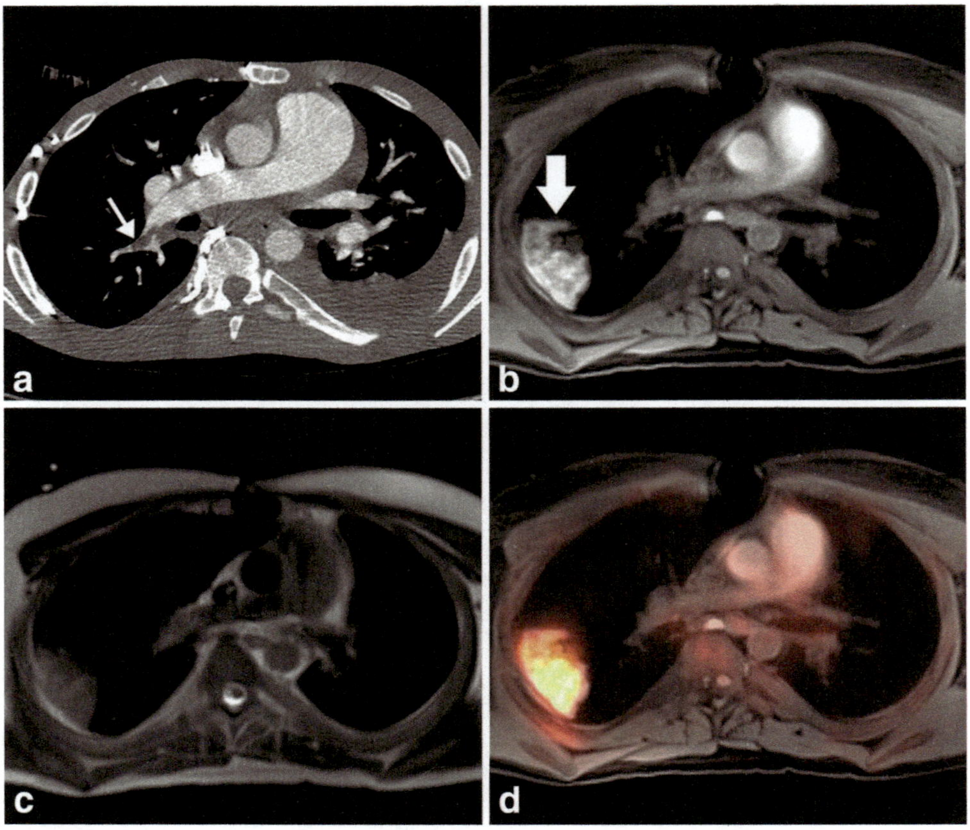

Fig. 30.1 CT chest angiogram (**a**), T1 radial VIBE axial with fat suppression (**b**), T2 HASTE axial (**c**), and PET/MR T1 radial VIBE axial with fat suppression fusion (**d**)

heal by cavitation, scarring, or forming bands. In the immediate stage of pulmonary infarct, the lesions are isointense on T1-weighted images and hyperintense on T2-weighted images. Between 1 and 7 days, the lesion becomes hyperintense on both T1- and T2-weighted images. Calcified infarcts showed greater T1 and T2 hypointensity.

PET/MR imaging characterization of an infarct exemplifies the complementary role of these modalities. Diffuse and somewhat heterogeneous FDG uptake on PET represents an inflammatory process, and the characteristic wedge-shaped lesion on MRI in a patient with known pulmonary embolism is consistent with an infarct.

Suggested Reading

Hochhegger B, Ley-Zaporozhan J, Marchiori E, Irion K, Souza AS Jr, Moreira J, et al. Magnetic resonance imaging findings in acute pulmonary embolism. Br J Radiol. 2011;84(999):282–7.

Nomori H, Horio H, Moringa S, Suemasu K. Multiple pulmonary infarctions associated with lung cancer. Jpn J Clin Oncol. 2000;30:40–2.

Wittram C, Scott JA. 18F-FDG PET of pulmonary embolism. AJR Am J Roentgenol. 2007;189(1): 171–6.

Case 31
Mediastinal Lymphoma

Rajesh Gupta

History

A 49-year-old male with HIV and lymphoma presents with right-sided neck pain. Ultrasound showed slow flow in the right subclavian vein (Fig. 31.1).

Diagnosis

Mediastinal lymphoma with mass effect on large veins

Findings

- Large conglomerate of lymph nodes forming a mass in the anterior mediastinum extending to the superior mediastinum and right lower neck that has heterogenous T1 hyperintense and T2 isointense signal (wide arrow).
- PET/MR fusion images show the large mass to have intense metabolic activity with an SUV 31.6.
- Formation of the superior vena cava from the left and right brachiocephalic veins is not visualized due to extrinsic compression of the large mass (thin arrow). Trachea is pushed to the left side.
- Collapse of the right internal jugular vein with prominent flow through the left internal jugular vein (asterisks) and enlargement of the azygos vein (curved arrow).
- Bilateral pleural effusions are also noted.

Discussion

Non-Hodgkin and Hodgkin lymphomas are hematologic malignances that arise from lymphocytes and lymphoblasts. They can present with nodal or, less commonly, extranodal disease. The mediastinum is a common location for lymphoma to manifest and can present as part of disseminated disease or rarely as the site of primary involvement. Diffuse large B-cell lymphoma (DLBCL) is a frequent histologic subtype of primary mediastinal lymphomas and typically presents at a younger age with a female predominance. Otherwise, large-cell lymphomas affecting other areas of the body present at a median age of 52 years with a male predominance. Plasmablastic lymphoma is considered a distinct aggressive subtype of DLBCL commonly seen in patients with HIV infection. Large-cell mediastinal lymphoma typically presents as a large anterior mediastinal mass which causes mass effect on adjacent structures leading to symptoms related to vascular compression resulting in superior vena cava syndrome and chest pain.

MRI is useful in evaluating the extent of mediastinal lymphoma, especially when assessing the thoracic wall, vascular, or bone marrow

R. Gupta et al., *PET/MR Imaging*, https://doi.org/10.1007/978-3-319-65106-4_31

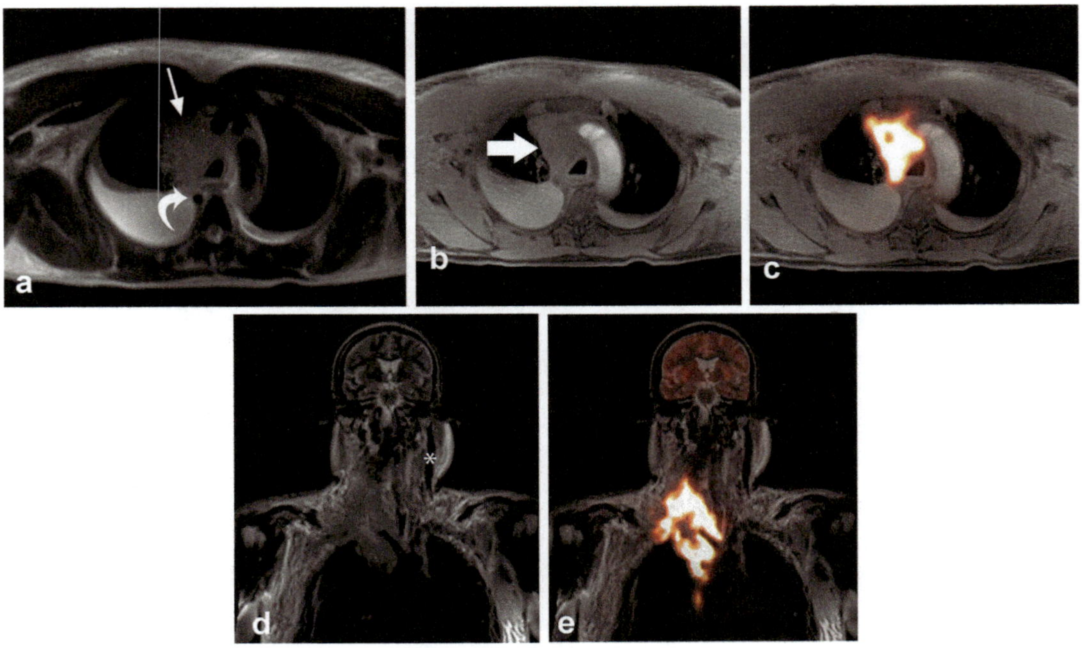

Fig. 31.1 T2-weighted axial (**a**), T1 radial VIBE with fat suppression axial (**b**), PET/MR T1 radial VIBE with fat suppression axial fusion (**c**), T2-weighted coronal (**d**), and PET/MR T2-weighted coronal fusion (**e**)

invasion. It provides excellent soft tissue resolution to evaluate the relationship between the tumor and intrathoracic structures such as the heart. MRI also provides excellent anatomical detail of the subcarinal and aortopulmonary window areas. Morphological changes of malignant lymph nodes that can be detected through MRI include enlarged size and a rounded configuration compared to their normal oval shape. Diffusion-weighted imaging has been shown to be sensitive to nodal disease and bone marrow involvement as apparent diffusion coefficient values have increased in successfully treated nodal disease.

The use of molecular imaging with FDG PET to evaluate large B-cell lymphoma has been well established. Lymphoma demonstrates avid FDG uptake, and therefore FDG PET combined with MR can provide information related to staging and response to treatment as well as prognosis. A reduction in the SUV maximum value by more than 66% after two cycles of chemotherapy indicates a satisfactory response to treatment and therefore a favorable prognosis. The intensity of the FDG uptake has been correlated with the aggressiveness of the lymphoma subtype. PET/MR has been shown to be particularly useful in identifying extranodal disease, especially bone marrow involvement which is often occult on CT or radiography.

Suggested Reading

Castillo JJ, Bibas M, Miranda RN. The biology and treatment of plasmablastic lymphoma. Blood. 2015;125(15):2323–30.

Heacock L, Weissbrot J, Raad R, Campbell N, Friedman KP, Ponzo F, et al. PET/MRI for the evaluation of patients with lymphoma: initial observations. AJR Am J Roentgenol. 2015;204(4):842–8.

Johnson SA, Kumar A, Matasar MJ, Schöder H, Rademaker J. Imaging for staging and response assessment in lymphoma. Radiology. 2015;276(2):323–38.

Shaffer K, Smith D, Kirn D, Kaplan W, Canellos G, Mauch P, et al. Primary mediastinal large-B-cell lymphoma: radiologic findings at presentation. AJR Am J Roentgenol. 1996;167(2):425–30.

Case 32 Inflammatory Breast Cancer

Elham Safaie

History

A 52-year-old female present with breast cancer and enlarged axillary lymph nodes (Fig. 32.1).

Diagnosis

Inflammatory breast cancer with lymph node metastases

Findings

- Right breast contains two adjacent spiculated masses that are isointense to muscle on T1-weighted image and hypointense on T2-weighted image (thin white arrows).
- Right breast skin thickening indicating an inflammatory response (white arrowheads).
- PET fusion image shows abnormal hypermetabolism within the two right breast masses compatible with malignancy.
- Increased mild FDG uptake corresponding to the thickened skin of the right breast and throughout the breast parenchyma compatible with an active inflammatory process.
- More superior images show enlarged hypermetabolic right axillary lymph nodes consistent with metastases (wide white arrow).
- PET MIP better depicts the diffuse inflammatory changes in the right breast as well as the multifocal malignancy (curved black arrow). Prominent hypermetabolic right axillary and cervical metastatic lymph nodes are present.

Discussion

Inflammatory breast cancer (IBC) is a rare and aggressive form of breast cancer accounting for 2–5% of breast cancers. IBC typically presents with skin erythema, edema, and an orange-peel appearance of the breast skin, instead of a lump. IBC affects young patients with an average age of 58 years at diagnosis, grows, and tends to spread rapidly, with an associated 20–40% rate of distant metastases at presentation.

The pathologic hallmark of IBC is dermal lymphatic involvement causing edema and erythema. Early tissue diagnosis with skin punch biopsy and clinical evidence is critical as IBC tends to grow rapidly. The key feature that differentiates IBC from other breast cancers is the locally advanced nature of inflammatory breast cancer at the onset of symptoms. Symptoms of IBC develop within 3 months or less, whereas symptoms of noninflammatory breast cancer typically develop over a more protracted period. The treatment course for inflammatory breast cancer includes preoperative chemotherapy, mastectomy, and radiation.

R. Gupta et al., *PET/MR Imaging*, https://doi.org/10.1007/978-3-319-65106-4_32

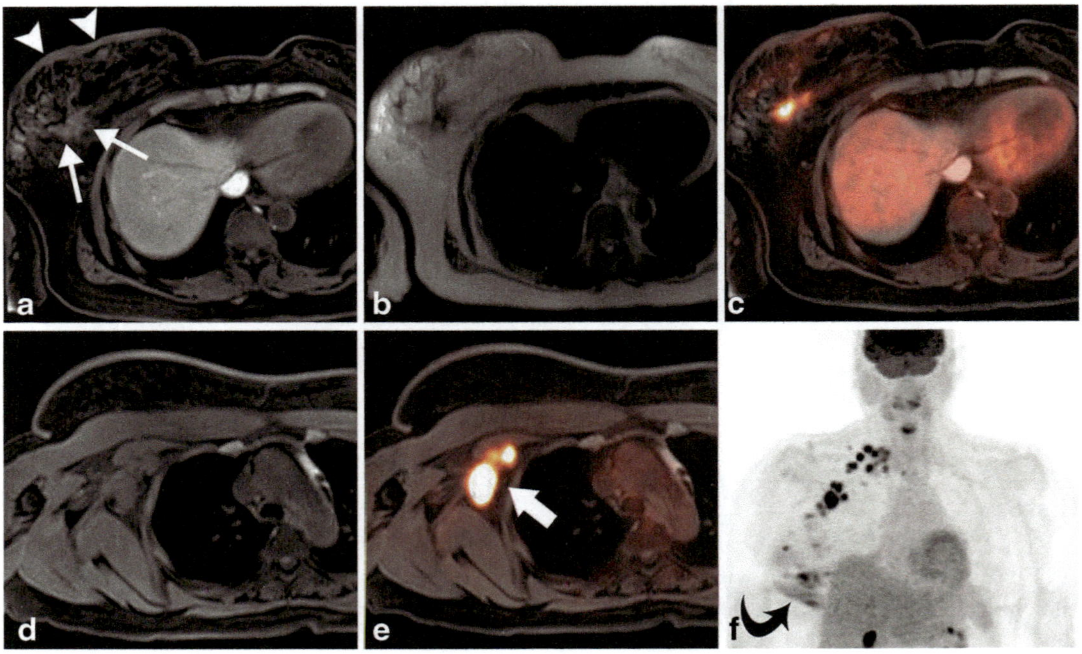

Fig. 32.1 T1 VIBE with fat suppression axial (**a**), T2 HASTE axial (inferior slice) (**b**), PET/MR T1 VIBE with fat suppression axial fusion (**c**), T1 VIBE with fat suppression axial, at more superior level (**d**), PET/MR T1 VIBE with fat suppression axial fusion, at more superior level (**e**), and PET MIP (**f**)

Typical mammographic findings include diffuse enlargement of the breast, stromal coarsening, diffuse increased density, skin thickening, and enlarged lymph nodes. If a mass or biopsy target is not detected at conventional imaging, MR is helpful to determine a biopsy target to confirm the diagnosis of IBC. Common findings of IBC on contrast-enhanced MR images are extensive or segmental non-mass like enhancement and diffuse skin thickening. Kinetics typically show initial rapid enhancement with washout or plateau curves. Because of the high likelihood of metastases at diagnosis, FDG PET/MRI can be extremely beneficial in the initial evaluation and staging of IBC.

PET/MR imaging also has a good ability to assess axillary lymph node involvement based on abnormal hypermetabolism. Lymphoscintigraphy in conjunction with surgical sampling is the most accurate method for detecting micrometastases within axillary lymph nodes. Normal axillary lymph nodes can be quite large on MR imaging, so size criteria is not reliable as in other locations. MRI features of metastases in axillary lymph nodes include an irregular margin, loss of the normal fatty hilum, and cortical thickening greater than 2–3 mm. The low T1 signal and intermediate T2 signal of a normal lymph node may remain present with early metastatic disease.

Suggested Reading

Chow CK. Imaging in inflammatory breast carcinoma. Breast Dis. 2005–2006;22:45–54.

Le-Petross HT, Cristofanilli M, Carkaci S, Krishnamurthy S, Jackson EF, Harrell RK, et al. MRI features of inflammatory breast cancer. AJR Am J Roentgenol. 2011;197(4):W769–76.

Girardi V, Carbognin G, Camera L, Bonetti F, Manfrin E, Pollini G, et al. Inflammatory breast carcinoma and locally advanced breast carcinoma: characterisation with MR imaging. Radiol Med. 2011;116(1):71–83.

Niikura N, Costelloe CM, Madewell JE, Hayashi N, Yu TK, Liu J, et al. FDG- PET/CT compared with conventional imaging in the detection of distant metastases of primary breast cancer. Oncologist. 2011;16(8):1111–9.

Case 33
Benign Loculated Pleural Effusion

Kavitha Yaddanapudi

History

A 52-year-old male with chronic lymphoid leukemia presents for restaging with PET/MRI (Fig. 33.1).

Diagnosis

Benign loculated pleural effusion

Findings

- Loculated fluid is heterogenously T1 and T2 hyperintense indicating exudative fluid (wide arrows). T2-weighted low-signal septations are identified (arrowheads).
- Areas of low T1 and T2-weighted signal globules represent areas of old hemorrhage (thin arrow).
- Moderate-sized loculated pleural effusion in the right lung base with no significant FDG uptake on PET imaging signifying a benign collection.
- Pleural thickening and atelectasis surrounding the loculated fluid collection with mild FDG activity indicate chronic inflammation.

Discussion

Pleural disease ranges from simple pleural effusions to complex effusions and pleural masses. A pleural effusion is an accumulation of fluid in the pleural space. Pleural effusions are broadly classified as transudative or exudative. Pleural fluid may become loculated within the fissures or between the visceral and parietal pleural layers. This most commonly occurs with exudative fluid, blood, and pus. When loculated pleural fluid becomes infected, it is termed an empyema, which can be potentially life-threatening, requiring prompt diagnosis and treatment. Often times, the lung parenchyma around the pleural fluid collapses, causing atelectasis that can lead to shortness of breath.

On cross-sectional axial images, pleural effusions appear as semicircular dependent fluid collections. MR imaging demonstrates simple transudative pleural effusions with homogenous hyperintense signal on T2-weighted imaging. On T1-weighted images, simple or transudative effusions are hypointense relative to the muscle, whereas complex and exudative effusions are hyperintense on T1-signifying proteinaceous material, chyle, or hemorrhagic products. MRI is

R. Gupta et al., *PET/MR Imaging*, https://doi.org/10.1007/978-3-319-65106-4_33

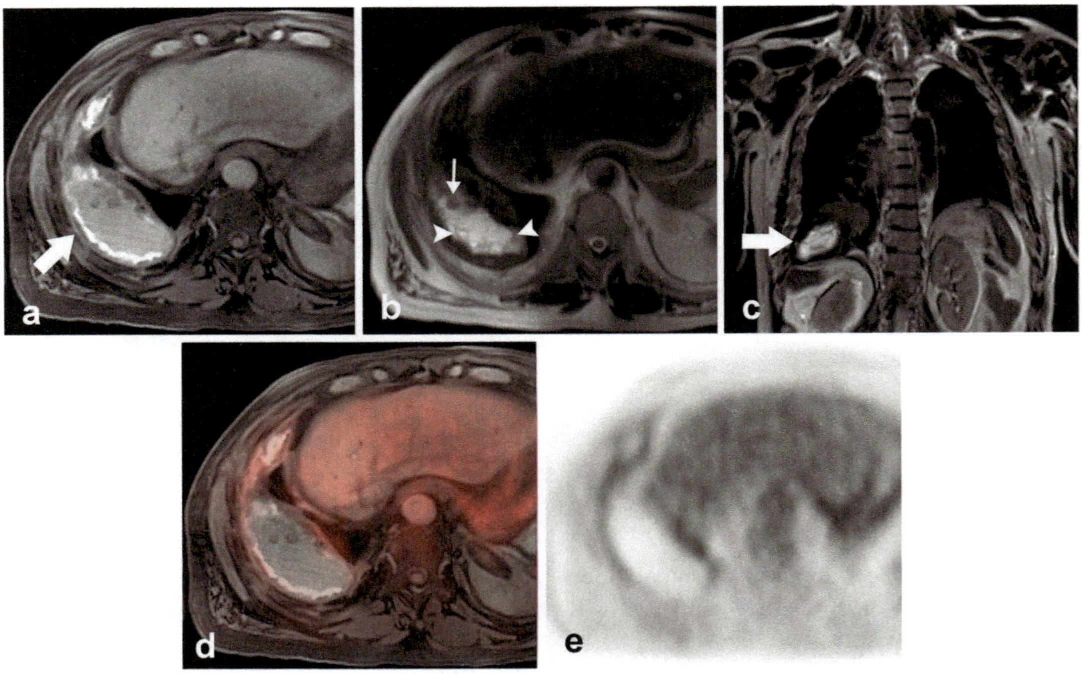

Fig. 33.1 T1 radial VIBE axial with fat suppression (**a**), T2 HASTE axial (**b**), T2 TSE coronal (**c**), PET/MR T1 radial VIBE with fat suppression axial fusion (**d**), and PET axial (**e**)

also helpful in identifying associated pleural thickening and nodularity including pleural metastases. Additionally, MRI is useful in identifying septa between the loculations and debris within the effusion. Thus, MRI offers better characterization of pleural effusions than CT. Recently diffusion-weighted imaging has been shown to be useful in differentiating transudative from exudative effusions.

FDG PET shows increased uptake in inflammatory, parapneumonic effusions and malignant effusions. Malignant effusions may be associated with more nodular or ringlike pleural FDG uptake especially in pleural metastases or malignant pleural mesothelioma. In patients with a known malignancy, FDG PET has been reported to have moderate accuracy in differentiating benign from malignant effusions. Visual and semiquantitative analysis can both be used to assess FDG uptake in effusions. FDG PET/MR imaging is useful in the assessment of complex effusions to further characterize and identify potential FDG-avid biopsy sites. FDG uptake can also be assessed prior to radiotherapy in malignant effusions to guide radiation treatment plan. The lack of significant FDG uptake and pleural thickening favors benign effusions.

Suggested Reading

Inan N, Arslan A, Akansel G, Arslan Z, Elemen L, Demirci A. Diffusion-weighted MRI in the characterization of pleural effusions. Diagn Interv Radiol. 2009;15(1):13–8.

Porcel JM, Hernández P, Martínez-Alonso M, Bielsa S, Salud A. Accuracy of fluorodeoxyglucose-PET imaging for differentiating benign from malignant pleural effusions: a meta-analysis. Chest. 2015;147(2):502–12.

Case 34
Chest Wall Metastasis from Renal Cell Carcinoma

Rajesh Gupta

History

A 65-year-old male with a history of renal cell carcinoma, post right nephrectomy, presents with palpable left posterior chest wall mass (Fig. 34.1).

Diagnosis

Chest wall metastasis from renal cell carcinoma (clear cell type)

Findings

- Hyperintense T2-weighted, isointense T1-weighted lesion within the inferior aspect of the left latissimus dorsi muscle of the posterior chest wall with avid FDG uptake (thin white arrow).
- PET MIP shows the lesion in the left latissimus muscle (thin black arrow). Notice only the left kidney is present (curved arrow).

Discussion

Renal cell carcinoma (RCC) is the most common renal neoplasm with the majority of cases having the clear cell histological subtype. Although renal cell carcinoma can metastasize to any site, spread to skeletal muscle is uncommon. In general, muscle metastases are quite rare from any primary malignancy. Metastatic pathways include hematogenous spread, lymphatic spread, and direct extension. Imaging plays an important role in detecting metastatic RCC, selecting patients for treatment, and monitoring response to therapy.

MRI allows for superior soft tissue details to discern a metastatic lesion and its relationship to adjacent soft tissue structures. Renal cell carcinomatous lesions are generally isointense on T1- and T2-weighted imaging and demonstrate avid arterial enhancement post gadolinium administration. MRI signal characteristics can change if the lesion contains areas of hemorrhage or necrosis. The clear cell subtype may be hyperintense on T2-weighted imaging and has been reported to have a greater propensity to metastasize compared to other cell types.

FDG PET alone without anatomical correlation has previously been shown to have a lower sensitivity for detecting primary or metastatic renal cell carcinoma, especially for primary lesions less than 2 cm in size since normal renal excretion of FDG masks the hypermetabolic lesion within the renal parenchyma. However, more recent reports have demonstrated increased sensitivity and specificity for FDG PET/CT in identifying metastatic RCC, of which the majority have increased metabolic

R. Gupta et al., *PET/MR Imaging*, https://doi.org/10.1007/978-3-319-65106-4_34

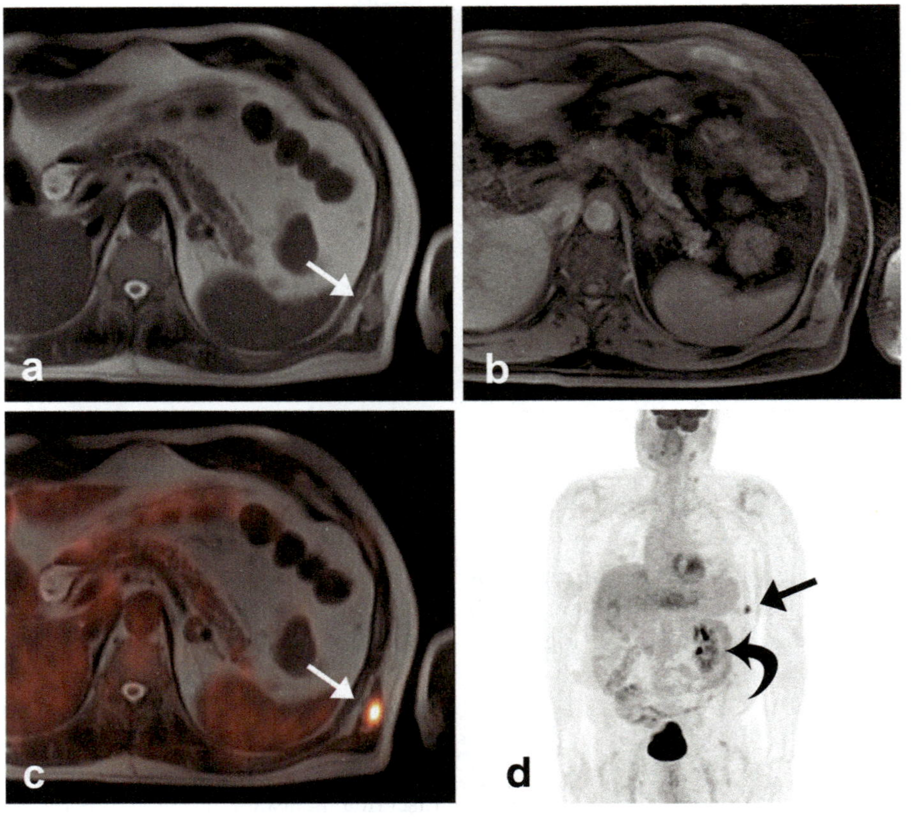

Fig. 34.1 T2 HASTE axial (**a**), T1 radial VIBE with fat suppression axial (**b**), PET/MR T2-weighted axial fusion (**c**), and PET MIP (**d**)

activity. FDG PET has also been shown to be promising in providing prognostic information as high SUV and increased number of positive lesions are associated with poorer outcomes. Treatment response can also be evaluated by showing decreasing metabolic activity following treatment. FDG PET/MRI provides increased accuracy for metastatic renal carcinoma detection and characterization, especially in unusual sites due to its combination of superior anatomic detail and functional information.

Suggested Reading

Griffin N, Gore ME, Sohaib SA. Imaging in metastatic renal cell carcinoma. AJR Am J Roentgenol. 2007;189(2):360–70.

Kayani I, Avril N, Bomanji J, Chowdhury S, Rockall A, Sahdev A, et al. Sequential FDG-PET/CT as a biomarker of response to Sunitinib in metastatic clear cell renal cancer. Clin Cancer Res. 2011;17(18):6021–8.

Oliva MR, Glickman JN, Zou KH, Teo SY, Mortelé KJ, Rocha MS, et al. Renal cell carcinoma: t1 and t2 signal intensity characteristics of papillary and clear cell types correlated with pathology. AJR Am J Roentgenol. 2009;192(6):1524–30.

Case 35
Non-small Cell Lung Cancer

Kavitha Yaddanapudi

History

A 67-year-old female presents for initial staging of right upper lobe lung cancer (Fig. 35.1).

Diagnosis

Non-small cell lung cancer

Findings

- A 3 cm right anterior upper lobe lung mass abutting the mediastinum that is homogenously intermediate hyperintense on both T1 and T2-weighted images (wide white arrow).
- Sagittal STIR image shows a hyperintense mass in the anterior right upper lung lobe that does not invade the chest wall (curved white arrow).
- PET/MR fusion shows that the lung mass has intense hypermetabolic activity compatible with malignancy.
- Note the esophagus with diffuse activity along its length that can be seen with inflammation, muscle spasm, and ingested radioactive saliva (thin white arrow).
- PET MIP shows the intense hypermetabolic mass (wide black arrow). There are severe small hypermetabolic mediastinal and hilar lymph nodes that are suspicious for malignancy (black arrowheads). The esophagus is well seen in its entirety on the MIP image.

Discussion

Lung cancer is one of the deadliest cancers with a 15% 5-year survival. The two major groups of lung cancer are small cell lung cancer and non-small cell lung cancer. Non-small cell lung cancer is the most common type of lung cancer accounting for 87% of cases. FDG PET/CT is the primary noninvasive staging modality in non-small cell lung cancer. The TNM Staging System using PET and other imaging modalities helps to determine proper therapy and management. Potential therapy includes surgery with or without chemotherapy and radiotherapy. The early stages of non-small cell cancer (stage 0 and IA) may require only surgery, while the most advanced stage IV usually relies on chemotherapy as the mainstay of treatment.

Some of the pitfalls of PET imaging include false-positive lung lesions and lymph nodes due to inflammation and infection. False-negative PET may be seen in early stage adenocarcinomas, carcinoid tumors, carcinomas in situ, and small-sized lung nodules (below the resolution of PET). Some lymph nodes with micrometastases are falsely negative and may be upstaged via bronchoscopic biopsy. FDG PET/CT is valuable

R. Gupta et al., *PET/MR Imaging*, https://doi.org/10.1007/978-3-319-65106-4_35

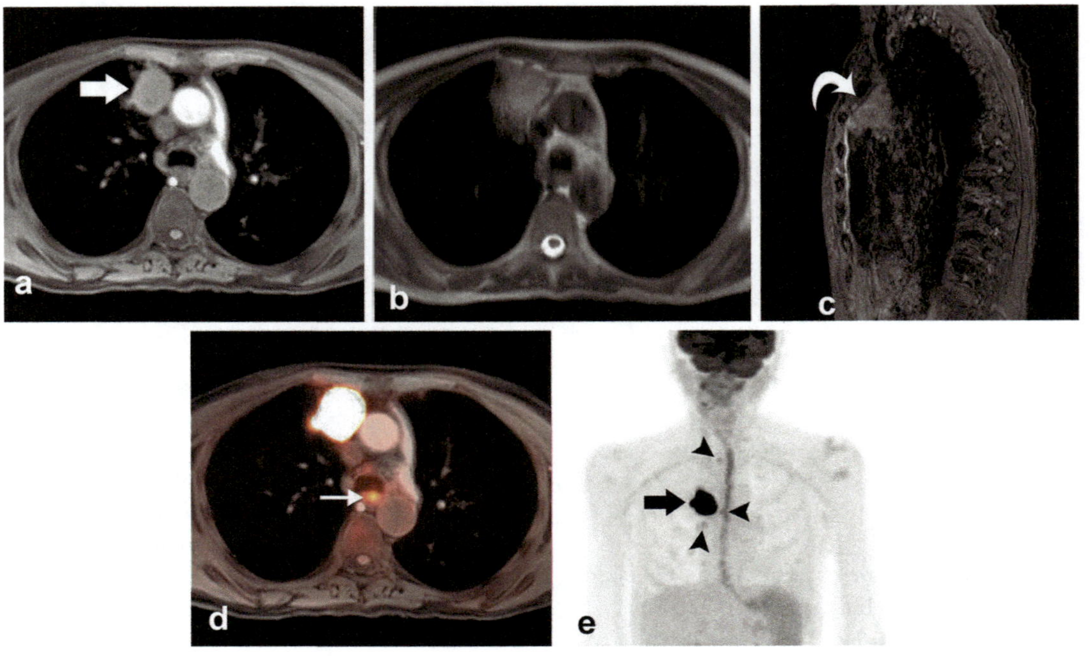

Fig. 35.1 T1 radial VIBE with fat suppression axial (**a**), T2 HASTE axial (**b**), STIR sagittal (**c**), PET/MR T1 radial VIBE with fat suppression axial fusion (**d**), and PET MIP (**e**)

in guiding biopsy and assessing treatment response especially to radiotherapy and chemotherapy and is extremely valuable in detecting local and distant metastases.

Although MRI has not been extensively used for lung cancer detection, several pilot studies have shown this to be useful in lung cancer detection. The main deterrent to the wider application of MR was the long acquisition times with older sequences. Some of the newer studies have shown the utility of radial VIBE which can be completed in 3 min or less and can detect lung nodules as small as 3–5 mm. Furthermore, MR can avoid the cumulative radiation from repeated CT scans. Primary lung cancer on MRI is usually low or intermediate signal on T1-weighted images and slightly hyperintense on T2-weighted images.

PET/MR has all the benefits of PET combined with the excellent soft tissue contrast and characterization of MR. It also avoids unnecessary radiation and contrast needed for CT characterization. Involvement of lymph nodes, chest wall including bone, mediastinal structures, and vessels is excellently delineated on noncontrast MRI. MRI is particularly helpful in the staging of superior sulcus tumors. Distant metastases in the adrenal glands, bones, and brain are also well evaluated on MRI. The added value of PET is in the ease of detection of small metastatic lesions and overall improvement in lesion identification. However, small subcentimeter lung metastasis may be missed on both PET/CT and PET/MR.

Suggested Reading

Kligerman S, Digumarthy S. Staging of non–small cell lung cancer using integrated PET/CT. AJR Am J Roentgenol. 2009;193(5):1203–11.

Schwenzer NF, Seith F, Gatidis S, Brendle C, Schmidt H, Pfannenberg CA, et al. Diagnosing lung nodules on oncologic MR/PET imaging: comparison of fast T1-weighted sequences and influence of image acquisition in inspiration and expiration breath-hold. Korean J Radiol. 2016;17(5):684–94.

Wu NY, Cheng HC, Ko JS, Cheng YC, Lin PW, Lin WC, et al. Magnetic resonance imaging for lung cancer detection: experience in a population of more than 10,000 healthy individuals. BMC Cancer. 2011;11:242.

Case 36
Cardiac Sarcoidosis

Robert Matthews

History

A 77-year-old female with sarcoidosis (Fig. 36.1).

Diagnosis

Cardiac sarcoidosis

Findings

- Short axis delayed-contrast enhancement image shows mid-wall enhancement in the anterior wall, septum, and inferior wall of the left ventricle (arrowheads).
- Short axis fusion image demonstrates more extensive abnormal FDG uptake in the anterior wall, septum, and inferior wall.
- Four-chamber delayed-contrast enhancement image shows mid-wall enhancement of the septum (curved arrow) with corresponding hypermetabolic activity.

Discussion

Sarcoidosis is a multisystem disease that is characterized by the formation of non-caseating granulomas in multiple tissues of the body. Cardiac involvement in sarcoidosis is frequently seen in as many as 25% of the patients. Sarcoid infiltration of the heart often involves the cardiac conduction system, causing various degrees of heart block, tachyarrhythmias, cardiac failure, and occasionally sudden death. Cardiac sarcoidosis has preference to involve the base of the left ventricle, but can involve the atriums, mitral valve, papillary muscles, and pericardium.

Contrast-enhanced cardiac MRI is highly effective in diagnosing and delineating cardiac sarcoid involvement. In the acute phase, myocardial inflammation is seen as focal areas of hyperintensity on T2-weighted images. There may be increased signal on early contrast-enhanced images, as well as areas of hypoperfusion. Myocardial abnormalities are often patchy, involving all portions of the myocardium, but are preferentially transmural or mid-myocardial. Gated MRI images show corresponding focal areas of wall motion abnormalities. Delayed contrast imaging is particularly useful in detecting post-inflammatory fibrotic changes and scarring with transmural and mid-myocardial enhancement. Overall, the pattern of cardiac involvement does not correspond to a specific coronary artery territory.

Dedicated cardiac FDG PET imaging offers greater sensitivity in detecting cardiac sarcoidosis when compared to contrast-enhanced MRI. Active sarcoid involvement shows intense

R. Gupta et al., *PET/MR Imaging*, https://doi.org/10.1007/978-3-319-65106-4_36

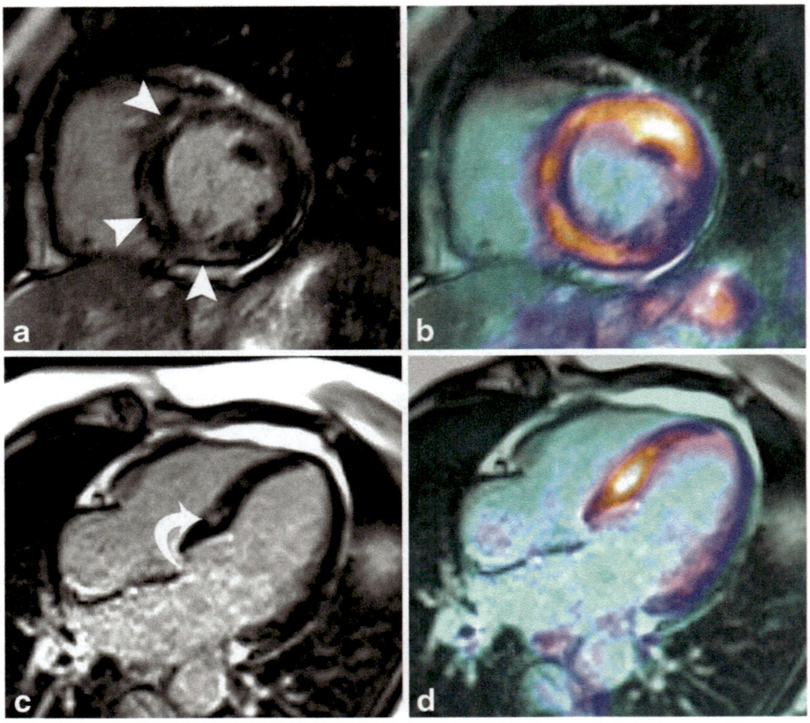

Fig. 36.1 True FISP post-delayed contrast enhancement, short axis (**a**), PET/MR True FISP post-delayed contrast enhancement (**b**), True FISP post-delayed contrast enhancement, four-chamber view (**c**), and PET/MR True FISP post-delayed contrast enhancement (**d**)

radiotracer uptake in affected portions of the heart on fasting PET protocols. The sensitivity of PET had been reported to be up to 100% with excellent detection of early lesions before the appearance of perfusion detects. When treated cardiac sarcoidosis FDG PET imaging is a leading indicator returning to low levels of uptake, despite the persistence of changes on MRI. However, PET imaging suffers from low specificity since the myocardium can have variable normal patterns of FDG uptake including diffusely homogenously intense uptake and patchy heterogeneous uptake, which may make sarcoid interpreting challenging. Heparin loading has been beneficial in suppressing FDG uptake in normal myocardium. Combined cardiac PET-MRI offers both high sensitivity and high specificity in the evaluation of cardiac sarcoidosis. The addition of whole-body PET/MR acquisition allows the detection of active sarcoidosis in the lung, mediastinum, and various lymph node regions.

Suggested Reading

Ohira H, Tsujino I, Ishimaru S, Oyama N, Takei T, Tsukamoto E, et al. Myocardial imaging with (18) F-fluoro-2-deoxyglucose positron emission tomography and magnetic resonance imaging in sarcoidosis. Eur J Nucl Med Mol Imaging. 2008;35:933–41.

Okumura W, Iwasaki T, Toyama T, Iso T, Arai M, Oriuchi N, et al. Usefulness of fasting 18F FDG PET in identification of cardiac sarcoidosis. J Nucl Med. 2004;45:1989–98.

Case 37
Internal Mammary Lymph Node Metastasis from Breast Cancer

Robert Matthews and Elham Safaie

History

A 71-year-old woman presents for staging of left breast cancer (Fig. 37.1).

Diagnosis

Metastatic breast cancer to internal mammary and axillary lymph nodes

Findings

- Small left internal mammary lymph node that is mildly hyperintense on T1-weighted image and mildly hypointense on T2-weighted image.
- PET/MR fusion shows the left internal lymph node to have abnormal FDG activity compatible with metastasis (thin arrow).
- Hypermetabolic left axillary lymph node is also seen that is hyperintense on T1-weighted image and hypointense on T2-weighted image (curved arrow).
- More inferior slice shows T1 hyperintense, hypermetabolic right breast malignancy (wide white arrow).
- Incidental metal induced susceptibility artifact from sternotomy wires.

Discussion

Internal mammary lymph node involvement is difficult to assess on both MRI and PET. Identification of these metastases is important in the staging of patients and may widen the radiation field used in radiotherapy following mastectomy. Internal mammary metastatic disease can arise from any breast quadrant. The larger the primary breast malignancy and the more axillary lymph nodes involved, the more likely there is to be internal mammary involvement. Deeper and medial breast lesions show a higher frequency of internal mammary node metastases. Younger patients also have a higher propensity to develop internal mammary lymphadenopathy. Because of the extensive lymphatic system around the sternum, internal mammary metastases can involve both sides. When the metastasis is large, there may be invasion of the chest wall and even erosion into the sternum.

On MR imaging, normal internal mammary lymph nodes usually measure between 1 and 5 mm in diameter and are confined to the intercostal space, although infrequently, normal internal mammary lymph nodes can be up to 9 mm in diameter. Therefore, visualization of an internal mammary lymph node can be a normal finding on MRI. The lymph node should lack

R. Gupta et al., *PET/MR Imaging*, https://doi.org/10.1007/978-3-319-65106-4_37

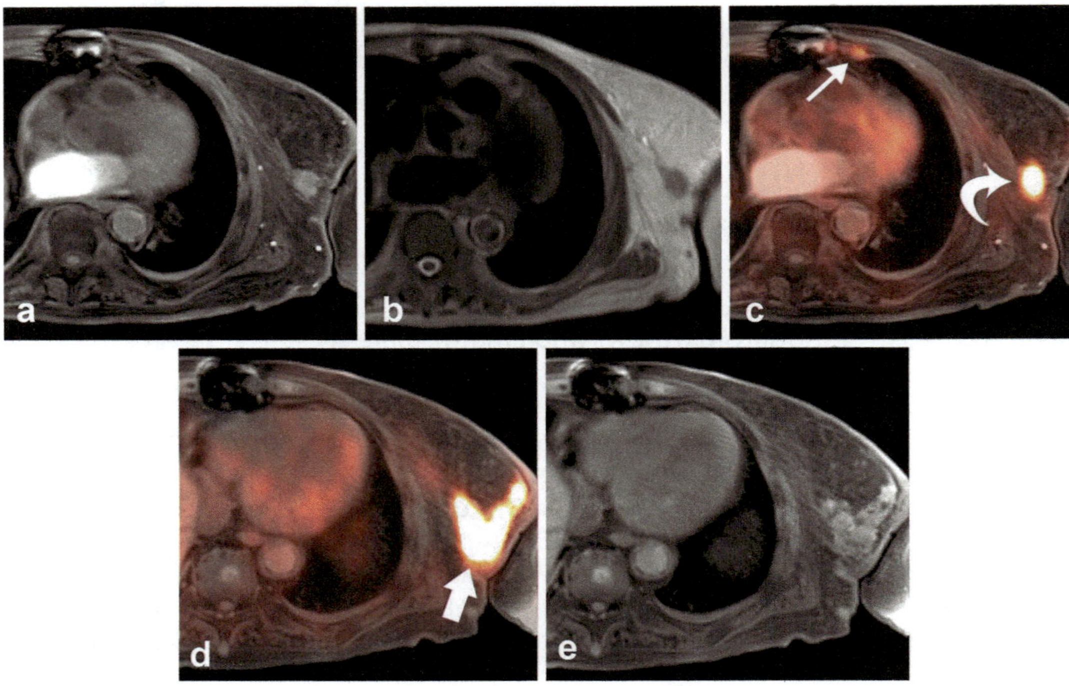

Fig. 37.1 T1 VIBE with fat suppression axial (**a**), T2 HASTE axial (**b**), PET/MR T1 VIBE with fat suppression axial fusion (**c**), PET/MR T1 VIBE with fat suppression axial fusion (more inferior slice) (**d**), and T1 VIBE with fat suppression axial fusion (more inferior slice) (**e**)

necrosis or a thickened cortex, and have a fatty hilum, a normal lobular or oval shape with a well-circumscribed margin. A normal lymph node should have low signal on T1-weighted images, intermediate signal on T2-weighted images, as well as a fatty hilum detected on non-fat saturated sequences.

On FDG PET/MR imaging, metastatic lymph nodes show increased metabolic activity. Mild activity is more commonly seen in cases of reactive lymph nodes that are associated with inflammatory breast cancer and in patients who have undergone lumpectomy or mastectomy. In the staging of breast cancer, the internal mammary lymph nodes are not routinely removed following lymphoscintigraphy, so the true pathological diagnosis is often not available unless there is gross lymph node enlargement or prominent FDG activity.

Suggested Reading

Mack M, Chetlen A, Liao J. Incidental internal mammary lymph nodes visualized on screening breast MRI. AJR. 2015;205:209–14.

Scatarige J, Boxen I, Smathers RL. Internal mammary lymphadenopathy: imaging of a vital lymphatic pathway in breast cancer. Radiographics. 1990;10:857–70.

Case 38
Lung Metastases

Kavitha Yaddanapudi

History

A 16-year-old female with adenoid cystic carcinoma of the left parotid gland presents for staging (Fig. 38.1).

Diagnosis

Lung metastases

Findings

- Widespread hypermetabolic pulmonary nodules throughout the bilateral lung fields consistent with lung metastases.
- Nodules are of varying size and signal intensity.
- PET/MR image at a more superior level shows physiological uptake in the thymus gland (thin arrow).
- Diffuse increased vertebral body FDG uptake consistent with bone marrow stimulation often associated with malignancy.

Discussion

The lungs are one of the most common organs for metastases to occur. Lung metastases are seen in 20–50% of cancer patients. Pulmonary metastases are typically from breast, colon, renal, endometrial and head and neck primaries. The most common pattern of lung metastases is nodules in a heterogeneous distribution. Other patterns such as endobronchial metastases and lymphangitic spread with interstitial thickening are much less common. Pulmonary metastases may occasionally have cavitation, calcification, and hemorrhage within them.

Computed tomography is very sensitive in the identification of pulmonary nodules, even as small as 1–2 mm; however, it is not very specific. FDG PET imaging is highly specific for detecting malignant nodules. However, PET by itself has a low sensitivity for identifying smaller nodules (<5 mm) due to limited resolution. MR imaging of pulmonary nodules is also fraught with difficulty including longer imaging times (due to the need for gating), lower resolution, and substantial artifacts. One of the major drawbacks

R. Gupta et al., *PET/MR Imaging*, https://doi.org/10.1007/978-3-319-65106-4_38

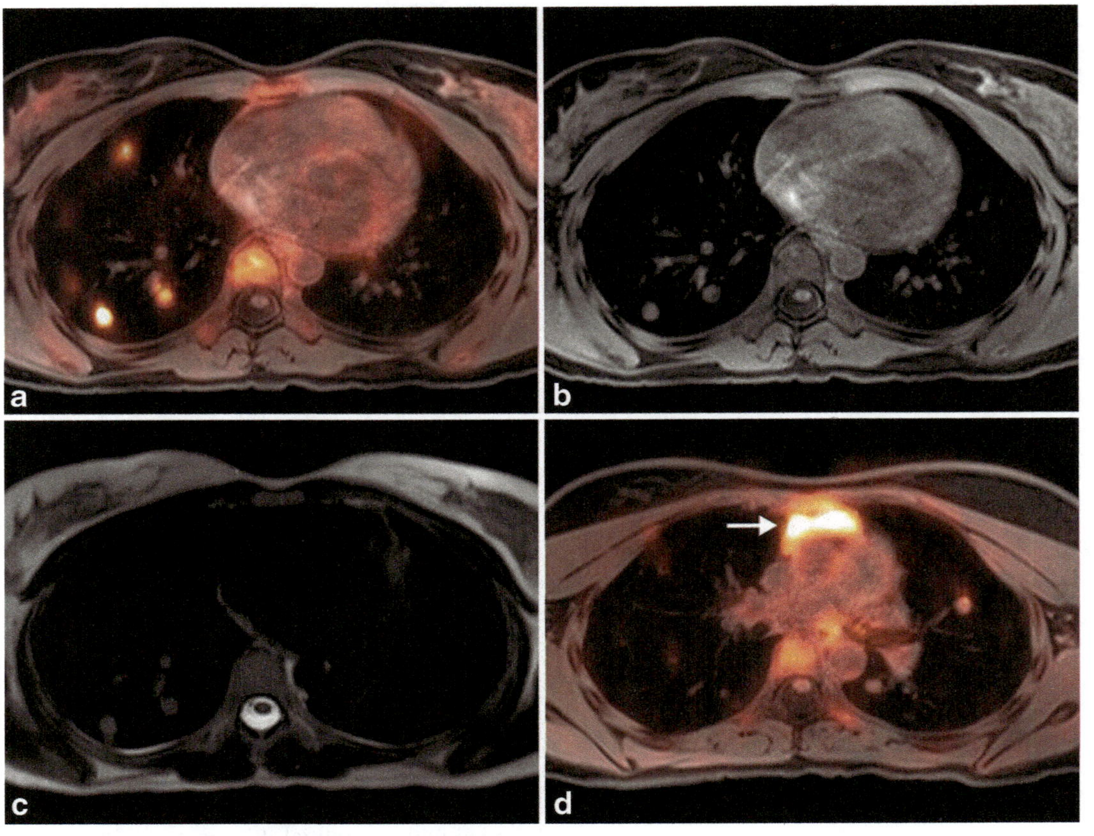

Fig. 38.1 PET/MR T1 radial VIBE with fat suppression axial fusion (**a**), T1 radial VIBE with fat suppression axial (**b**), T2 HASTE axial (**c**), and PET/MR T1 radial VIBE with fat suppression axial fusion, more superior level (**d**)

in using PET/MR oncological imaging is the difficulty in detecting pulmonary metastases. The addition of gadolinium contrast does not provide any additional benefit to lung nodule or metastases detection. However, newer MRI scanners have stronger gradients where free breathing sequences such as T1-weighted radial VIBE have been shown to overcome some of the problems with detecting small pulmonary nodules.

Metastases are usually FDG avid and readily identifiable on MRI when larger than 5 mm in size. Although FDG PET/CT remains a more sensitive modality for the detection of tiny pulmonary metastases, PET/MRI will play a greater role in cancer imaging even with suspected pulmonary metastases due to its significantly decreased radiation and overall advantage for the evaluation of certain malignancies in the abdomen and pelvis.

Suggested Reading

Chandarana H, Heacock L, Rakheja R, LR DM, Bonavita J, Block TK, et al. Pulmonary nodules in patients with primary malignancy: comparison of hybrid PET/MR and PET/CT imaging. Radiology. 2013;268(3):874–81.

Lee KH, Park CM, Lee SM, Lee JM, Cho JY, Paeng JC, et al. Pulmonary nodule detection in patients with a primary malignancy using hybrid PET/MRI: is there value in adding contrast-enhanced MR imaging? PLoS One. 2015;10(6):e0129660.

Case 39
Pleural Metastases from Invasive Thymoma

Kavitha Yaddanapudi

History

A 72-year-old female with thymic neoplasm presents with a left pleural mass (Fig. 39.1).

Diagnosis

Pleural metastases from invasive thymoma

Findings

- Large hypermetabolic, lobulated, solid lesion in the left posterior pleural space is isointense on T1 and heterogeneously hyperintense on a T2.
- Pleural mass is relatively hypointense compared to the tiny pleural effusion that is higher in signal on a T2-weighted image (thin arrow).

Discussion

Pleural metastases commonly originate from lung cancer, breast cancer, and lymphoma. Extra thoracic neoplasms that metastasize to the pleura include ovarian, uterine, and gastrointestinal neoplasms. Invasive thymoma, although usually localized at diagnosis, when it metastasizes, predominantly spreads to the pleura as diffuse widespread pleural thickening or discrete multiple masses. Pleural metastatic disease usually manifests as pleural effusions with associated pleural thickening, nodular implants, or masses. Isolated pleural masses deposit along the costal or mediastinal pleura. Metastases can also involve the interlobar fissures.

Pleural metastases and malignant pleural mesothelioma have identical imaging features. On MRI, they present as isointense to muscle on T1 weighting and heterogeneously hyperintense pleural implants or masses on T2-weighted sequences. MRI provides excellent soft tissue contrast to discern pleural lesions in the presence of an effusion. The T2-weighted properties of fluid allow for the detection of pleural deposits, which are relatively hypointense compared to the high T2-weighted signal of an effusion. After the administration of gadolinium contrast, pleural metastases will enhance avidly.

FDG PET is a very useful modality in detecting pleural metastases with a reported sensitivity of 80–100%. On PET imaging, malignant pleural effusions have increased FDG uptake compared to background mediastinal uptake. Additionally, discrete pleural metastases have intense FDG uptake, which highlights the extent of disease, compared to CT alone. However, the pitfall of

R. Gupta et al., *PET/MR Imaging*, https://doi.org/10.1007/978-3-319-65106-4_39

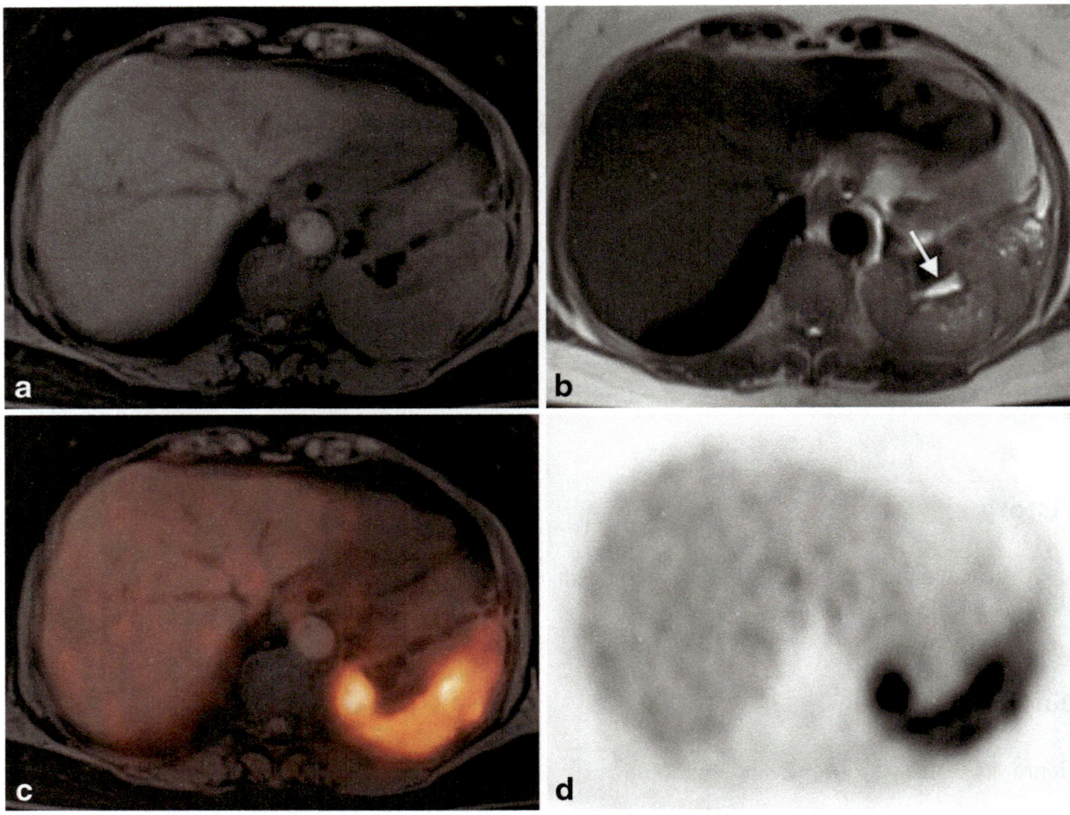

Fig. 39.1 T1 radial VIBE with fat suppression axial (**a**), T2 HASTE axial (**b**), PET/MR T1 radial VIBE with fat suppression axial (**c**), and PET axial (**d**)

PET imaging is that inflammatory pleural lesions such as empyema, parapneumonic effusion, and thickening can have significantly increased FDG uptake. Therefore, history and correlation with pleural fluid cytology play a crucial role. PET/MR imaging improves the detection of malignant pleural disease by combining excellent soft tissue contrast and metabolic information. It can therefore guide biopsy sites, concurrently evaluate for local and distant metastatic disease, and assess response to therapy.

Suggested Reading

Erasmus JJ, HP MA, Rossi SE, Goodman PC, Coleman RE, Patz EF. FDG PET of pleural effusions in patients with non-small cell lung cancer. AJR Am J Roentgenol. 2000;175(1):245–9.

Jeong YJ, Kim S, Kwak SW, Lee NK, Lee JW, Kim KI, et al. Neoplastic and nonneoplastic conditions of Serosal membrane origin: CT findings. Radiographics. 2008;28(3):801–17.

Nishino M, Ashiku SK, Kocher ON, Thurer RL, Boiselle PM, Hatabu H. The thymus: a comprehensive review. Radiographics. 2006;26(2):335–48.

Case 40
Thoracic Aortic Aneurysm

Kavitha Yaddanapudi and Rajesh Gupta

History

A 79-year-old female with a lung nodule referred for PET/MR evaluation (Fig. 40.1). She has a history of an abdominal aortic aneurysm that underwent endovascular repair.

Diagnosis

Thoracic aortic aneurysm

Findings

- Aneurysmal dilation of the aortic arch and descending thoracic aorta with tortuosity.
- Small foci of low T1 and T2-weighted signal in the wall of the aneurysm (white arrowhead) represents atherosclerotic calcification.
- Heterogeneous T2-weighted signal is seen in the aneurysmal thoracic aorta due to turbulent arterial blood flow (curved white arrow). Usually, moving blood should demonstrate a dark T2-weighted flow void.
- Metal-induced susceptibility artifact is seen from sternotomy wires.
- Moderate mediastinal FDG uptake localized to the dilated aortic arch corresponds to the calcific atherosclerotic changes (thin white arrow).
- PET MIP images show extensive aortic arch disease (wide black arrow). The malignant lung nodule is seen in the right lung field (black arrowhead).

Discussion

Thoracic aortic aneurysms are less common than abdominal aortic aneurysms. They most commonly occur in the 50–60 year old age group, with a male predominance. The ascending aorta is the most frequent segment to be involved, followed by the descending aorta and then the aortic arch. The major etiology is atherosclerotic plaque causing remodeling due to luminal stenosis and compensatory changes.

MRI is a good imaging modality for thoracic aortic aneurysm diagnosis and follow-up. The aortic size can be assessed even on non-contrast MRI, thereby avoiding harmful radiation and contrast in young patients who are followed up annually. MRI measurements are highly reproducible and can reliably monitor aneurysm expansion rate over time. Aortic dissection and atherosclerotic aortic aneurysms can also be assessed on MRI with detailed evaluation of lumen, root, valve involvement, and regurgitative flow. Slow, turbulent flow can mimic thrombus and limit evaluation of the lumen on conventional MR sequences. Contrast-enhanced MR angiography and bright blood techniques can provide

R. Gupta et al., *PET/MR Imaging*, https://doi.org/10.1007/978-3-319-65106-4_40

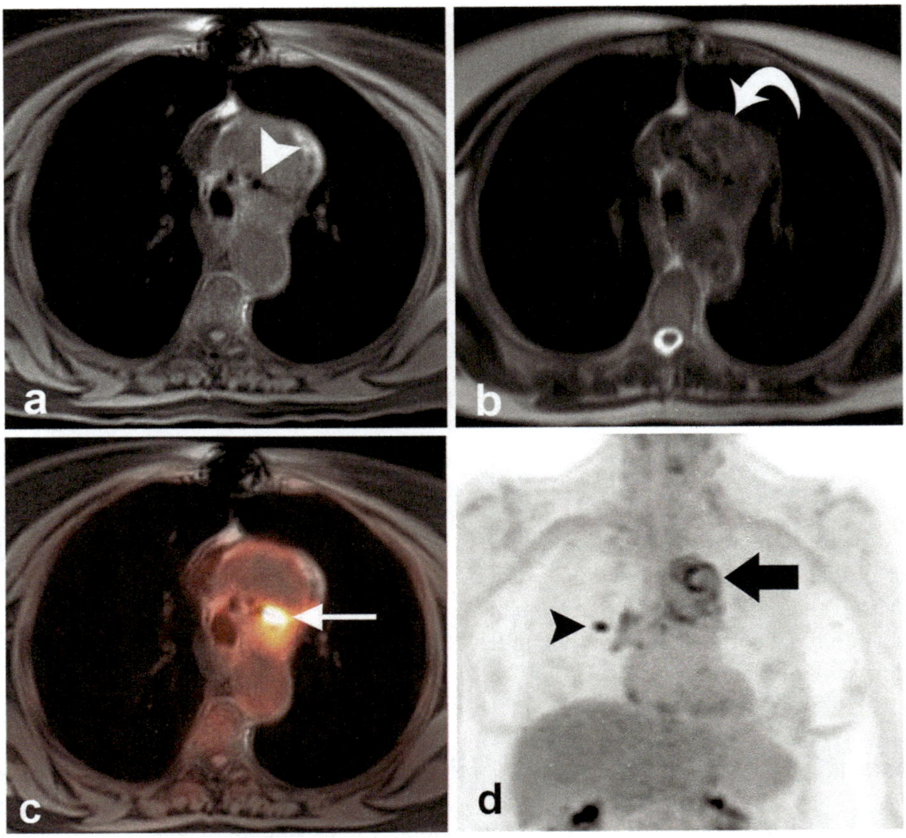

Fig. 40.1 T1 radial VIBE axial with fat suppression axial (**a**), T2 HASTE axial (**b**), PET/MR T1 radial VIBE with fat suppression axial fusion (**c**), and PET MIP (**d**)

superior evaluation of the aortic lumen, even when there is slow flow. MRI, however, has longer acquisition times and is not the modality of choice in patients with acute aortic pathology who are hemodynamically unstable.

FDG PET uptake has been noted in atherosclerotic aneurysms and is attributed to the inflammatory changes in the atherosclerotic plaques. These findings have been more commonly demonstrated in abdominal aortic aneurysms and studies have also linked the FDG uptake to the risk of rupture in abdominal aortic aneurysms. In addition to atherosclerotic aneurysm, infected or mycotic aneurysms also have increased FDG uptake. Arteritis can be differentiated from atherosclerotic changes in that arteritis has usually diffuse concentric uptake compared to patchy, heterogeneous uptake exhibited by atherosclerotic aneurysms. Arteritis also usually has normal caliber or a narrowed aortic lumen and tends to involve proximal arch branch vessels. Combining PET and MRI can provide more thorough evaluation both of aortic aneurysm morphology and flow as well as of inflammation.

Suggested Reading

Litmanovich D, Bankier AA, Cantin L, Raptopoulos V, Boiselle PM. CT and MRI in diseases of the aorta. AJR Am J Roentgenol. 2009 Oct;193(4):928–40.

Timur UT, van Herwaarden JA, Mihajlovic D, De Jong P, Mali W, Moll FL. 18F-FDG PET scanning of abdominal aortic aneurysms and correlation with molecular characteristics: a systematic review. EJNMMI Res. 2015;5:76.

Case 41
Mediastinal Sarcoidosis

Kavitha Yaddanapudi

History

A 79-year-old female with sarcoidosis presents for restaging of colon cancer (Fig. 41.1).

Diagnosis

Mediastinal sarcoidosis

Findings

- Bilateral enlarged hilar and subcarinal adenopathy that are hyperintense on T1-weighted image as compared with muscle and isointense on T2-weighted image.
- Prominent FDG uptake in the hilar and subcarinal lymph nodes compatible with active sarcoidosis.
- PET MIP demonstrates extensive hypermetabolic mediastinal and hilar adenopathy.

Discussion

Mediastinal and hilar lymphadenopathy is the most common and typical manifestations of sarcoidosis. In the Siltzbach's classification of radiographic findings, stages I and II demonstrate lymphadenopathy without and with pulmonary opacities respectively. Right paratracheal and symmetric bilateral hilar lymphadenopathy is seen in 95% of sarcoidosis patients. Prevascular, subcarinal, and left paratracheal lymph nodes are among the other groups of mediastinal lymph nodes involved in sarcoidosis. Although bilateral hilar lymphadenopathy may be seen in patients with lymphoma and tuberculosis, the presence of bilateral hilar lymphadenopathy in an asymptomatic individual is highly suggestive of sarcoidosis. Atypical manifestations, more common in older patients, include mediastinal adenopathy without hilar lymphadenopathy, or the presence of paravertebral, retrocrural, or internal mammary lymphadenopathy. Lymph nodes in sarcoidosis can calcify and a characteristic "egg shell pattern" has been described, which can also be seen in silicosis. Amorphous and punctate forms of calcification are also seen.

On cross-sectional imaging, an enlarged mediastinal lymph node is defined as a node larger than 1 cm in short axis with loss of the normal fatty hilum. MRI provides excellent inherent soft tissue contrast between blood vessels and nodes to detect mediastinal and hilar abnormalities, even without the use of gadolinium contrast. However, a disadvantage of MRI compared to CT is that small individual lymph nodes may appear as a large conglomerate mass on MRI due to partial volume averaging. Additionally, scattered calcifications within lymph nodes can go undetected on MRI.

FDG PET is highly sensitive, and shows moderate specificity in detecting pathologic lymph

R. Gupta et al., *PET/MR Imaging*, https://doi.org/10.1007/978-3-319-65106-4_41

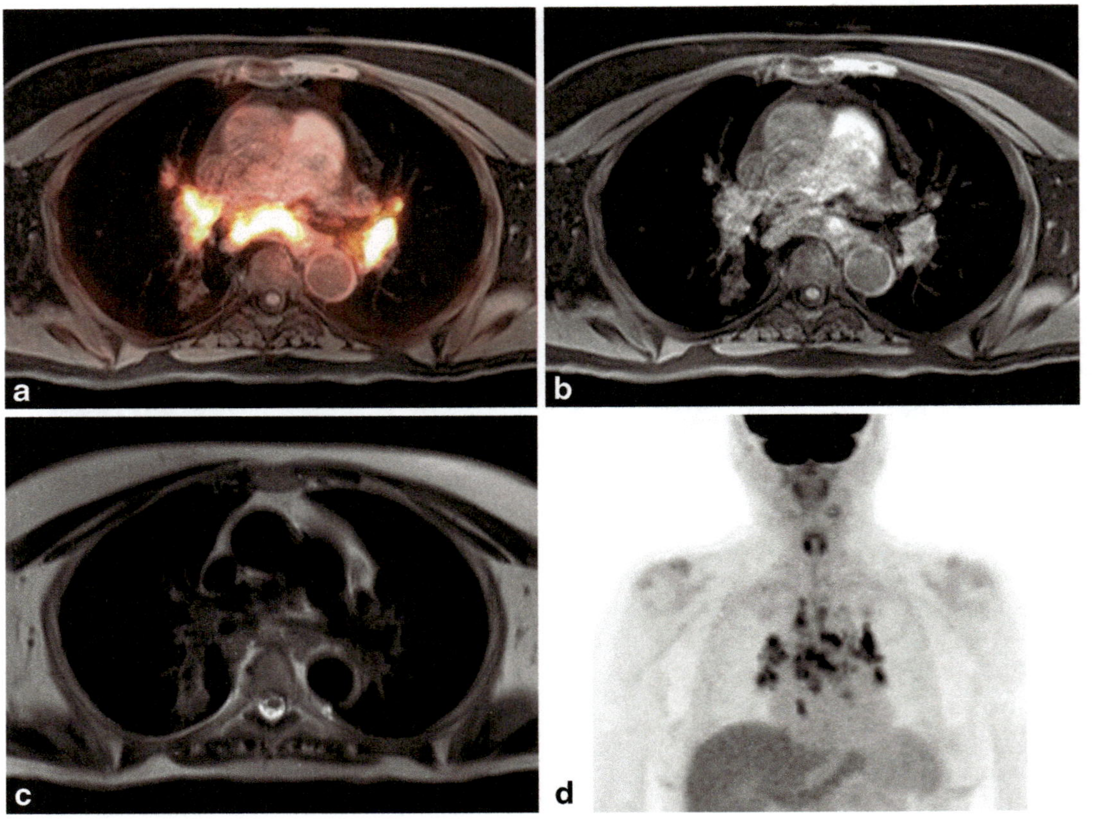

Fig. 41.1 PET/MR T1 radial VIBE with fat suppression axial fusion (**a**), T1 radial VIBE with fat suppression axial (**b**), T2 HASTE axial (**c**), and PET MIP (**d**)

nodes. This is advantageous over size criteria which is not always accurate in differentiating benign from malignant lymph nodes. On the other hand, specificity of PET is decreased as neoplastic, inflammatory, or infectious lymphadenopathy can all be hypermetabolic due to increased glucose utilization. Evaluating mediastinal lymphadenopathy with PET/MR imaging combines the sensitivity of PET with the superior anatomic detail and image contrast resolution possible with MRI. Therefore, this modality is helpful in identifying the ideal site for biopsy, evaluating whole body disease burden in sarcoidosis, and assessing treatment response.

Suggested Reading

Criado E, Sánchez M, Ramírez J, Arguis P, de Caralt TM, Perea RJ, et al. Pulmonary sarcoidosis: typical and atypical manifestations at high-resolution CT with pathologic correlation. Radiographics. 2010;30(6):1567–86.

Torabi M, Aquino SL, Harisinghani MG. Current concepts in lymph node imaging. J Nucl Med. 2004;45(9):1509–18.

Case 42
Metastatic Breast Cancer to the Liver

Elham Safaie and Robert Matthews

History

A 51-year-old female with metastatic breast cancer to lymph nodes and liver (Fig. 42.1).

Diagnosis

Metastatic breast cancer to liver and multiple lymph nodes

Findings

- Extensive metastatic involvement of the liver showing multiple T1 hypointense, T2 hyperintense lesions that are hypermetabolic on FDG PET.
- Large exophytic right breast mass that is isotense on T1 with intense hypermetabolic activity consistent with primary breast malignancy (thin arrow). This mass demonstrates central necrosis on PET with a photopenic center.
- Hepatic dome is noted on the thoracic images with intense FDG activity (curved arrow).
- PET MIP show multiple metastatic mediastinal and hilar lymph nodes, extensive liver metastases, right breast lesion, and right axillary lymph nodes.
- Note that large malignant tumor burden may cause decreased FDG activity in the brain.

Discussion

The liver is the most frequent site of hematogenous metastatic spread from many cancers including those in the gastrointestinal tract, breast, lung, and melanomas. Liver metastases from breast cancer are associated with a poorer prognosis. The subgroup of these patients with no dissemination to organs other than the liver may benefit from surgery. However, only in exceptional cases do these patients survive more than 2 years even when given chemotherapy and hormonal treatment. A variety of local ablative therapies are available and may be performed including radiofrequency ablation, thermal ablation, and yttrium-90 microspheres therapy.

PET/MR whole body imaging, because of its large field of view, is limited in the assessment of both primary breast cancers and their local axillary lymph node metastases when compared with traditional imaging modalities. However, it is an excellent modality for the evaluation of distant metastases to the lung, bone, brain, and liver. PET/MR imaging can characterize liver lesions with greater conspicuity and with less radiation dose compared to PET/CT. It also allows for the accurate detection of other sites of distant metastases. The appearance of breast metastases in the liver on PET/MR can be quite variable, but is avidly FDG positive. Typically, the lesion is

R. Gupta et al., *PET/MR Imaging*, https://doi.org/10.1007/978-3-319-65106-4_42

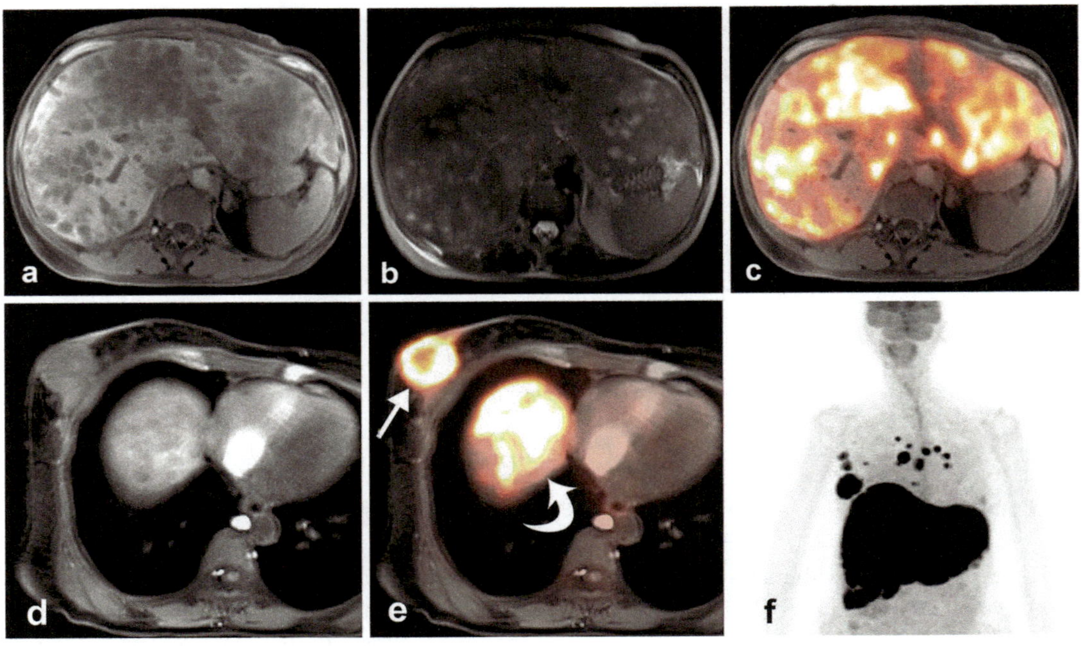

Fig. 42.1 T1 VIBE with fat suppression axial, abdomen (**a**), T2 HASTE axial, abdomen (**b**), PET/MR T1 VIBE with fat suppression axial fusion, abdomen (**c**), T1 VIBE with fat suppression axial, thorax (**d**), PET/MR T1 VIBE with fat suppression axial fusion, thorax (**e**), and PET MIP (**f**)

hypointense on T1-weighted images, hyperintense on T2-weighted images, and shows post gadolinium contrast enhancement.

Suggested Reading

Bhattacharya R, Rao S, Kowdley KV. Liver involvement in patients with solid tumors of nonhepatic origin. Clin Liver Dis. 2002;6(4):1033–43.

Hustinx R, Paulus P, Jacquet N, Jerusalem G, Bury T, Rigo P. Clinical evaluation of whole-body 18F-fluorodeoxyglucosepositron emission tomography in the detection of liver metastases. Ann Oncol. 1998;9(4):397–401.

Rosenkrantz AB, Friedman K, Chandarana H, Melsaether A, Moy L, Ding YS, et al. Current status of hybrid PET/MRI in oncologic imaging. AJR Am J Roentgenol. 2016;206(1):162–72.

Sacks A, Peller PJ, Surasi DS, Chatburn L, Mercier G, Subramaniam RM. Value of PET/CT in the management of liver metastases, part 1. AJR Am J Roentgenol. 2011;197(2):W256–9.

Case 43
Multifocal Pneumonia

Rajesh Gupta

History

An 88-year-old male with multiple myeloma presents for restaging (Fig. 43.1).

Diagnosis

Multifocal pneumonia

Findings

- Images at the level of the tracheal bifurcation demonstrate an ill-defined T1 isointense consolidation in the posterior right upper lung lobe. This consolidation is better defined on the T2 image, where it is hyperintense (thin arrow).
- On PET/MR fusion, the consolidation has diffusely heterogeneous FDG activity indicating infection.
- More inferiorly, at the level of the heart, images show a multifocal right lung consolidation that is hyperintense on T2 (arrowheads). This is also associated with heterogeneous diffuse FDG activity.

Discussion

Pneumonia is an inflammation of the lung, primarily affecting the alveoli, and usually caused by infection with bacteria, viruses, or fungi. Traditional imaging to diagnose pneumonia relies on chest radiography and occasionally high-resolution chest CT. However, MRI also has the ability to detect lung infection and has been shown to have a sensitivity of 94% and specificity of 98%, when compared to CT. Although, not a first choice test to diagnose pneumonia, MR may detect it incidentally when a patient is undergoing evaluation for another pathology and MR may occasionally play a first line role in pediatric and pregnant patients in whom radiation exposure is of high concern.

Chest imaging with MRI has vastly improved with modern sequences, including VIBE sequence that produces high-resolution 3D T1-weighted images in under a 30 s breath-hold. Breath-hold sequences help to eliminate artifact from respiratory motion. Pneumonia consists of inflammatory and infectious cells, with a high water content, filling the alveoli. Therefore, pneumonia appears as isointense T1 signal against a background of

R. Gupta et al., *PET/MR Imaging*, https://doi.org/10.1007/978-3-319-65106-4_43

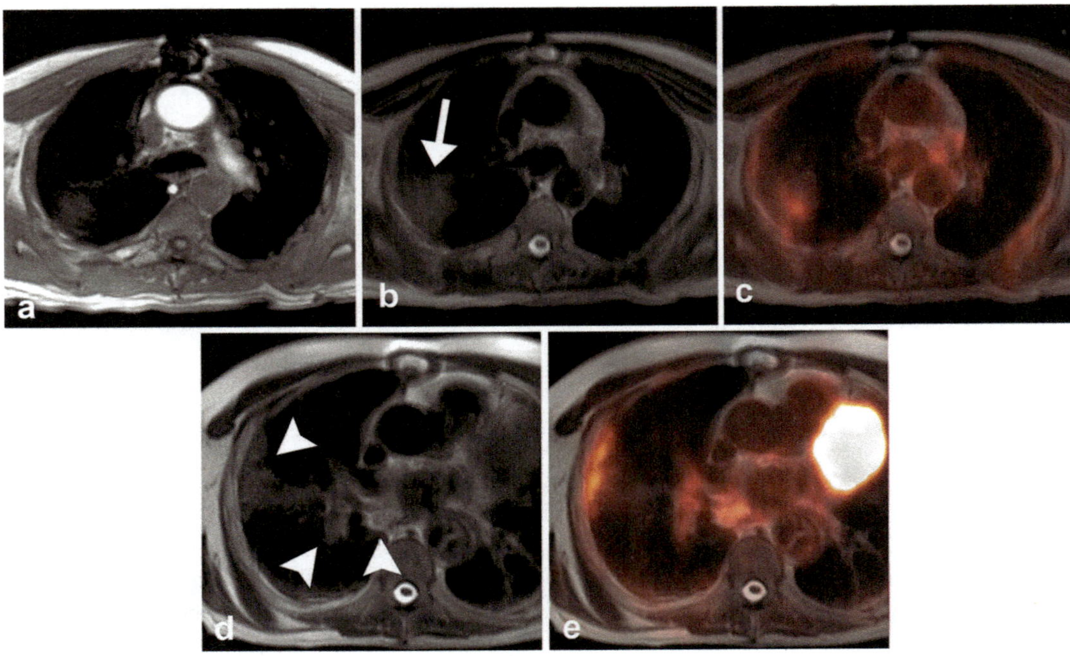

Fig. 43.1 T1 VIBE axial, at carinal angle (**a**), T2 HASTE axial, at carinal angle (**b**), PET/MR T2 HASTE axial fusion, at carinal angle (**c**), T2 HASTE axial, at cardiac level (**d**), and PET/MR T2 HASTE axial fusion, at cardiac level (**e**)

hypointense signal from the normally aerated lung parenchyma. Because T2 sequences are sensitive to water accumulation, they detect pneumonia as a mildly hyperintense consolidation against a hypointense background of the normal lung.

PET imaging with FDG is highly sensitive for infectious processes, since active inflammatory cells demonstrate increased glucose utilization. Pneumonia typically show diffuse radiotracer distribution and less FDG uptake, as compared to malignancy. However, higher SUV values are not uncommon in acute inflammation. In these cases, MR findings of consolidation should be relied upon for the diagnosis. In some cases, the lung infectious process is detected on PET first with only subtle changes on CT or MR, and clinical and laboratory data can help in the diagnosis. Follow-up imaging should demonstrate improvement or clearance of the pulmonary consolidation after therapy in typical cases of pneumonia. Identifying lung infection on PET/MR imaging is important as it can be found incidentally, especially in cancer patients as they are prone to infection due to their compromised immune status.

Suggested Reading

Kapucu LO, Meltzer CC, Townsend DW, Keenan RJ, Luketich JD. Fluorine-18-fluorodeoxyglucose uptake in pneumonia. J Nucl Med. 1998;39(7):1267–9.

Syrjala H, Broas M, Ohtonen P, Jartti A, Pääkkö E. Chest magnetic resonance imaging for pneumonia diagnosis in outpatients with lower respiratory tract infection. Eur Respir J. 2017;49(1):pii: 1601303.

Case 44
Invasive Lobular Breast Cancer

David Capaldi

History

A 60-year-old female with left lobular breast cancer (Fig. 44.1).

Diagnosis

Invasive lobular breast cancer with metastases

Findings

- Left medial breast density with mild FDG activity consistent with known lobular breast cancer (wide arrow). Two tiny T1 hypointense signals within the breast density are markers from biopsy.
- Mildly hyperintense T2 and isointense T1 uterine mass with only mild FDG activity that on surgery was found to be lobular breast cancer metastasis (arrowhead).
- Hyperintense STIR signal in T11 vertebral body with no significant FDG activity representing a non-FDG avid metastasis (thin arrow).

Discussion

Invasive lobular breast cancer (ILC) originates in the milk-producing lobules of the breast and is the second most common form of breast cancer, accounting for 10–15% of all breast cancers. ILC is more likely to occur in older post-menopausal females, averaging 65 years in age. ILC is associated with a higher rate of multiple lesions and bilateral lesions than other types of breast cancer. It usually presents as large breast lesions with 14% of tumors greater than 5 cm in diameter at presentation. ILC can also be difficult to detect clinically, as lesions often do not form palpable discrete masses. In its earliest stages, ILC may cause no signs and symptoms. As it grows larger, ILC may cause breast thickening, breast fullness or swelling, and changes in the texture or appearance of the skin overlying the breast lesion.

At the time of diagnosis, 60% of patients with ILC will have lymph node or distant organ metastases, and about 30–80% of patients will develop metastatic disease following the initiation of therapy. The most common sites of metastases for ILC are similar to those of invasive ductal carcinoma (IDC) including lymph nodes, bone, and a variety of other soft tissues. ILC is three times more likely than invasive ductal cancer, to metastasize to the peritoneum, gastrointestinal tract, and ovaries (6.7% ILC vs. 1.8% IDC). ILC is less likely than IDC to affect the lungs, pleura, and CNS.

At MR imaging, the most common manifestation of ILC is a solitary irregular or angular mass with spiculated, ill-defined margins (31–43% of cases). Additional manifestations include a dominant lesion surrounded by multiple small enhancing foci, enhancing foci with interconnecting

R. Gupta et al., *PET/MR Imaging*, https://doi.org/10.1007/978-3-319-65106-4_44

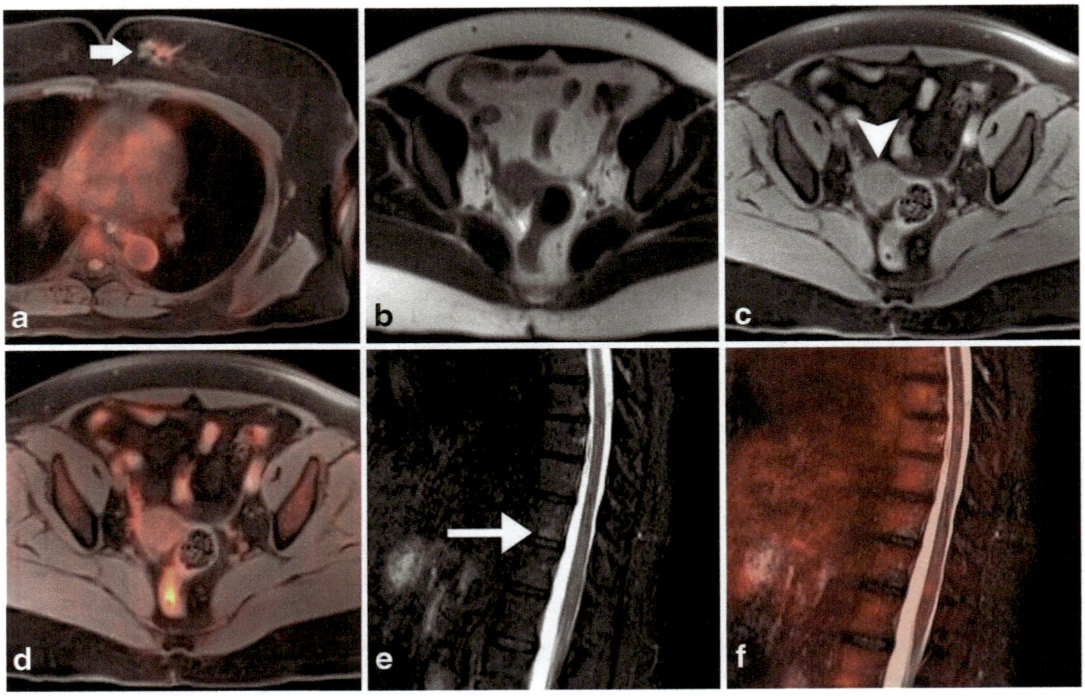

Fig. 44.1 PET/MR T1 radial VIBE axial fusion, chest (**a**), T2 HASTE, pelvis (**b**), T1 radial VIBE axial, pelvis (**c**), PET/MR T1 radial VIBE axial fusion, pelvis (**d**), STIR sagittal spine (**e**), and PET/MR STIR sagittal spine fusion (**f**)

enhancing strands, architectural distortion, regional or focal heterogeneous enhancement, enhancing septa, or rarely normal findings. The findings of ILC at dynamic contrast-enhanced breast MR imaging suggest that, unlike most invasive breast carcinomas with a classic pattern of rapid enhancement and washout, ILC often demonstrates delayed maximum enhancement, with washout shown only in a minority of lesions.

The results of most studies show that the capability of PET to depict lesions smaller than 1 cm in diameter is constrained by limited spatial resolution without a dedicated positron emission mammography camera. PET also is of limited use for identifying tumors that are well differentiated histologically, such as ductal carcinoma in situ, and slow-growing cancers such as tubular carcinoma. PET is less sensitive for the detection of invasive lobular carcinoma than it is for invasive ductal carcinoma. The SUV measurements are usually considerably lower in ILC, in both the primary breast lesion and metastatic disease. Osseous lesions are usually sclerotic appearing with low or no FDG uptake. Certain biologic properties of invasive lobular carcinoma, such as low tumor cell density and diffuse infiltration of the surrounding tissue, may help explain its lower FDG uptake.

Suggested Reading

Lim HS, Yoon W, Chung TW, Kim JK, Park JG, Kang HK, et al. FDG PET/CT for the detection and evaluation of breast diseases: usefulness and limitations. Radiographics. 2007;27(Suppl 1):S197–213.

Lopez JK, Bassett LW. Invasive lobular carcinoma of the breast: Spectrum of mammographic, US, and MR imaging findings. Radiographics. 2009;29(1):165–76.

Rosen EL, Eubank WB, Mankoff DA. FDG PET, PET/CT, and breast cancer imaging. Radiographics. 2007;27(Suppl 1):S215–29.

Case 45
Hodgkin's Lymphoma of the Lung

Rajesh Gupta

History

A 17-year-old female with relapsing Hodgkin lymphoma presents for restaging (Fig. 45.1).

Diagnosis

Hodgkin's lymphoma of the lung (nodular sclerosing type on biopsy)

Findings

- Heterogeneously isointense T1 and moderate hyperintense T2-weighted masslike consolidation involving the right middle and lower lobes of the lung (curved arrows).
- Masslike consolidation is intensely FDG avid.
- T2 hyperintense small right pleural effusion is also noted without hypermetabolic activity.

Discussion

Hodgkin's lymphoma is a predominantly nodal malignancy that accounts for 1% of all cancers, with the most common age of diagnosis between 30 and 40 years. It spreads contiguously along lymphatic channels. Although extranodal disease is much less common in Hodgkin disease than in non-Hodgkin lymphomas, intrathoracic manifestations are more common. Hodgkin lymphoma can affect the pleura, heart, pericardium, thymus, and chest wall. Parenchymal lung involvement is relatively rare, accounting for 6–12% of cases, and is usually accompanied by hilar and mediastinal node disease. However, it is commonly seen in treated patients with a relapse involving the chest.

Primary pulmonary Hodgkin disease is usually a direct extension from hilar nodes to the lung. Nodular lung lesions are often peripheral with poorly defined borders and favor the upper lobes. Imaging patterns also include mass or masslike consolidation and atelectasis of a lobe or lung segment. Interstitial disease spreading along the lymphatic channels of the pulmonary lobule is a less common pattern. High-resolution CT is usually the modality of choice to evaluate lung parenchyma, especially for tiny nodules. However, MR protocols that apply fast breath-hold sequences have been able to provide a radiation-free evaluation of the lungs. Mass-like lung consolidation will show heterogeneous T1 and T2-weighted signal characteristics that reflect the cellular properties of the primary malignancy.

FDG PET is a proven tool for the detection, staging, and assessment of treatment response in Hodgkin disease and other types of lymphoma. Extranodal Hodgkin disease is metabolically active and will have intense FDG uptake. Hybrid PET/MR imaging is an excellent modality in the initial evaluation and staging of Hodgkin disease

R. Gupta et al., *PET/MR Imaging*, https://doi.org/10.1007/978-3-319-65106-4_45

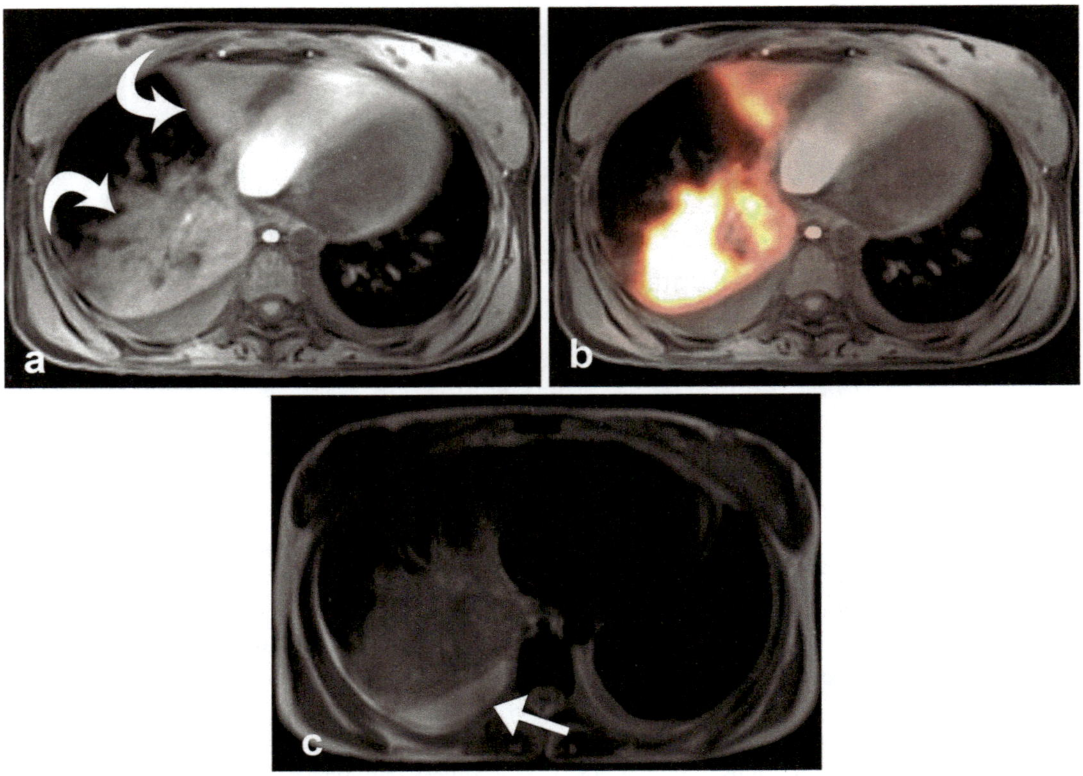

Fig. 45.1 T1 radial VIBE axial (**a**), PET/MR T1 radial VIBE axial fusion (**b**), and T2 HASTE axial (**c**)

as it can thoroughly evaluate masses and lesions throughout the body. PET/MRI provides the ability to restage disease and exclude the presence of persistent or recurrent Hodgkin lymphoma after therapy. However, in treated patients, biopsy of hypermetabolic pulmonary disease may still be required to avoid false-positive cases that include benign conditions such as infection, radiation pneumonitis, or drug-induced lung disease. The decreased radiation compared to PET/CT makes PET/MR favorable for pediatric and younger patients who may require multiple follow-up examinations.

Suggested Reading

Guermazi A, Brice P, de Kerviler EE, Fermé C, Hennequin C, Meignin V, et al. Extranodal Hodgkin disease: spectrum of disease. Radiographics. 2001;21(1):161–79.

Schaefer NG, Taverna C, Strobel K, Wastl C, Kurrer M, Hany TF. Hodgkin disease: diagnostic value of FDG PET/CT after first-line therapy–is biopsy of FDG-avid lesions still needed? Radiology. 2007;244(1):257–62.

Part III

Gastrointestinal

Case 46
Liver Metastases from Colon Cancer

Robert Matthews

History

A 79-year-old male with colon cancer and new liver lesions (Fig. 46.1).

Diagnosis

Liver metastases from colon cancer

Findings

- Multiple large heterogenous liver masses that are T1 hypointense and T2 hyperintense relative to the liver.
- Contrast enhanced T1 image with gadolinium shows delayed enhancement of the liver masses.
- PET/MR fusion image demonstrates intense hypermetabolic activity within the liver masses. Decreased FDG activity within the center of the masses reflect central necrosis.
- DWI shows increased signal intensity within the lesions and decreased signal on the corresponding ADC maps compatible with malignancy.

Discussion

Of all malignant lesions occurring in the liver, metastases are far more frequent than primary liver malignancy. In patients with metastatic liver disease, complete surgical resection or treatment of the liver lesions increases overall survival in most cancer patients. Therefore, the accurate detection of liver metastases is essential in cancer workup, especially the detection of small metastatic lesions. In addition, imaging is vital to avoid unnecessary diagnostic workup of benign tumors and other incidental hepatic lesions.

Most metastases encountered in the liver are hypointense to isointense on T1-weighted images and isointense to hyperintense on T2-weighted images. Contrast enhanced T1-weighted images with gadolinium contrast are essential in detecting liver metastases on MRI. Liver lesions may be either hypervascular with enhancement on the arterial dominant phase of contrast or hypovascular with slower less intense enhancement on the portal venous phase imaging. Hypervascular metastases are common with renal cell carcinoma, neuroendocrine tumors, thyroid carcinoma, and sometimes melanoma. Hypovascular metastases are often seen with colorectal cancer, lung cancer, and gastric cancer. Necrotic metastases may appear hypovascular, even when they are not. Breast cancer metastases can be either hyper or hypovascular. Regardless of the type of metastases, both the hypervascular and hypovascular lesions usually exhibit a continuous rim of enhancement. T2 hypointensity that often accompanies T1 hyperintensity reflects hemorrhage or melanin. The addition of newer MRI sequences such as diffusion-weighted imaging and hepatobiliary contrast agents can be useful.

R. Gupta et al., *PET/MR Imaging*, https://doi.org/10.1007/978-3-319-65106-4_46

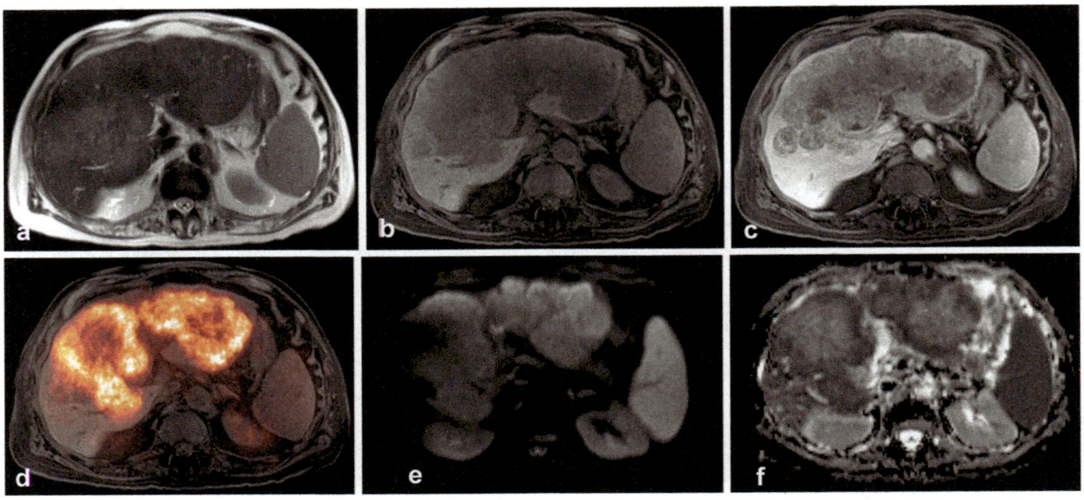

Fig. 46.1 T2 HASTE axial (**a**), T1 VIBE with fat suppression axial (**b**), T1 VIBE with fat suppression post-delayed contrast enhancement with gadolinium axial (**c**), PET/MR T1 VIBE with fat suppression axial fusion (**d**), diffusion-weighted image axial (**e**), and apparent diffusion coefficient axial (**f**)

In comparing contrast enhanced CT with non-contrast PET/CT in the detection of liver metastases, PET/CT imaging has been shown to be slightly more sensitive. Contrasted enhanced CT may miss metastatic liver lesions in up to 7% of patients and may overestimate metastatic involvement of the liver. Combined PET/MR leads to a high degree of sensitivity and accuracy in detecting liver metastases and offers better lesion delineation. PET/MR imaging with the inclusion of diffusion-weighted imaging showing increased signal with corresponding low signal restricted diffusion on ADC maps leads to even higher accuracy in metastatic detection.

Suggested Reading

Beiderwellen K, Geraldo L, Ruhlmann V, Heusch P, Gomez B, Nensa F, et al. Accuracy of [18F]FDG PET/MRI for the detection of liver metastases. PLoS One. 2015;10(9):e0137285.

Brendle C, Schwenzer NF, Rempp H, Schmidt H, Pfannenberg C, la Fougère C, et al. Assessment of metastatic colorectal cancer with hybrid imaging: comparison of reading performance using different combinations of anatomical and functional imaging techniques in PET/MRI and PET/CT in a short case series. Eur J Nucl Med Mol Imaging. 2016;43:123–32.

Namasivayam S, Martin DR, Saini S. Imaging of liver metastases: MRI. Cancer Imaging. 2007;7:2–9.

Case 47
Esophageal Adenocarcinoma

Robert Matthews

History

A 71-year-old male with esophageal adenocarcinoma and an esophageal stent (Fig. 47.1).

Diagnosis

Esophageal adenocarcinoma with lymph node metastasis

Findings

- Distal esophagus shows wall thickening that is isointense on T1-weighted image and mildly hyperintense on T2-weighted image (arrowheads).
- PET/MR fusion image shows abnormal hypermetabolic activity corresponding to the distal esophagus.
- More inferior slices show an enlarged T1 hypointense gastrohepatic lymph node that has high signal on DWI and low signal on ADC maps compatible with metastasis (arrows).

Discussion

Esophageal cancer represents 1% of all cancers in the United States, but is much more common in parts of China, India, and southern Africa. The two major types of esophageal cancer are adenocarcinoma that occurs in the distal esophagus, and squamous cell carcinoma that is found in the upper and middle portions of the esophagus. The initial diagnosis of esophageal cancer is made by upper endoscopy and biopsy. Afterward, endoscopic ultrasonography (EUS) is used to determine primary tumor depth involvement by identifying layers of the esophageal wall. Cross-sectional imaging with CT, MRI, and PET is performed for advanced esophageal cancer to aid in the detection of local spread of disease and distant metastases. FDG PET/MRI is rapidly demonstrating advantages in initial staging of esophageal cancer due to its superior soft tissue resolution and FDG avidity.

Up until about 8 years ago, MRI had difficulty imaging esophageal cancer due to normal peristaltic movement. With newer, faster sequences, MRI has shown to be able to identify esophageal wall layers. On T2-weighted images, the submucosa has high signal intensity compared to the mucosal and muscularis propria layers. With malignancy high-resolution T2-weighted images demonstrates esophageal wall thickening with mildly increased signal at the location of the lesion. Diffusion-weighted images aid in the detection of malignancy which show restricted diffusion. Esophageal cancer is isointense to the wall of the esophagus on T1-weighted images and shows enhancement following the administration of gadolinium contrast.

R. Gupta et al., *PET/MR Imaging*, https://doi.org/10.1007/978-3-319-65106-4_47

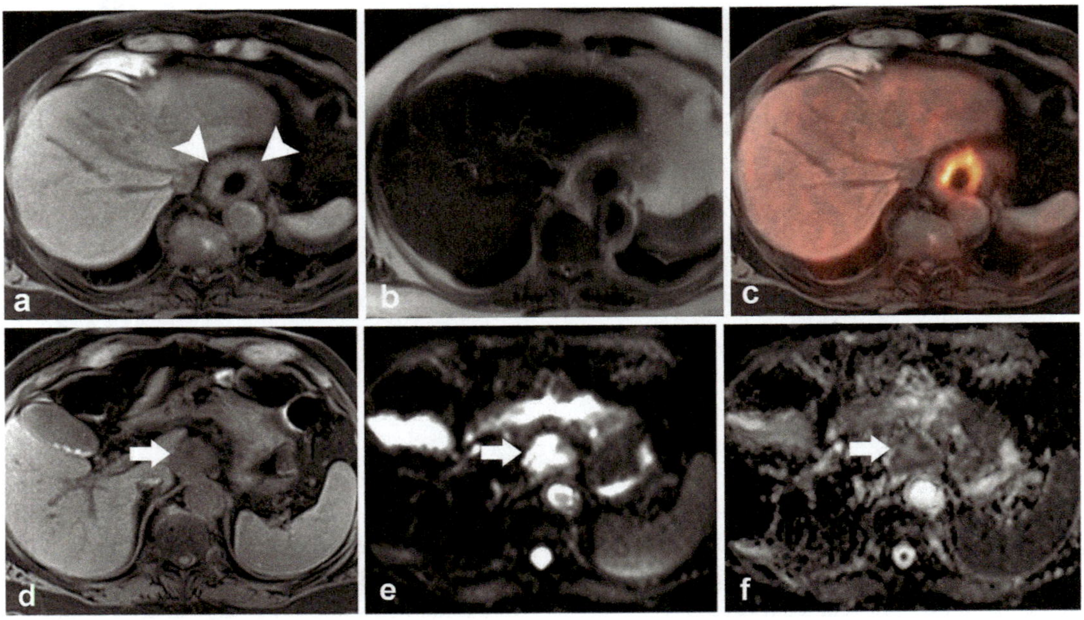

Fig. 47.1 T1 VIBE with fat suppression axial (**a**), T2 HASTE axial (**b**), PET/MR T1 VIBE with fat suppression axial fusion (**c**), T1 VIBE with fat suppression axial, at more inferior level (**d**), Diffusion-weighted image axial, at more inferior level (**e**), and apparent diffusion coefficient axial, at more inferior level (**f**)

Esophageal cancer demonstrates intense metabolic activity on PET imaging. However, PET has a limited role in making the initial diagnosis of esophageal cancer since many benign etiologies in the same anatomic location also have increased FDG uptake including leiomyomas, esophageal spasm, candida infection, radiation inflammation, swallowed secretions, and reflux disease. Although PET/CT has a limited ability to detect regional lymph nodes, PET/MRI demonstrates superiority at paraesophageal lymph node detection compared to EUS, contrast enhanced CT, or PET/CT. The addition of diffusion-weighted images and contrast enhancement on MRI improves metastatic detection. PET/MRI is also advantageous in detecting regional spread and distant metastatic disease.

Suggested Reading

Kim TJ, Kim HY, Lee KW, Kim MS. Multimodality assessment of esophageal cancer: preoperative staging and monitoring of response to therapy. Radiographics. 2009;29(2):403–21.

Lee G, Hoseok I, Kim SJ, Jeong YJ, Kim IJ, Pak K, et al. Clinical implication of PET/MR imaging in preoperative esophageal cancer staging: comparison with PET/CT, endoscopic ultrasonography, and CT. J Nucl Med. 2014;55(8):1242–7.

van Rossum PS, van Lier AL, Lips IM, Meijer GJ, Reerink O, van Vulpen M, et al. Imaging of oesophageal cancer with FDG-PET/CT and MRI. Clin Radiol. 2015;70(1):81–95.

Case 48
Focal Colonic Activity

Robert Matthews

History

A 79-year-old male with head and neck cancer presenting for restaging (Fig. 48.1).

Diagnosis

Benign focal colonic activity

Findings

- Prominent hypermetabolic focus in the right colon.
- MRI demonstrates no corresponding abnormality within the right colon.
- No evidence of mesenteric metastases.
- No pathology encountered on colonoscopy.

Discussion

Within the upper and lower gastrointestinal tracts, there can be highly variable radiotracer uptake especially in the colon. The uptake can be diffuse, focal, or segmental in distribution. There are many causes of focal uptake in bowel including lymphatic tissue, infection, microbacteria uptake, swallowed secretions, inflammatory polyps, and benign or malignant tumors. An incidental focus of FDG uptake in the colon or rectum has an approximately 50% chance of representing an underlying adenoma or malignant lesion on colonoscopy. Overall, only 10% of focal uptake is due to colonic malignancy. Although malignancies usually have a higher SUV value compared with other lesions, there is no SUV cutoff value that can reliably distinguish between benign and malignant lesions.

In the post-surgical patient, colonic staples or sutures following bowel resection can elicit an inflammatory or granulomatous reaction with scar formation that can mimic the appearance of local recurrence. These changes can persist months after surgery. In addition, highly dense material such as metal, IV contrast, or barium can artificially increase signal on PET. Variable gas in the colon or rectum will produce an attenuation artifact with increased PET signal. Chemotherapy and radiation can also produce inflammatory change in the bowel as well as the mesentery with lymphadenopathy. All these changes may be difficult for PET/MRI to interpret when focal colonic uptake is encountered. Usually definite diagnosis requires colonoscopy.

R. Gupta et al., *PET/MR Imaging*, https://doi.org/10.1007/978-3-319-65106-4_48

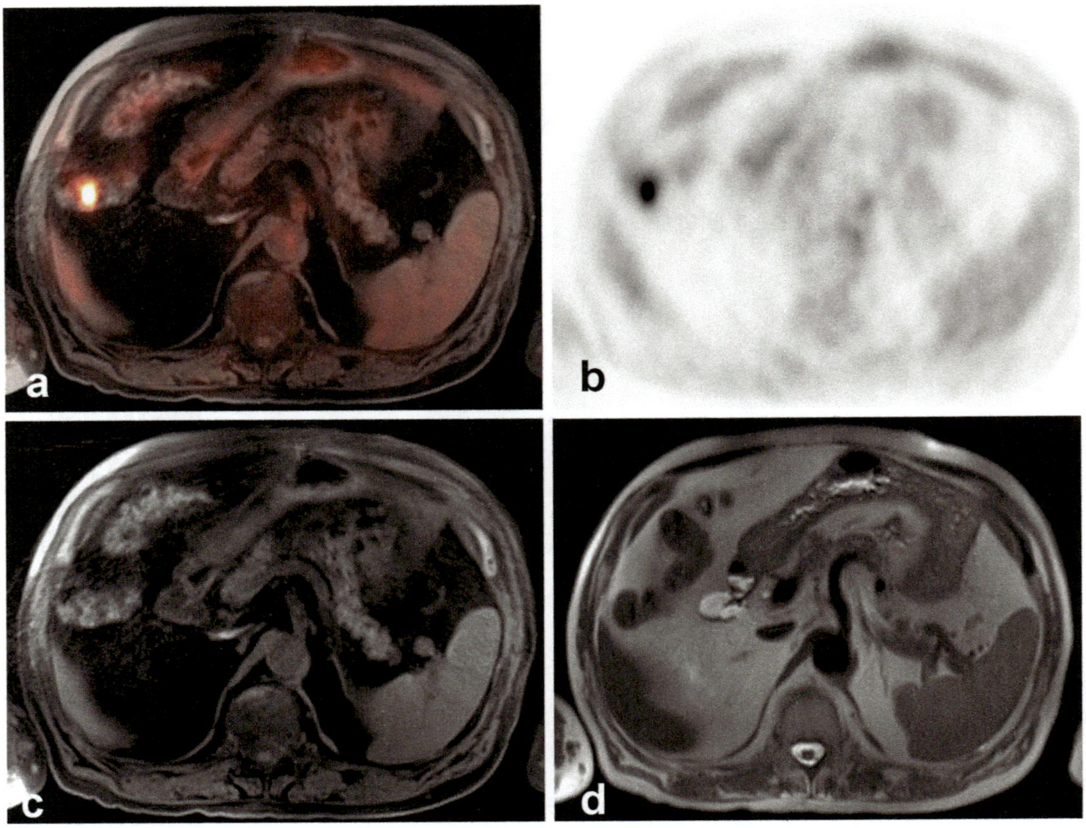

Fig. 48.1 PET/MR T1 radial VIBE with fat suppression axial fusion (**a**), PET axial (**b**), T1 radial VIBE with fat suppression axial (**c**), and T2 HASTE axial (**d**)

Suggested Reading

Corrigan AJ, Schleyer PJ, Cook GJ. Pitfalls and artifacts in the use of PET/CT in oncology imaging. Semin Nucl Med. 2015;45:481–99.

Safaie E, Matthews R, Bergamaschi R. PET scan findings can be false positive. Tech Coloproctol. 2015;19:329–30.

Case 49
Diffuse Fatty Liver

Robert Matthews

History

A 56-year-old male with elevated metanephrines to evaluate for pheochromocytoma (Fig. 49.1).

Diagnosis

Diffuse fatty liver (hepatic steatosis)

Findings

- No focal areas of increased FDG uptake on the PET images to suggest malignancy.
- No gross abnormalities on the T1 or T2-weighted images.
- Drop in signal on the out-of-phase images in comparison to the in-phase images.

Discussion

Non-alcoholic fatty liver disease is the most common chronic liver disease that includes a wide spectrum of disorders including benign macrovesicular hepatic steatosis, non-alcoholic steatohepatitis (NASH), hepatic fibrosis, cirrhosis of the liver, and hepatocellular carcinoma. Fatty liver disease may involve up to 12–24% of the general population with a significantly higher incidence in obese and diabetic patients. The incidence of this disorder has markedly increased, even in the pediatric population in the last 2 decades. Its presence is associated with a higher incidence of cardiovascular disease and atherosclerosis. NASH is associated with inflammation that can progress to fibrosis and ultimately to cirrhosis. NASH is estimated to account for 20% of liver failures leading to transplantation.

Inflammatory cells especially neutrophils are metabolically active and can show increased FDG uptake. Normal hepatocytes have an enzyme glucose-6-phophatase that helps to maintain blood glucose levels and therefore have the capacity to export FDG back into the blood. During active inflammatory stages of NASH, usually the maximum SUV is not affected although changes in the medium SUV have been reported in the literature.

It can be difficult to detect hepatic steatosis on routine T1 and T2-weighted MRI sequences. Chemical shift imaging using T1-weighted in-phase and out-of-phase sequences has a high sensitivity in detecting fatty infiltration, and is routinely used clinically. A lesion that has microscopic fat and water that is contained in normal tissue will have a drop in signal on the out-of-phase images in comparison to the in-phase image. Thus, the out-of-phase image will appear darker than the in-phase images. Usually, mild hepatomegaly accompanies hepatic steatosis. Fatty infiltration may diffusely involve the liver, but can also be geometric in pattern. Areas of focal fatty sparing called pseudolesions may

R. Gupta et al., *PET/MR Imaging*, https://doi.org/10.1007/978-3-319-65106-4_49

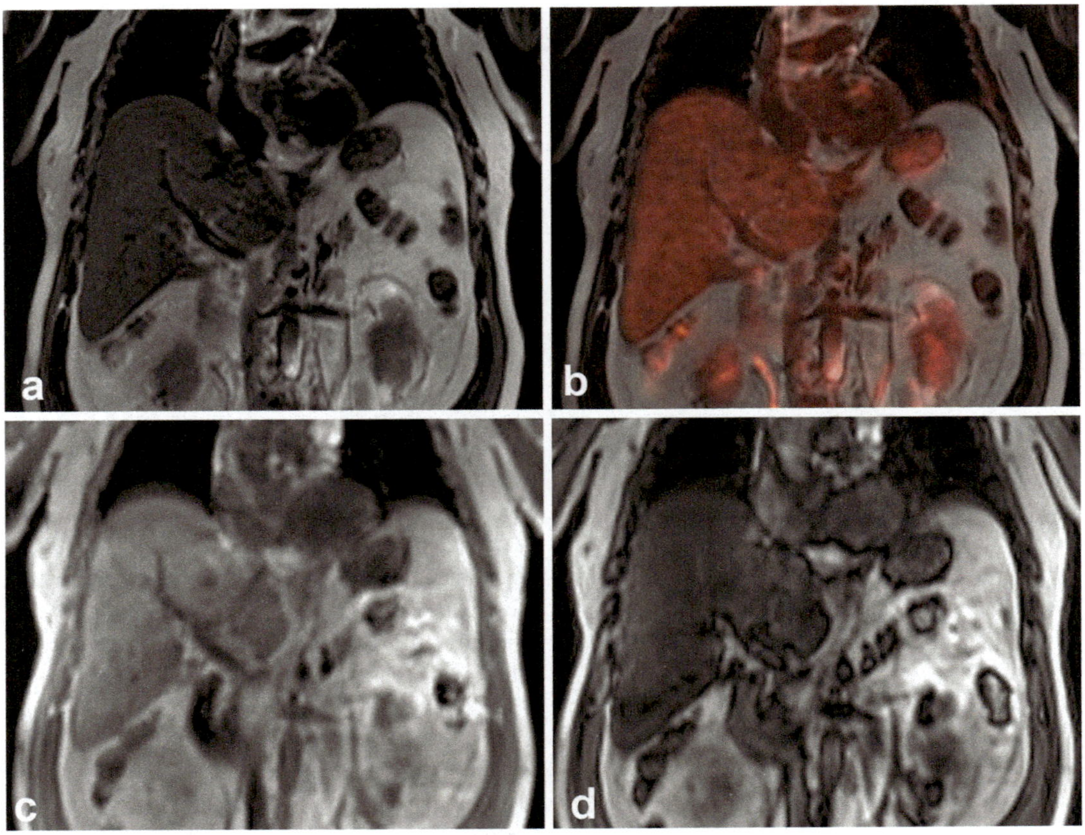

Fig. 49.1 T2 TSE coronal (**a**), PET/MR T2 TSE coronal fusion (**b**), Dixon T1-weighted in-phase coronal (**c**), and Dixon T1-weighted out-of-phase coronal (**d**)

occur adjacent to the porta hepatitis, gallbladder, falciform ligament, and in the subcapsular region. An important feature to distinguish focal fatty sparing from mass lesion on PET/MRI is the absence of mass effect with the presence of normal appearing vessels through that region and lack of focal FDG uptake.

Suggested Reading

Décarie PO, Lepanto L, Billiard JS, Olivié D, Murphy-Lavallée J, Kauffmann C, et al. Fatty liver deposition and sparing: a pictorial review. Insights Imaging. 2011;2:533–8.

Keramida G, Potts J, Bush J, Verma S, Dizdarevic S, Peters AM. Accumulation of 18F-FDG in the liver with hepatic steatosis. AJR Am J Roentgenol. 2014 Sep;203(3):643–8.

Case 50 Pancreatic Ductal Adenocarcinoma

Robert Matthews

History

A 62-year-old male presents with pancreatic mass seen on CT performed for evaluating abdominal pain (Fig. 50.1).

Diagnosis

Pancreatic ductal adenocarcinoma

Findings

- Irregular ill-defined mass in the pancreatic body that is mildly heterogeneously isointense on T1 and with mildly decreased signal on T2-weighted images (wide arrow).
- PET images show abnormal hypermetabolic activity within the pancreatic body mass.
- T2-weighted image demonstrates posterior extension of the mass with obliteration of the splenic vein (thin arrow).
- Distal pancreatic duct dilatation demonstrating high T2 intensity (arrowheads).

Discussion

Pancreatic ductal adenocarcinoma is ranked fourth in cancer-causing deaths. Because of its late presentation, most cases of pancreatic cancer are advanced and unresectable at the time of diagnosis. Surgical resection is the mainstay of therapy which may be withheld if there is evidence of liver metastases, distant lymph node involvement, arterial encasement, or more than 50% major venous structure encasement.

MRI has superior soft tissue resolution and is more suitable for evaluating findings of pancreatic cancer invasion. MRI is superior at identifying main pancreatic duct dilatation, encasement of adjacent vessels, cystic and necrotic changes, and fibrotic changes. The normal pancreas has high signal intensity on unenhanced T1-weighted images with fat suppression and shows homogenous arterial enhancement that becomes isointense on delayed imaging. Pancreatic adenocarcinoma is usually mildly hypointense on fat-suppressed T1 fat images due to the desmoplastic reaction, but can be isointense or even slightly hyperintense. Contrast enhanced T1-weighted imaging is the most useful in characterizing pancreatic lesions showing gradual enhancement on delayed images. T2 and FLAIR signal intensity can be variable depending on the amount of desmoplastic reaction, necrosis, inflammation, and hemorrhage. However, T2-weighted imaging is valuable in assessing dilatation of the common bile duct and pancreatic duct.

Most malignant cancers of the pancreas show increased FDG activity on PET imaging, especially if the lesion exceeds 1 cm in size. PET/CT and PET/MR imaging demonstrate high sensitivity and specificity in lesion detection compared

R. Gupta et al., *PET/MR Imaging*, https://doi.org/10.1007/978-3-319-65106-4_50

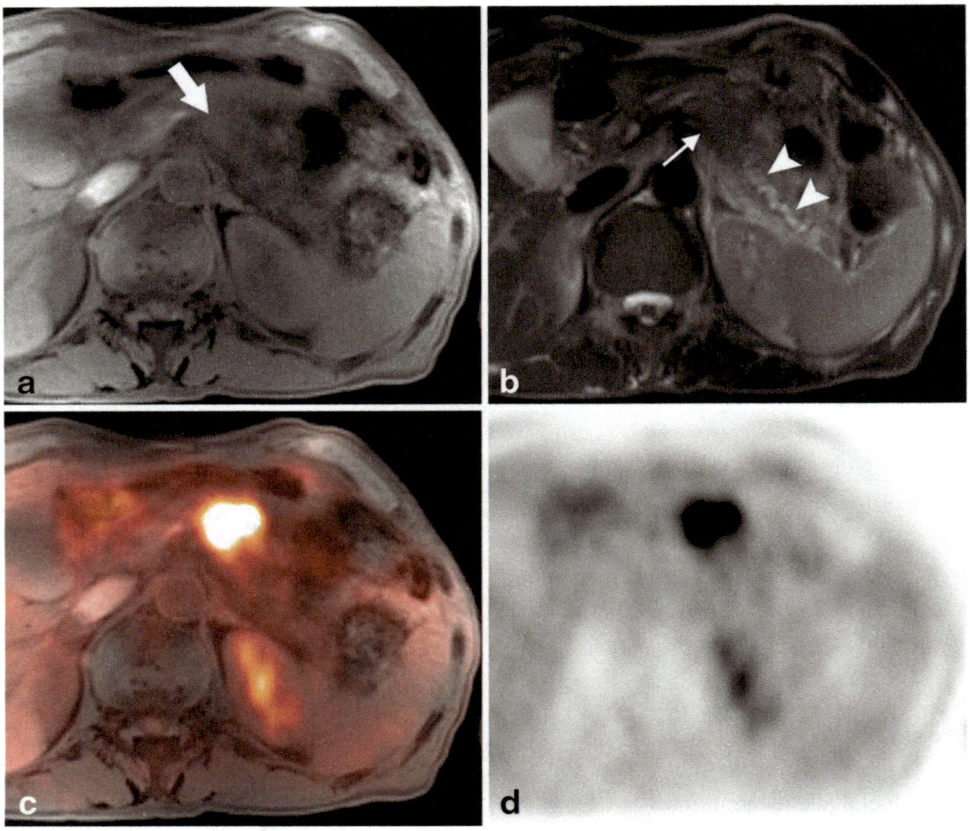

Fig. 50.1 T1 radial VIBE with fat suppression axial (**a**), T2 HASTE axial (**b**), PET/MR T1 radial VIBE with fat suppression axial fusion (**c**), and PET axial (**d**)

to contrast enhanced CT scan. Some false positive findings can occur with inflammatory lesion demonstrating focal FDG uptake that may be difficult to distinguish from malignant lesions. Overall, the degree of FDG uptake in terms of maximum SUV value correlates with pathological grade, tumor size, and staging.

Suggested Reading

Jha P, Bijan B, Melendres G, Shelton DK. Hybrid imaging for pancreatic malignancy. Clin Nucl Med. 2015;40:206–13.

Miller FH, Rini NJ, Keppke AL. MRI of adenocarcinoma of the pancreas. AJR Am J Roentgenol. 2006;187(4):W365–74.

Nagamachi S, Nishii R, Wakamatsu H, Mizutani Y, Kiyohara S, Fujita S, et al. The usefulness of (18) F-FDG PET/MRI fusion image in diagnosing pancreatic tumor: comparison with (18)F-FDG PET/CT. Ann of Nucl Med. 2013;27:554–63.

Case 51
Diffuse Splenic Uptake

Robert Matthews

History

A 39-year-old female with metastatic breast cancer with radiation to brain who is currently undergoing chemotherapy (Fig. 51.1).

Diagnosis

Diffuse splenic uptake

Findings

- Normal homogenous T1 and T2-weighted signal on MRI in a normal-size spleen.
- PET shows homogenous increased FDG uptake without focal lesions.
- Increased bone marrow FDG activity.

Discussion

The spleen is a lymphoid organ that is involved in humoral and cell-mediated immune response, as well as destruction of old or damaged red blood cells. Normal FDG uptake in the spleen is equal to, or slightly less than, liver intensity. In a patient undergoing chemotherapy, granulocyte colony-stimulating factor and erythropoietin can stimulate FDG uptake in the spleen, as well as the bone marrow. Chemotherapy, especially platinum-based agents, can also cause increased splenic and bone marrow activity on PET. When this occurs the spleen usually remains unchanged in size and there are no focal lesions identified on MRI. Hematologic diseases like anemia, especially thalassemia, can cause diffusely increased splenic FDG uptake without concomitant bone marrow stimulation. When there is diffuse hypermetabolism within the spleen and splenomegaly, especially with the absence of bone marrow hypermetabolic activity, there is a higher probability of pathological involvement. The differential diagnosis of increased PET activity includes a wide variety of diseases including malignancy, infection, or inflammation. Specific pathological diseases found to have diffuse splenic hypermetabolism include diffuse microscopic lymphomatous involvement of the spleen, systemic lupus erythematous, acute Epstein-Barr virus infection, Castleman's disease, leukemia, glycogen storage diseases, among other diseases.

MRI has an improved ability to detect both focal splenic lesions and diffuse involvement compared to CT due to improved tissue contrast. Typically, on T1-weighted images the spleen demonstrates a lower signal intensity than the liver and on T2-weighted images the signal intensity is brighter. On gadolinium contrast enhanced images the spleen may have initial serpentine pattern from variable circulation that becomes more homogenous after the first minute.

Extramedullary hematopoiesis is typically seen with long-standing anemia, and demonstrates

R. Gupta et al., *PET/MR Imaging*, https://doi.org/10.1007/978-3-319-65106-4_51

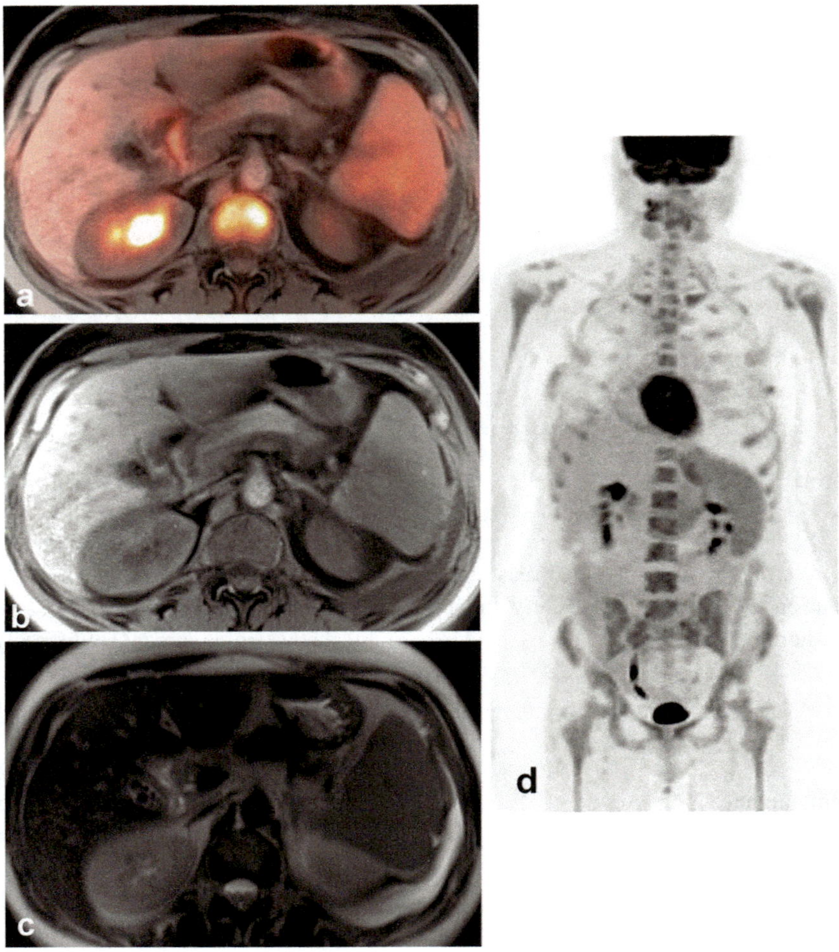

Fig. 51.1 PET/MR T1 radial VIBE with fat suppression axial fusion (**a**), T1 radial VIBE with fat suppression axial (**b**), T2 HASTE axial (**c**), and PET MIP (**d**)

diffuse homogenous infiltration of the spleen on MRI. When extramedullary hematopoiesis is severe, the spleen shows intermediate to high signal on T1-weighted images, high signal on T2-weighted images, and mild gadolinium contrast enhancement. Diffuse liver diseases such as glycogen storage disease would show low signal on T1-weighted images and intermediate to high signal on T2-weighted images. Typically, MRI does not readily demonstrate changes following the administration of erythropoietin, granulocyte colony-stimulating factors, and chemotherapy that can be visualized on PET.

Suggested Reading

Abouzied MM, Crawford ES, Nabi HA. 18F-FDG imaging: pitfalls and artifacts. J Nucl Med Technol. 2005;33:45–155.

Elsayes KM, Narra VR, Mukundan G. MR imaging of the spleen: spectrum of abnormalities. Radiographics. 2005;25:967–82.

Case 52
Simple Hepatic Cyst and Hemorrhagic Hepatic Cyst

Robert Matthews

History

A 72-year-old male with colon cancer for restaging (Fig. 52.1).

Diagnosis

Simple hepatic cyst and hemorrhagic hepatic cyst

Findings

- Focal liver lesion that is T1 hypointense and T2 hyperintense consistent with fluid density containing a thin wall, without internal septations or solid components (arrow).
- No contrast enhancement and no hypermetabolic activity within this simple hepatic cyst.
- The more inferior focal liver lesion shows peripheral T1 hypointense cystic signal and more complex central hemorrhagic component with T1 ring like hyperintensity (curved arrow). T2 signal is hyperintense.
- The more inferior hemorrhagic hepatic cyst shows no contrast enhancement or hypermetabolic activity on the fusion image.
- Hemorrhagic hepatic cyst is located adjacent to the gallbladder (thin arrow).

Discussion

Cystic liver lesions are one of the most common findings in abdominal imaging. These are fluid contained lesions that may be the result of a variety of benign and malignant pathologies as well as being the sequelae of certain therapies. The most common etiology encountered on PET/MR imaging is the simple liver cyst. This lesion is hypointense on T1-weighted images, hyperintense on T2-weighted images, and demonstrates no contrast enhancement. Simple cysts have smooth walls with no septum or wall nodularity, and can be solitary or multiple. These benign lesions demonstrate absence of FDG uptake. Rarely, complications may occur with simple cysts such as infection or hemorrhage. Hemorrhagic cysts usually have hyperintense T1 contents and at times can have fluid levels. They lack contrast enhancement, although occasionally may have mild enhancement. No FDG uptake is seen in hemorrhagic cysts. On the other hand, infected hepatic cysts demonstrate increased FDG uptake.

Complex cysts are fluid containing lesions that can have wall thickening, internal nodularity, septas, calcification, hemorrhage, or proteinaceous content. Biliary cystadenoma and biliary cystadenocarcinoma are solitary complex cyst masses

R. Gupta et al., *PET/MR Imaging*, https://doi.org/10.1007/978-3-319-65106-4_52

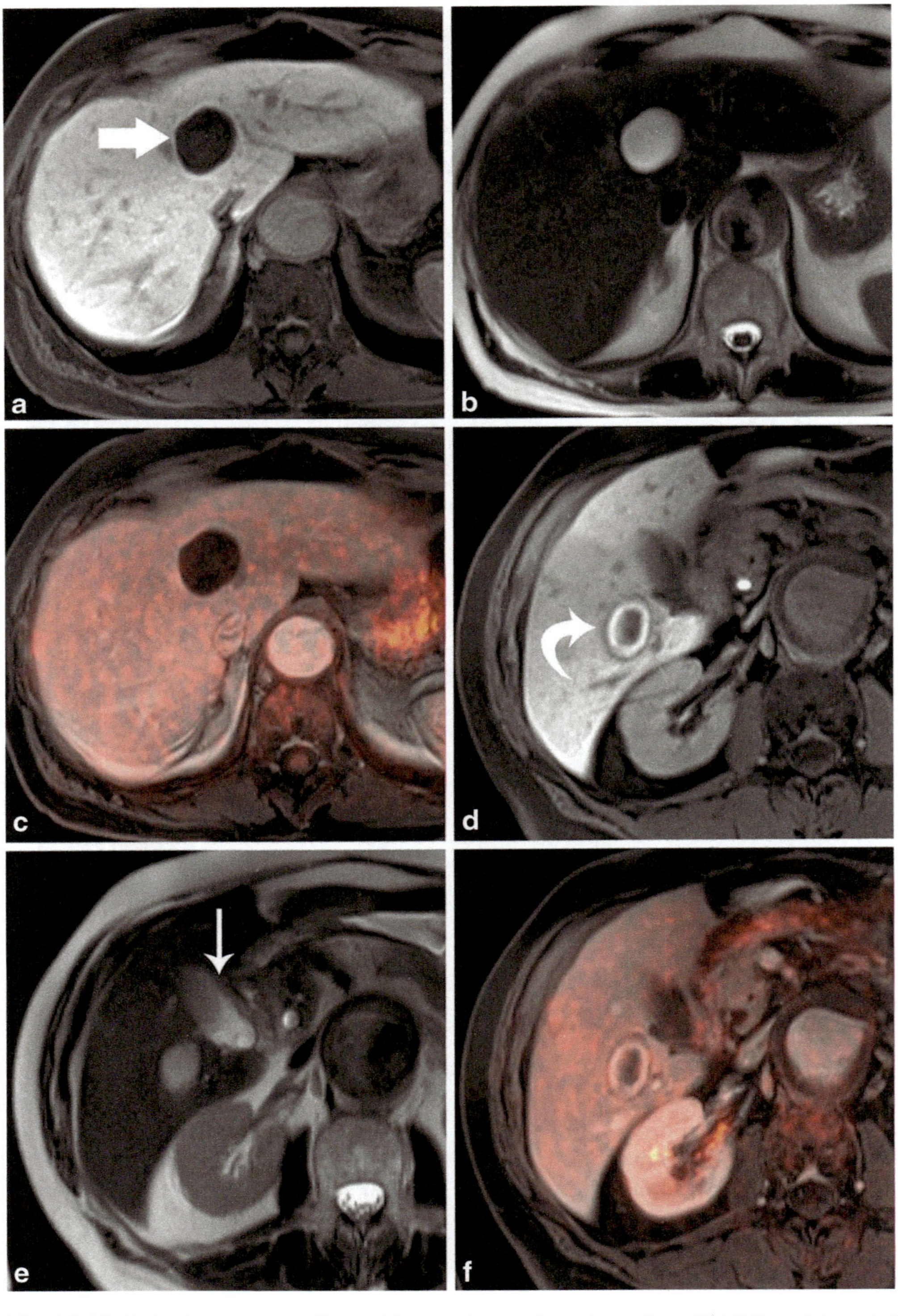

Fig. 52.1 T1 VIBE with fat suppression 15 min delayed contrast enhancement axial (**a**), T2 HASTE axial (**b**), PET/MR T1 VIBE with fat suppression with early contrast enhancement axial fusion (**c**), T1 VIBE with fat suppression 15 min delayed contrast enhancement axial (more inferior level) (**d**), T2 HASTE axial (more inferior level) (**e**), and PET/MR T1 VIBE with fat suppression with early contrast enhancement axial fusion (more inferior level) (**f**)

with a thick fibrous capsule, internal septations, and wall nodularity. MRI signal characteristics are widely variable depending on its contents which may contain hemorrhage, solid components, and proteinous material. The cystic "fluid" usually has low signal on T1-weighted images and homogenous high signal on T2-weighted images. Biliary cystadenocarcinoma shows contrast enhancement and FDG uptake.

Cystic metastases may be encountered on PET/MR imaging. These cystic metastases are often the result of necrosis in hypervascular tumors such as metastatic melanoma, neuroendocrine tumor, sarcoma, and some breast and lung cancers. Mucinous metastatic tumors may also appear cystic, as seen in some ovarian and colon cancers. On MRI the lesions appear as single or multiple with thick irregular walls, septations, and internal debris. Cystic metastases demonstrate less T2 hyperintensity compared to the simple cysts and show contrast enhancement with gadolinium contrast. Cystic metastases reveal FDG avidity on PET/MR imaging. Treated metastatic lesions may also appear cystic due to their degeneration, do not enhance, and have little FDG activity. Hepatocellular carcinoma (HCC) may rarely be necrotic or cystically degenerated. The solid components have characteristic findings of HCC including T2 hyperintensity, T1 hypointensity, and early contrast enhancement followed by washout. Cystic lesions are commonly seen on PET/MRI following liver surgery and biopsy due to seromas, hematomas, bilomas, or infected collections. No optimal SUV cutoff value is available to determine if a cystic lesion is malignant.

Suggested Reading

Mortelé KJ, Ros PR. Cystic focal liver lesions in the adult: differential CT and MR imaging features. Radiographics. 2001;21(4):895–910.

Xia Q, Feng Y, Wu C, Huang G, Liu J, Chen T. Differentiation between malignant and benign solitary lesions in the liver with (18)FDG PET/CT: accuracy of age-related diagnostic standard. J Cancer. 2015;6(1):40–7.

Case 53
Carcinoid Tumor with Gallium DOTATATE

Joseph R. Stein

History

A 48-year-old male with mesenteric root mass and MEN syndrome (Fig. 53.1).

Diagnosis

Metastatic carcinoid tumor detected with gallium DOTATATE

Findings

- Superior slice showing a mildly hyperintense T2, isointense T1 endoluminal mass within a proximal loop of ileum (thin white arrow).
- PET/MR fusion image shows abnormal radiotracer activity corresponding to the endoluminal mass representing the primary carcinoid tumor.
- Inferior level images demonstrate a mildly hyperintense T2, hypermetabolic mesenteric lymph node (curved white arrow) compatible with carcinoid metastasis.
- PET MIP shows the hypermetabolic endophytic mass (black arrowhead) and the hypermetabolic mesenteric lymph node (wide black arrow). A cluster of smaller hypermetabolic lymph nodes is seen associated with the inferior aspect of the mass.

Discussion

Carcinoid tumor is a type of neuroendocrine tumor (NET) that can arise in various locations, with those found in the gastrointestinal tract accounting for 60–85% of all carcinoids. They are slow growing tumors but are capable of metastasis. On MR imaging, submucosal small bowel carcinoid tumors are isointense on T1-weighted images and hyperintense to isointense on T2-weighted images. On T1 post contrast imaging, small bowel carcinoid tumors demonstrate a moderately intense enhancement pattern, which is typically homogenous.

Gallium-68 (Ga-68) is a generator-produced positron emitter that allows for on-site on-demand availability. DOTATATE is a positron emitting somatostatin analogue that binds to somatostatin receptors with a much higher affinity for type 2 receptors (SST2), which are overexpressed in NETs. It is also the peptide most commonly used for radionuclide therapy with lutetium-177 and yttrium-90. The uptake of DOTATATE correlates with the density of somatostatin receptors in NETs. In 2016, the FDA approved Ga-68 DOTATATE for PET imaging of neuroendocrine tumors. When compared to gamma camera imaging using Indium-111 octreotide, advantages of DOTATATE are lower radiation dose, improved lesion detectability, and shorter and faster exam.

R. Gupta et al., *PET/MR Imaging*, https://doi org/10.1007/978-3-319-65106-4_53

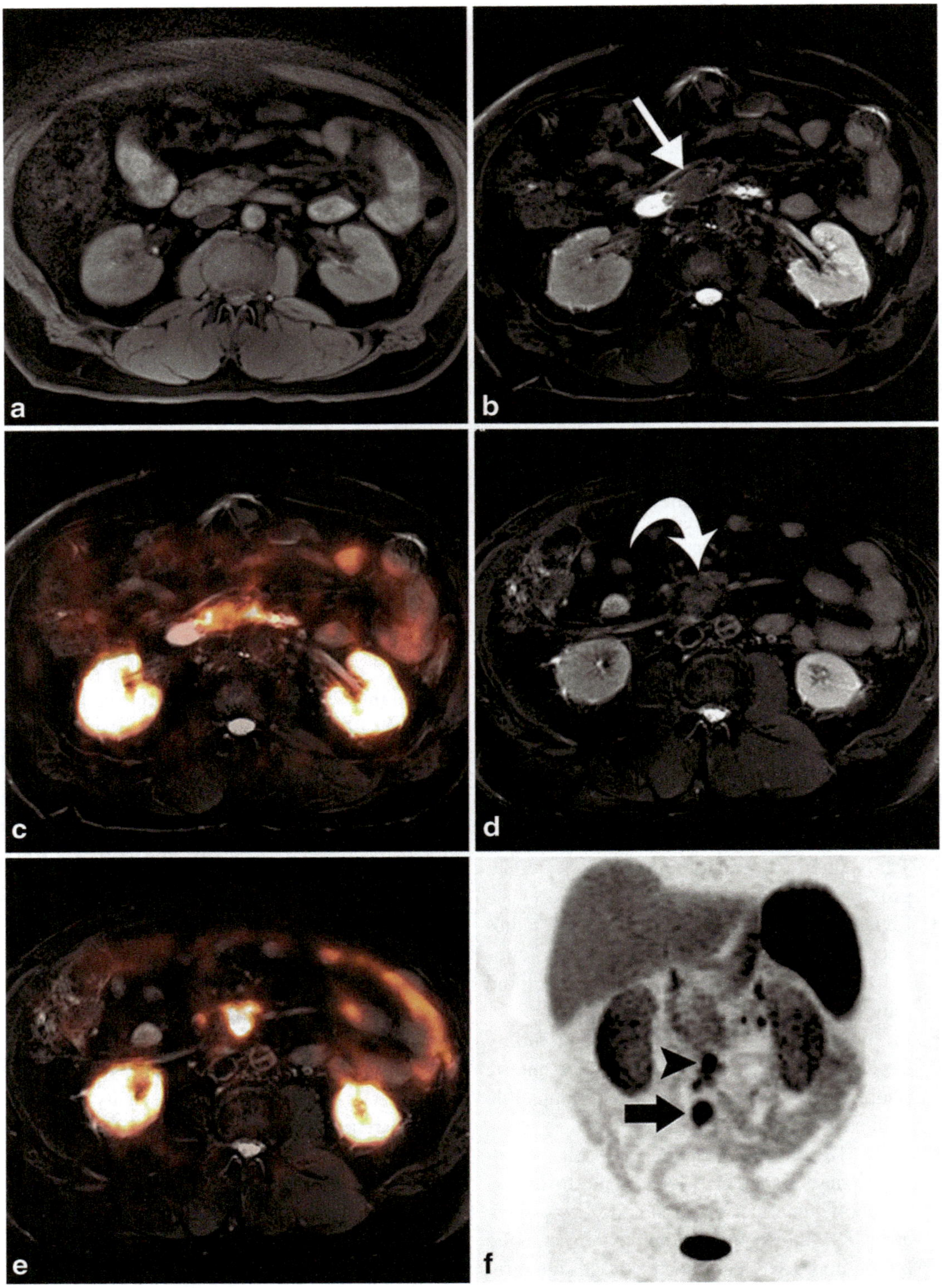

Fig. 53.1 T1 radial VIBE with fat suppression axial, at superior level (**a**), T2 BLADE with fat suppression axial, at superior level (**b**), DOTATATE PET/MR T2 BLADE with fat suppression axial fusion, at superior level (**c**), T2 BLADE with fat suppression axial, at inferior level (**d**), DOTATATE PET/MR T2 BLADE with fat suppression axial fusion, at inferior level (**e**), and DOTATATE PET MIP (**f**)

DOTATATE has minimal background activity in the muscles and soft tissue which leads to a high tumor-to-background contrast. The normal uptake pattern of DOTATATE can be seen in SST2-expressing organs such as the pituitary, salivary glands, thyroid gland, head and uncinate process of the pancreas, and adrenals. The highest intensity physiological uptake of DOTATATE occurs in the spleen, followed by the adrenal glands, kidneys, and pituitary. Less intense activity can be seen in the liver, salivary glands, thyroid, and pancreas. Interpreting physicians must be aware of normal physiologic and other pathologic processes that have increased Ga-68 DOTATATE uptake. Up to one third of patients will demonstrate moderately prominent pancreatic uncinate process uptake. Splenosis can be a common finding during restaging that can be mistaken for peritoneal metastases in a patient with a previous pancreatic NET who underwent a splenectomy. Another pitfall is physiologic uptake in the adrenal glands which can interfere with the diagnosis of adrenal NETs. Meningiomas are frequent incidental findings on gallium-68 DOTATATE PET. These tiny lesions, often sub centimeter, do not require additional workup. Inflammatory uptake is commonly observed in reactive axillary, hilar, and mediastinal lymphadenopathy as well as prostatitis and post radiation changes.

Gastroenteropancreatic NETs, carcinoid tumors, pheochromocytomas, pancreatic islet cell tumors, and medullary carcinoma of the thyroid are all DOTATATE positive. Uptake of Ga-68 DOTATATE has been shown in a wide range of other tumors of neuroendocrine origin including pituitary adenoma, hemangioblastoma, meningioma, and melanoma. It has also been shown to be effective at localizing the primary tumor in patients with metastatic NET with an unknown primary. For the detection of NETs, Ga-68 DOTATATE PET has sensitivity and specificity that ranges from 88 to 90% and from 80 to 100%, respectively.

Suggested Reading

Bader TR, Semelka RC, Chiu VC, Armao DM, Woosley JT. MRI of carcinoid tumors: spectrum of appearances in the gastrointestinal tract and liver. J Magn Reson Imaging. 2001;14(3):261–9.

Levy AD, Sobin LH. From the archives of the AFIP: gastrointestinal carcinoids: imaging features with clinicopathologic comparison. Radiographics. 2007;27(1):237–57.

Mojtahedi A, Thamake S, Tworowska I, Ranganathan D, Delpassand ES. The value of ^{68}Ga-DOTATATE PET/CT in diagnosis and management of neuroendocrine tumors compared to current FDA approved imaging modalities: a review of literature. Am J Nucl Med Mol Imaging. 2014;4(5):426–34.

Case 54
Large Gallstone and Sludge

Christopher Shackles and Amit Gupta

History

An 86-year-old female presents for restaging of breast cancer (Fig. 54.1). She complains of right upper quadrant abdominal pain.

Diagnosis

Large gallstone and sludge

Findings

- Large calcified stone in the gallbladder with hypointense signal on both T1 and T2 images (thin arrow).
- T1 hypointensity within the posterior aspect of the gallbladder representing layering sludge (arrowhead).
- Mildly enlarged gallbladder seen on coronal image (curved arrow).
- No FDG uptake is seen associated with the gallbladder.

Discussion

Cholelithiasis is a common cause of symptomatic gallbladder disease. Clinical symptoms are often vague, but tend to include right upper quadrant to mid-epigastric pain and nausea. While initial evaluation is usually performed with ultrasound or CT, MRI is often performed to evaluate the biliary system in cases with a concern for biliary obstruction.

Gallstones will appear on MR as hypointense foci on T1 and T2 sequences and are usually particularly conspicuous against the background of T2 hyperintense bile. Calcified stones will also bloom on gradient echo or susceptibility-weighted sequences. In chronic cholecystitis, which is often associated with cholelithiasis, the gallbladder will typically appear contracted with irregularly thickened walls. Following gadolinium administration, a gallbladder with chronic cholecystitis will demonstrate uniform, mild enhancement, to a lesser degree than that seen in acute cholecystitis. Although MR cholangiography and functional MR cholangiography have also been suggested, their utility in chronic cholecystitis remains unclear.

PET has no significant role in the workup of cholelithiasis or other benign gallbladder diseases, even though there are case reports suggesting the role of PET in diagnosing acute cholecystitis. However, PET may have a role in differentiating benign from malignant gallbladder wall thickening. While polypoid gallbladder malignancies are easier to identify, those that simply appear as diffuse gallbladder wall thickening can be difficult to differentiate from benign entities such as cholecystitis. FDG is known to be taken up by both activated inflammatory cells and malignant cells. However, by stratifying

R. Gupta et al., *PET/MR Imaging*, https://doi.org/10.1007/978-3-319-65106-4_54

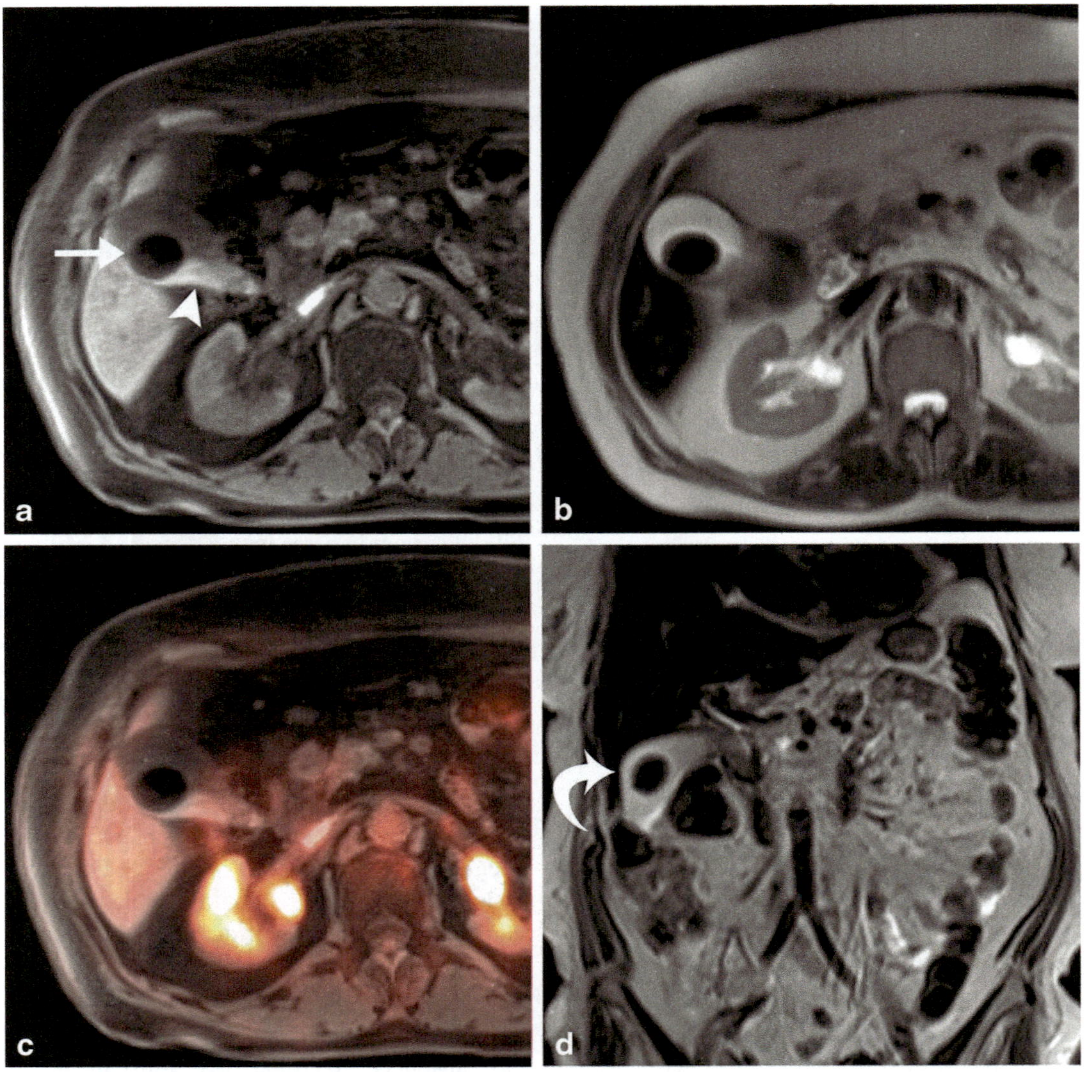

Fig. 54.1 T1 radial VIBE with fat suppression axial (**a**), T2 HASTE axial (**b**), FDG PET/MR T1 radial VIBE with fat suppression axial fusion (**c**), and T2 TSE coronal (**d**)

these patients with blood markers for acute inflammation such as elevated C-reactive protein, increased SUV levels can be used to differentiate a malignant from a benign process with a sensitivity and specificity up to 75–100%, respectively.

Suggested Reading

Aparici CM, Win AZ. Acute calculous cholecystitis missed on computed tomography and ultrasound but diagnosed with fluorodeoxyglucose-positron emission tomography/computed tomography. J Clin Imaging Sci. 2016;6:31.

Catalano OA, Sahani DV, Kalva SP, Cushing MS, Hahn PF, Brown JJ, et al. MR imaging of the gallbladder: a pictorial essay. Radiographics. 2008;28(1):135–55. quiz 324

Oe A, Kawabe J, Torii K, Kawamura E, Higashiyama S, Kotani J, et al. Distinguishing benign from malignant gallbladder wall thickening using FDG-PET. Ann Nucl Med. 2006;20(10):699–703.

Case 55
Cecal Cancer

Robert Matthews

History

A 45-year-old female presents for initial staging of colon cancer (Fig. 55.1).

Diagnosis

Cecal cancer with lymph node involvement

Findings

- T1 image shows a hyperintense heterogeneous mass in the cecum that is dark on T2 (arrows).
- There are multiple T1-weighted heterogenous hyperintense, T2-weighted hypointense, enlarged lymph nodes extending from the mass to the right paraaortic region (arrowheads).
- PET images show intense hypermetabolic activity within the cecal mass and lymph nodes consistent with malignancy.

Discussion

Colorectal cancer is the third most common malignancy in the United States. At the time of diagnosis, liver metastases are seen in up to 25% of patients. The initial diagnosis of colon cancer usually requires colonoscopy with biopsy. Often contrast enhanced CT of the abdomen and pelvis is routinely performed to look for metastatic lesions in lymph nodes, liver, and peritoneal cavity. Colorectal cancer involving the cecum has been associated with advanced tumor growth before symptoms and signs like pain, anemia, and palpable mass are elicited.

On MRI colon cancer and large lymph node metastases are iso to hyperintense on T1-weighted images and hypointense to isointense on T2-weighted images. Contrast enhanced MRI and use of diffusion-weighted images improve lesion detection by showing avid contrast enhancement and restricted diffusion. On PET imaging colon cancer and lymph node metastases demonstrate well-defined increased radiotracer uptake.

Traditional anatomic imaging defines metastatic mesenteric lymph nodes on the basis of size and shape criteria, with 5 mm being the cutoff in size. Early metastatic lymph nodes may not show contrast enhancement or change in MRI signal, especially loss of central fat. MRI can easily detect changes in size, due to improved contrast as compared to CT. However, reactive lymph nodes are common and these mildly enlarged lymph nodes may be misinterpreted as metastases. The absence or presence of hypermetabolic activity within these indeterminate mesenteric lymph nodes on PET/MRI images can lead to a more accurate assessment of

R. Gupta et al., *PET/MR Imaging*, https://doi.org/10.1007/978-3-319-65106-4_55

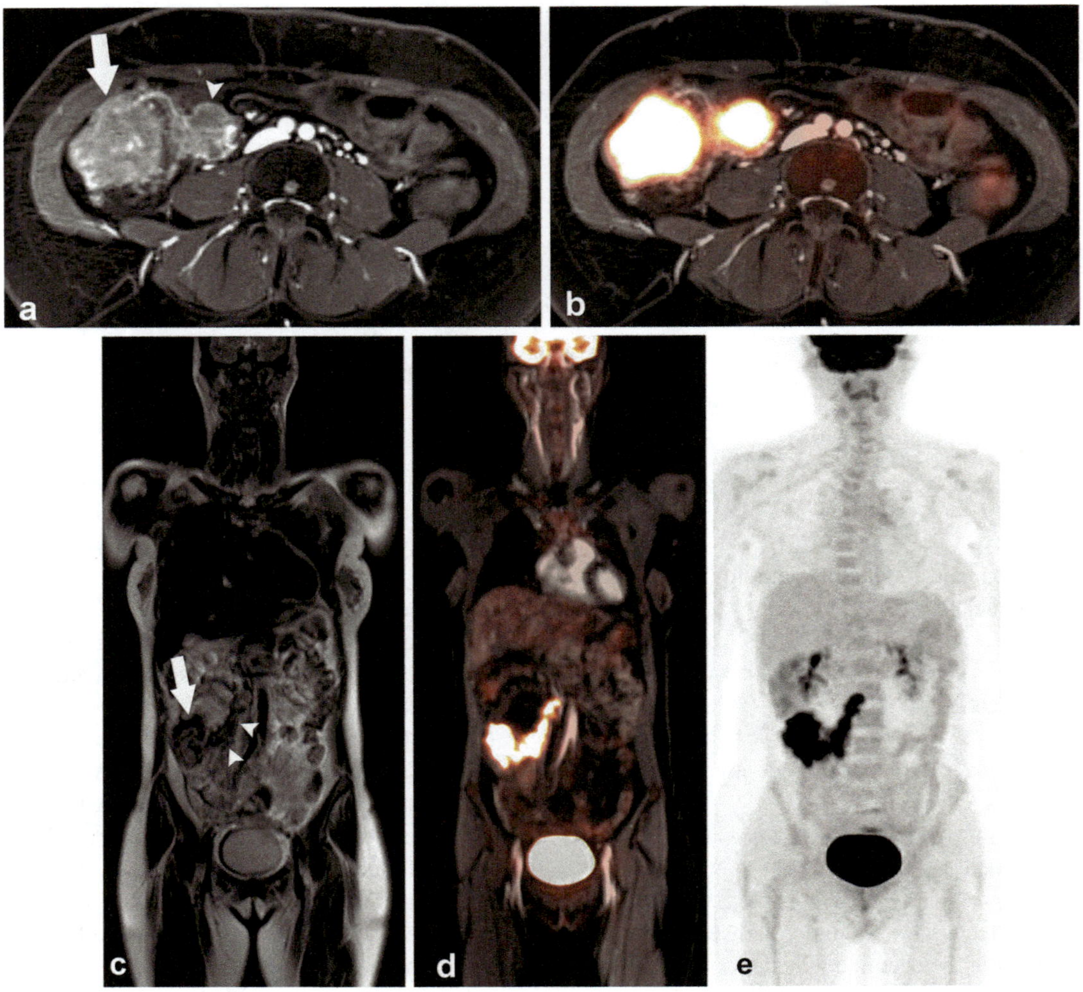

Fig. 55.1 T1 radial VIBE with fat suppression axial (**a**), PET/MRI T1 radial VIBE with fat suppression axial fusion (**b**), T2 TSE coronal (**c**), PET/MRI Dixon T1-weighted water sequence coronal fusion (**d**), and PET MIP (**e**)

regional metastases. Since anatomic registration of lymph nodes, especially abdominal nodes, is difficult, simultaneous PET/MR has distinct staging advantages.

Suggested Reading

Kang B, Lee JM, Song YS, Woo S, Hur BY, Jeon JH, et al. Added value of integrated whole body PET/MRI for evaluation of colorectal cancer: comparison with contrast-enhanced MDCT. AJR Am J Roentgenol. 2016;206:W10–20.

Mainenti PP, Romano F, Pizzuti L, Segreto S, Storto G, Mannelli L, et al. Non-invasive diagnostic imaging of colorectal liver metastases. World M Radiol. 2015;28:157–69.

Case 56 Non-FDG Avid Hepatocellular Carcinoma

Robert Matthews

History

A 69-year-old male with cirrhosis and suspected hepatocellular carcinoma (Fig. 56.1).

Diagnosis

Non-FDG Avid Hepatocellular Carcinoma

Findings

- Large mass in the dome of the liver that is T1 mildly hyperintense and T2 isointense (wide arrow).
- T1 hyperintense tumor thrombosis in right main portal vein (curved arrow).
- PET fusion image shows no significant radiotracer uptake within the mass.
- Mass surrounded by T2 hyperintense dilated intrahepatic bile ducts (arrowheads).
- Small cirrhotic appearing liver that has low T2-weighted signal, compatible with iron deposition.

Discussion

Hepatocellular carcinoma (HCC) is the most common primary form of liver cancer, and most commonly occurs in patients with chronic liver disease, especially cirrhosis. The pathogenesis of liver cancer is repeated liver damage followed by inflammation and parenchymal repair. The most frequent causes of the long-term damage are hepatitis B, hepatitis C, alcohol abuse, autoimmune disease, and iron overload from hemochromatosis. Hepatocellular carcinoma should be assessed on CT or MRI screening studies in patients with chronic liver disease and elevated serum alpha-fetoprotein levels.

Typically, hepatocellular carcinoma begins as a dysplastic nodule that is at least 1 cm in size and is T1 hyperintense and T2 hypointense in comparison to the liver. Dysplastic nodules have an enhancement pattern similar to normal hepatic tissue. As the dysplastic nodule transforms into hepatocellular carcinoma, it becomes T1 hypointense and T2 hyperintense, growing in size to 2 cm or larger. HCC enhances on the arterial phase appearing hyperintense on T1-weighted images. During the portal venous and delayed phases, HCC washes out and becomes hypointense to the background liver. However, any new or enlarging space occupying mass in a cirrhotic liver should be suspected as hepatocellular carcinoma even in the absence of the characteristic MRI signal intensities. When using hepatobiliary MRI contrast agents, there is no uptake on the delayed hepatocyte phase due to lack of functional hepatocytes in HCC. HCC is unique among malignancies in that it can be diagnosed with imaging criteria alone.

R. Gupta et al., *PET/MR Imaging*, https://doi.org/10.1007/978-3-319-65106-4_56

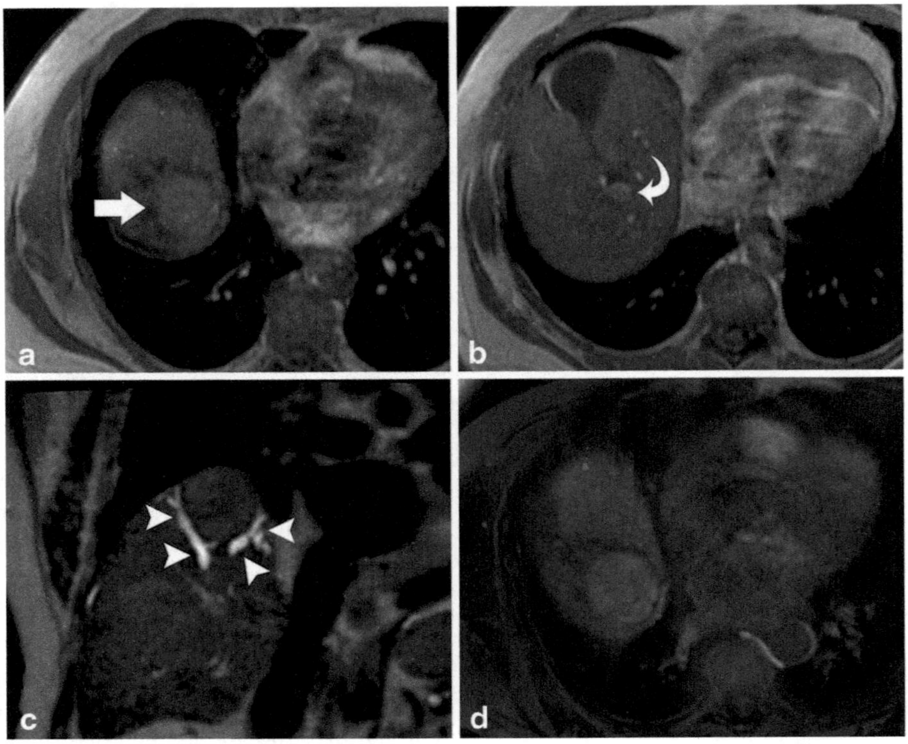

Fig. 56.1 T1 GRE axial (**a**), T1 GRE axial, at more inferior level (**b**), T2 HASTE coronal (**c**), and PET/MR T1 VIBE with fat suppression axial fusion (**d**)

FDG uptake in hepatocellular carcinoma depends on the aggressiveness of the tumor. Well-differentiated HCC, similar to normal liver hepatocytes, has low hexokinase activity and increased glucose-6-phosphatase activity resulting in less trapping of FDG into the cell and more dephosphorylation of FDG, allowing it to escape. This results in decreased or normal FDG uptake in well-differentiated HCC as compared with surrounding liver activity. As the tumor becomes more aggressive, there is an increase in hexokinase activity with trapping of FDG and decrease in glucose-6-phosphatase activity. Overall only about 50–60% of HCC are hypermetabolic on PET imaging. With PET/MR imaging, HCC can be better characterized as high or low grade malignancy with the higher SUV corresponding to more aggressive tumors. PET/MRI is even more valuable in detecting extrahepatic disease since aggressive lesions are the ones that metastasize, and the FDG uptake of the metastases parallel the primary tumor.

Suggested Reading

Chou CT, Chou JM, Chang TA, Huang SF, Chen CB, Chen YL, et al. Differentiation between dysplastic nodule and early-stage hepatocellular carcinoma: the utility of conventional MR imaging. World J Gastroenterol. 2013 Nov 14;19(42):7433–9.

Sacks A, Peller PJ, Surasi DS, Chatburn L, Mercier G, Subramaniam RM. Value of PET/CT in the management of primary hepatobiliary tumors, part 2. AJR Am J Roentgenol. 2011 Aug;197(2):W260–5.

Case 57
Metformin Induced Bowel Uptake

Amit Gupta and Robert Matthews

History

A 64-year-old male presents for evaluation of a lung nodule (Fig. 57.1).

Diagnosis

Diffuse FDG uptake in the bowel secondary to metformin use

Findings

- Diffuse intense FDG uptake throughout the sigmoid colon (wide white arrow). The sigmoid colon is collapsed without any MRI signal abnormalities.
- Transverse colon also shows prominent diffuse increased FDG uptake without corresponding wall thickening or signal changes on the MR (curved white arrows).
- PET MIP shows intense FDG uptake throughout the entire colon (black arrowheads) with several loops of small bowel also with increased FDG uptake (thin black arrow).

Discussion

Metformin is an oral anti-diabetic medicine that is commonly used in the treatment of type II diabetes. Metformin has been shown to cause intense diffuse FDG uptake in the colon although this uptake may be more variable. The small intestines are less affected, with portions showing diffuse uptake of lesser intensity. Several different hypotheses for this uptake have been proposed, including FDG uptake by the smooth muscles of the bowel, FDG uptake by lymphoid tissue, bowel inflammation, luminal excretion of FDG, and direct increased cellular kinase activity. However, the exact mechanism involved is likely a combination of these theories.

The most common side effects of metformin are digestive symptoms such as diarrhea and vomiting, which occurs in 30% of patients. Evaluation of bowel by MR is generally challenging unless an imaging study is optimized for bowel evaluation with measures such as bowel distension with oral contrast agents, fast acquisition and use of antispasmodics to reduce the artifact from peristalsis. It becomes even more challenging to evaluate bowel on PET/MR

R. Gupta et al., *PET/MR Imaging*, https://doi.org/10.1007/978-3-319-65106-4_57

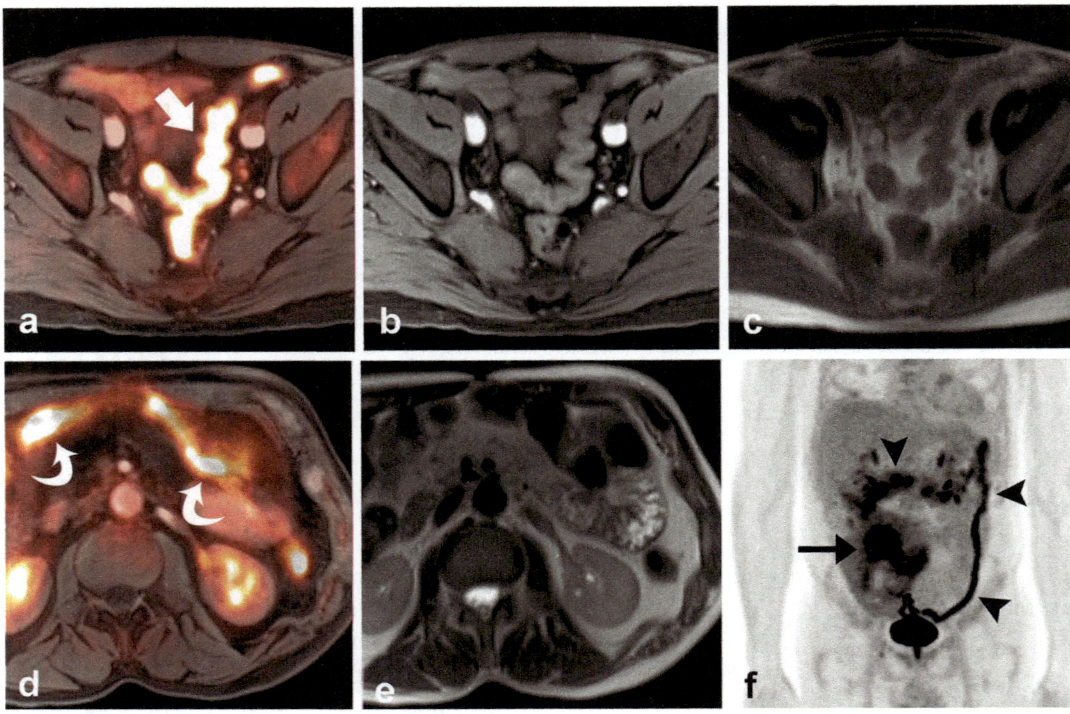

Fig. 57.1 PET/MR T1 radial VIBE with fat suppression axial fusion (pelvis) (**a**), T1 radial VIBE with fat suppression axial (pelvis) (**b**), T2 HASTE axial (pelvis) (**c**), PET/MR T1 radial VIBE with fat suppression axial fusion (abdomen) (**d**), T2 HASTE axial (abdomen) (**e**), and PET MIP (**f**)

imaging if the patient is on metformin due to diffuse FDG uptake in bowel. Some groups have suggested that withholding metformin should be considered when PET studies are planned, especially if the patients have history of bowel cancer. MR imaging may have some role in such patients in whom metformin cannot be withheld, due to its better soft tissue resolution.

On PET/MR routine body imaging, one of the main difficulties is distinguishing bowel thickening from underdistention. The normal small bowel wall thickness measures up to 2 mm when imaged using an oral contrast agent. Bowel wall edema from inflammation or infection causes an increase signal on T2-weighted images, which can be distinguished from fat by the use of fat suppression images. There is generally some degree of enhancement with gadolinium on T1-weighted images within the small and large bowel. Hyperenhancement to a given bowel segment may be seen with ischemia, inflammatory disease, adhesions, and tumors. Other sequences that can be used for small bowel assessment are diffusion-weighted imaging and cine imaging. If the patient has history of bowel cancer or inflammatory bowel disease, withholding metformin would clearly improve the diagnostic accuracy of PET/MR imaging.

Suggested Reading

Cronin CG, Delappe E, Lohan DG, Roche C, Murphy JM. Normal small bowel wall characteristics on MR enterography. Eur J Radiol. 2010;75(2):207–11.

Gontier E, Fourme E, Wartski M, Blondet C, Bonardel G, Le Stanc E, et al. High and typical 18F-FDG bowel uptake in patients treated with metformin. Eur J Nucl Med Mol Imaging. 2008;35(1):95–9.

Kavaliauskiene G, Ziech MLW, Nio CY, Stoker J. Small bowel MRI in adult patients: not just Crohn's disease—a tutorial. Insights Imaging. 2011;2(5):501–13.

Case 58
Splenic Hemangioma

Robert Matthews

History

A 79-year-old male with head and neck cancer involving the scalp (Fig. 58.1).

Diagnosis

Splenic hemangioma

Findings

- Hyperintense T2 and isointense T1 lesion in the spleen reflecting hemangioma (arrow).
- No corresponding abnormal FDG activity within the lesion.
- Accessory spleen (curved arrow).

Discussion

Lesions within the spleen are occasionally found on PET/MR imaging. There are a variety of solid benign tumors encountered in the spleen including hemangiomas, hamartomas, littoral cell angiomas, lymphangiomas, and inflammatory pseudotumors. Malignant tumors are most commonly lymphomas. Although the spleen is a vascular organ, metastatic lesions within the spleen are surprisingly infrequent. Cystic lesions within the spleen include neoplastic masses, pseudocysts, congenital cysts, and parasitic cysts such as echinococcal disease. The most common type of cystic neoplastic disease in the spleen is lymphoma, metastases, and hemangiomas. Pseudocysts are secondary to trauma, hemorrhage, infarction, or inflammation.

FDG PET imaging is an excellent tool for evaluating indeterminate splenic lesions. In patients with known cancer, FDG PET has a high negative predictive value for solid splenic lesions. PET imaging can have false positive results for splenic lesions with both inflammatory and infectious etiologies such as sarcoidosis and bacterial infections. When metastatic lesions occur in the spleen, there are usually multiple splenic lesions and other sites of metastatic disease in the abdomen and elsewhere. Pseudotumor can accumulate FDG in its early stages but its activity resolves over time. Benign tumors such as hemangiomas, hamartomas, littoral cell angioma, and lymphangioma do not demonstrate increased FDG uptake within the spleen.

Hemangiomas are the most common benign tumors found within the spleen, which are detected incidentally on imaging in an otherwise asymptomatic patient. Most lesions are less than 2 cm in size, but lesions can be much larger than this. Large lesions may spontaneously rupture and hemorrhage. On T2-weighted MRI images, hemangiomas show homogenous high T2 signal and isointense to hypointense signal on T1-weighted images. On contrast enhanced T1

R. Gupta et al., *PET/MR Imaging*, https://doi.org/10.1007/978-3-319-65106-4_58

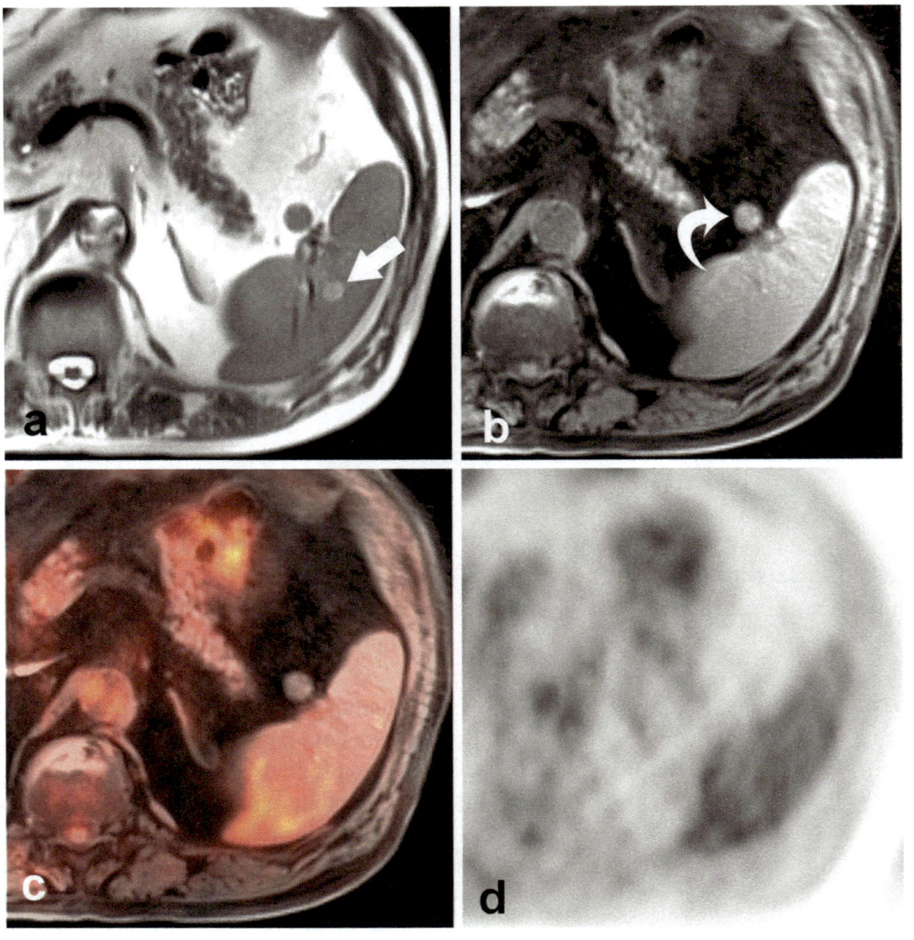

Fig. 58.1 T2 HASTE axial (**a**), T1 radial VIBE with fat suppression axial (**b**), PET/MR T1 radial VIBE with fat suppression axial fusion (**c**), and PET axial (**d**)

images, there is peripheral nodular enhancement that persists on delayed imaging.

Hamartoma is a much rarer benign tumor that is usually less than 3 cm in size. These may contain cystic and necrotic components as well as calcifications. Hamartomas if large can also become ruptured. On T2-weighted images, hamartomas are well defined and slightly hyperintense while isotense to normal splenic tissue on T1-weighted images with early heterogenous contrast enhancement. Metastatic lesions are usually isointense on T1 and T2-weighted images, but may become T2 hyperintense when necrosis or cystic changes occur. Metastases are usually initially T1 hypointense following contrast enhanced and then isointense on delayed imaging.

Suggested Reading

Elsayes KM, Narra VR, Mukundan G, Lewis JS Jr, Menias CO, Heiken JP. MR imaging of the spleen: spectrum of abnormalities. Radiographics. 2005;25:967–82.

Metser U, Miller E, Kessler A, Lerman H, Lievshitz G, Oren R, et al. Solid splenic masses: evaluation with 18F-FDG PET/CT. J Nucle Med. 2005;46:52–9.

Case 59
Invasive Anal Cancer

Robert Matthews

History

A 71-year-old female present for staging of anal cancer (Fig. 59.1).

Diagnosis

Invasive anal cancer with lymph node metastases

Findings

- Large mass in the anorectal region with mildly low T1 and moderately high T2 signal. There are small lymph nodes in its posterior aspect (arrowheads).
- This focus of primary anal cancer has intense hypermetabolic activity consistent with malignancy. The normal bladder is marked with an asterisk.
- On the more superior slices there are multiple hypermetabolic lymph nodes and nodules in the perirectal fat and peritoneum (thin arrows). One right external iliac lymph node has centrally low T1 signal and high T2 signal characteristic of necrosis (curved arrow).

Discussion

The majority of invasive anal cancers are squamous cell carcinomas that originate from the squamous cell mucosa lining the anal canal and anal margin. Anal cancer demonstrates both wall invasion and spread through the lymphatic system. The latter occurs via the inguinal, internal iliac, and perirectal lymph nodes. More superior anal cancers may spread to the lymph nodes adjacent to the inferior mesenteric vessels, while more inferior tumors have a predilection for spread to the inguinal and femoral lymph nodes.

Anal cancer on MRI shows low to intermediate signal on T1-weighted sequences. On T2-weighted and STIR images, the tumor has intermediate signal that is higher than skeletal muscle, but lower than intramuscular fat. Anal cancers show strong enhancement following gadolinium contrast. As the lesions become larger, the MRI signal may become more heterogeneous. Increased T2 signal of the tumor can be seen in metastatic involvement of the sphincter complex, vagina, bladder, and urethra, as well as the skin and subcutaneous tissue. Deeper structures such as skeletal muscle can be well delineated on MRI. MRI is useful in assessing lymph

R. Gupta et al., *PET/MR Imaging*, https://doi.org/10.1007/978-3-319-65106-4_59

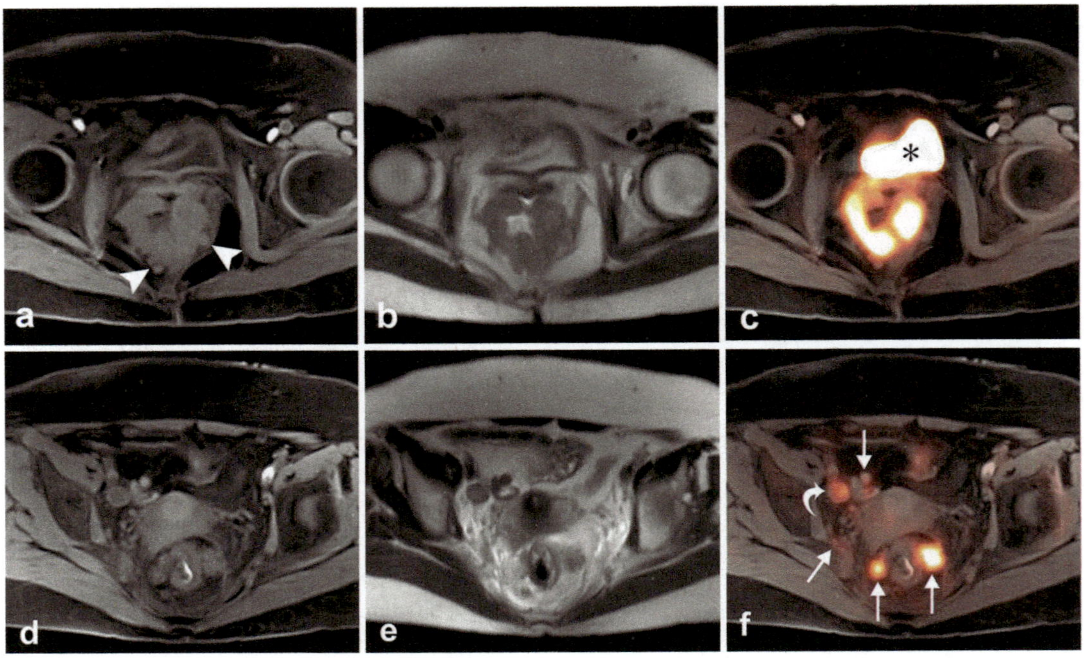

Fig. 59.1 T1 radial VIBE with fat suppression axial of pelvis (**a**), T2 HASTE axial pelvis (**b**), PET/MR T1 radial VIBE with fat suppression axial fusion of pelvis (**c**), T1 radial VIBE with fat suppression axial (more superior slice) (**d**), T2 HASTE axial (more superior slice) (**e**), and PET/MR T1 radial VIBE with fat suppression axial fusion (more superior slice) (**f**)

node involvement, although using nodal size criteria alone does not always accurately evaluate for malignancy. The use of contrast enhancement improves determination of lymph node involvement. Often anal tumors are associated with proctitis and abscesses that can be detected by MRI as well.

Anal cancer shows prominent hypermetabolic activity within the tumor. PET/MR imaging aids in the detection and helps to determine local metastatic spread of the tumor in neighboring structures. It is also useful in delineating the extent of tumor involvement of the rectum when proctitis is associated with the tumor. PET is useful in detecting early lymph node involvement before anatomical changes appear on MRI. It has a high detection rate of early inguinal lymph nodes involvement compared to MRI. However, small reactive lymph nodes that are commonly seen with mild FDG activity may be challenging for PET/MRI interpretations. Anal cancer can spread to the liver, lungs, and bone that may be unrecognized if only a pelvic examination is performed. Full-body PET/MR imaging allows the evaluation of distant metastatic disease.

Suggested Reading

Grigsby PW. FDG-PET/CT: new horizons in anal cancer. Gastroenterol Clin Biol. 2009;33(5):456–8.

Tonolini M, Bianco R. MRI and CT of anal carcinoma: a pictorial review. Insights Imaging. 2013;4(1):53–62.

Uronis HE, Bendell JC. Anal cancer: an overview. Oncologist. 2007;12(5):524–34.

Case 60
Liver Iron Deposition

Robert Matthews

History

A 62-year-old female presents for restaging of lymphoma and breast cancer. She has received multiple blood transfusions during therapy (Fig. 60.1).

Diagnosis

Liver iron deposition (due to multiple blood transfusions)

Findings

- Diffusely decreased T2-weighted signal in the liver compared to the skeletal muscle.
- T1-weighted image detects no abnormal signal in the liver.
- Normal homogeneous FDG activity throughout the liver on PET images.
- In-phase sequence shows a signal drop in the liver compared to the out-of-phase sequence (arrows).

Discussion

Iron is an important component in the body, found in muscle and red blood cells in the form of hemoglobin and myoglobin. The normal small intestines absorb 1–2 mg of dietary iron per day to replenish lost iron in the form of epithelial desquamation, menstruation, and other forms of blood loss. When old erythrocytes are destroyed by the spleen, the iron is recycled. Humans have no active way of eliminating iron. Iron instead is stored within the liver, spleen, and other organs of the reticuloendothelial system. Hence, iron overload is not infrequent. Iron overload can occur as a result of primary hemochromatosis, cirrhosis, anemia, and multiple transfusions.

Many benign lesions on PET have normal FDG uptake relative to background liver activity. Although there have been a few case reports of iron deficiency and overload mildly affecting liver FDG activity, in the vast majority of cases no measurable changes are seen in the liver SUV. Other lesions such as focal nodular hyperplasia, hepatic adenomas, and hemangiomas have FDG uptake similar to background liver uptake on PET images.

MRI is highly sensitive at detecting iron overload within the liver and spleen. Because of the paramagnetic properties of iron in the magnetic field, both T1 and T2-weighted images can show a loss of signal in proportion to the amount of iron deposition. Normally, T2-weighted images of the liver and spleen have a higher signal compared to neighboring paraspinal skeletal muscle signal. When there is iron overload, the T2-weighted images of the liver and spleen show a drop in signal intensity in comparison to skeletal muscle signal, thus appearing darker. This is

R. Gupta et al., *PET/MR Imaging*, https://doi.org/10.1007/978-3-319-65106-4_60

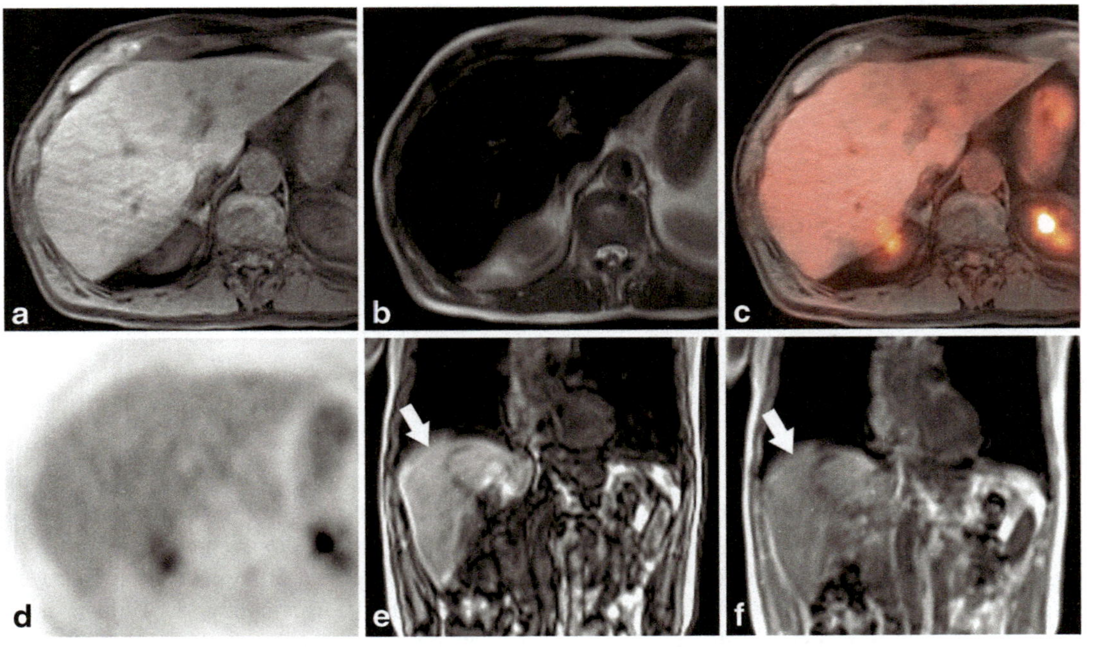

Fig. 60.1 T1 radial VIBE with fat suppression axial (**a**), T2 HASTE axial (**b**), PET/MRI T1 radial VIBE with fat suppression axial fusion (**c**), PET axial (**d**), Dixon T1-weighted out-of-phase coronal (**e**), and Dixon T1-weighted in-phase coronal (**f**)

the basis of susceptibility-weighted imaging, an MRI sequence particularly sensitive in detecting blood products. Paramagnetic compounds such as deoxyhemoglobin, ferritin, and hemosiderin interact with the local magnetic field and alter the phase of local tissues resulting in loss of signal. Chemical shift imaging using in-phase and out-of-phase sequences will also show a drop in signal on the in-phase sequence in comparison to the out-of-phase sequence, due to susceptibility changes caused by the iron. This is opposite to the effect of hepatic steatosis which shows a relative drop in signal on the out-of-phase sequence.

Suggested Reading

Delbeke D, Martin WH, Sandler MP. Evaluation of benign vs malignant hepatic lesions with positron emission tomography. Arch Surg. 1998;133(5):510–5.

Queiroz-Andrade M, Blasbalg R, Ortega CD. MR imaging findings of iron overload. Radiographics. 2009;29(6):1575–89.

Tong KA, Ashwal S, Obenaus A. Susceptibility-weighted MR imaging: a review of clinical applications in children. AJNR Am J Neuroradiol. 2008;29(1):9–17.

Case 61
Peritoneal Metastases from Colon Cancer

Robert Matthews

History

A 75-year-old female with colon cancer treated by right hemicolectomy, presents with a new density inferior to the liver (Fig. 61.1).

Diagnosis

Peritoneal metastases from colon cancer

Findings

- Peritoneal nodule with indistinct margins below the right hepatic lobe, isointense on T1 and mildly hyperintense on T2 relative to muscle (wide arrows).
- Intense hypermetabolic activity in the peritoneal nodule below the right hepatic lobe consistent with metastasis.
- More superior images show an additional mildly hypointense T1 and mildly hyperintense T2 metastatic mesenteric nodule with hypermetabolic activity consistent with a metastatic deposit (curved arrows).
- The infiltrative aspect of the nodule with an irregular shape distinguishes this peritoneal metastasis from a lymph node.

Discussion

Peritoneal metastases represent spread of malignant cells through the serosal membranous peritoneum that lines the abdominal and pelvic cavities. The peritoneum includes the parietal peritoneum that lines the anterior abdominal wall and retroperitoneum, the visceral peritoneum that covers the abdominal and pelvic organs, mesentery, and the lesser and greater omenta. The most common cancers that spread directly through intraperitoneal seeding include ovarian, gastric, esophageal, colorectal, pancreatic, and gallbladder cancer. Hematologic spread to the peritoneum occurs with breast cancer, lung cancer, and malignant melanoma. When the peritoneal involvement is more extensive, the term peritoneal carcinomatosis is used. Frequently, patients with peritoneal metastases also have distant metastatic disease.

Peritoneal spread is seen as thickened peritoneum that may be either smooth, nodular, or ill-defined. There may be multiple small nodules or there may be several large lesions. Usually, the peritoneal metastases are seen as parietal peritoneal thickening, frequently near the liver or as a seeding of the greater omentum. There is often concomitant bowel involvement with wall thickening or distortion. On MRI peritoneal

R. Gupta et al., *PET/MR Imaging*, https://doi.org/10.1007/978-3-319-65106-4_61

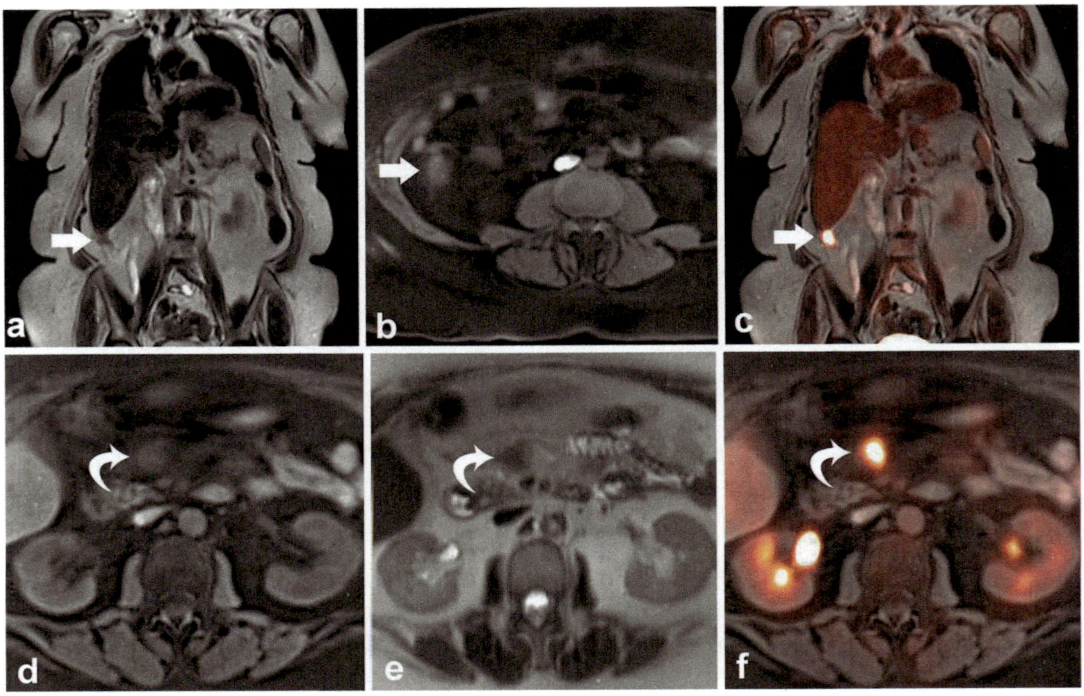

Fig. 61.1 T2 TSE coronal (**a**), T1 radial VIBE with fat suppression axial (**b**), PET/MR T2 TSE coronal fusion (**c**), T1 radial VIBE with fat suppression axial, at more superior level (**d**), T2 HASTE axial, at more superior level (**e**), and PET/MR T1 radial VIBE with fat suppression axial fusion, at more superior level (**f**)

metastases have low signal on T1-weighted images and show mild to moderate intensity on T2-weighted images. Smaller metastases are often best seen with T2 fat-suppressed sequences. The peritoneal lesions avidly enhance with gadolinium contrast. Diffusion-weighted imaging has been shown to be helpful in detecting small peritoneal lesions.

PET imaging is effective in detecting peritoneal metastases, especially in combination with MRI. FDG uptake in small peritoneal metastases, as well as mucinous tumors, may be low. False positive PET findings may be seen in the case of inflammatory lesions that have increased metabolic activity, such as post-surgical changes or fat necrosis which can be readily identified with MRI. Ascites is the most common feature associated with peritoneal metastases which demonstrates high T2 signal from its fluid content and may hide small peritoneal metastases on MRI. PET is useful in elucidating these small lesions hidden within the fluid. It also can help to identify peritoneal spread overlying large and small bowel that MRI has difficulty detecting.

Suggested Reading

Healy JC. Detection of peritoneal metastases. Cancer Imaging. 2001;1(2):4–12.

Patel CM, Sahdev A, Reznek RH. CT, MRI and PET imaging in peritoneal malignancy. Cancer Imaging. 2011;11:123–39.

Case 62
Malignant Gallbladder Polyp

Robert Matthews

History

A 50-year-old male with colorectal cancer treated 2 years ago presents for surveillance PET scan (Fig. 62.1).

Diagnosis

Malignant gallbladder polyp with colon cancer lymph node metastases

Findings

- Small polypoid lesion within the gallbladder wall that is mildly T1 hypointense and mildly T2 hyperintense compared to the liver (curved arrow).
- PET fusion image shows hyperintense activity in the polypoid lesion found to be primary gallbladder cancer.
- Multiple small hypermetabolic abdominal lymph nodes consistent with metastases from colon cancer (arrows).

Discussion

Gallbladder polyps and related lesions are usually discovered incidentally. In most cases, the patients are asymptomatic, rarely there may be nausea, vomiting, and right upper quadrant abdominal pain from gallbladder luminal obstruction. Polyps are found in 5% of gallbladders on autopsy and they have a variety of etiologies and variable malignant potential. The most common type of gallbladder polyps are cholesterol polyps, usually multiple, less than 1 cm and have no malignant potential. Cholesterol polyps are best characterized on MRI by an absence of enhancement and the presence of fat. The latter are detected by a drop in signal on out-of-phase imaging.

Inflammatory polyps are composed of granulation and fibrous tissue, and are associated with chronic cholecystitis. These lesions are less than 1 cm in size, show mild T2 hyperintensity, and may demonstrate slow gradual mild contrast enhancement. Overall the MRI characteristics are similar to the thickened wall of chronic cholecystitis. On PET these lesions are similar to chronic cholecystitis and may have mild FDG uptake. Adenomyomas are precancerous polyps that are usually single, less than 1 cm, and located in the fundus. They comprise 25% of gallbladder polyps and appear as a polypoid ingrowth from the gallbladder wall with similar MRI signal and no contrast enhancement. Gallbladder adenomas are benign lesions less than 2 cm in size, and may show some degree of contrast enhancement. They are not reliably distinguished from early gallbladder adenocarcinoma and therefore must be followed up with imaging. Adenomas, especially with high grade dysplasia, may show mild FDG uptake.

R. Gupta et al., *PET/MR Imaging*, https://doi.org/10.1007/978-3-319-65106-4_62

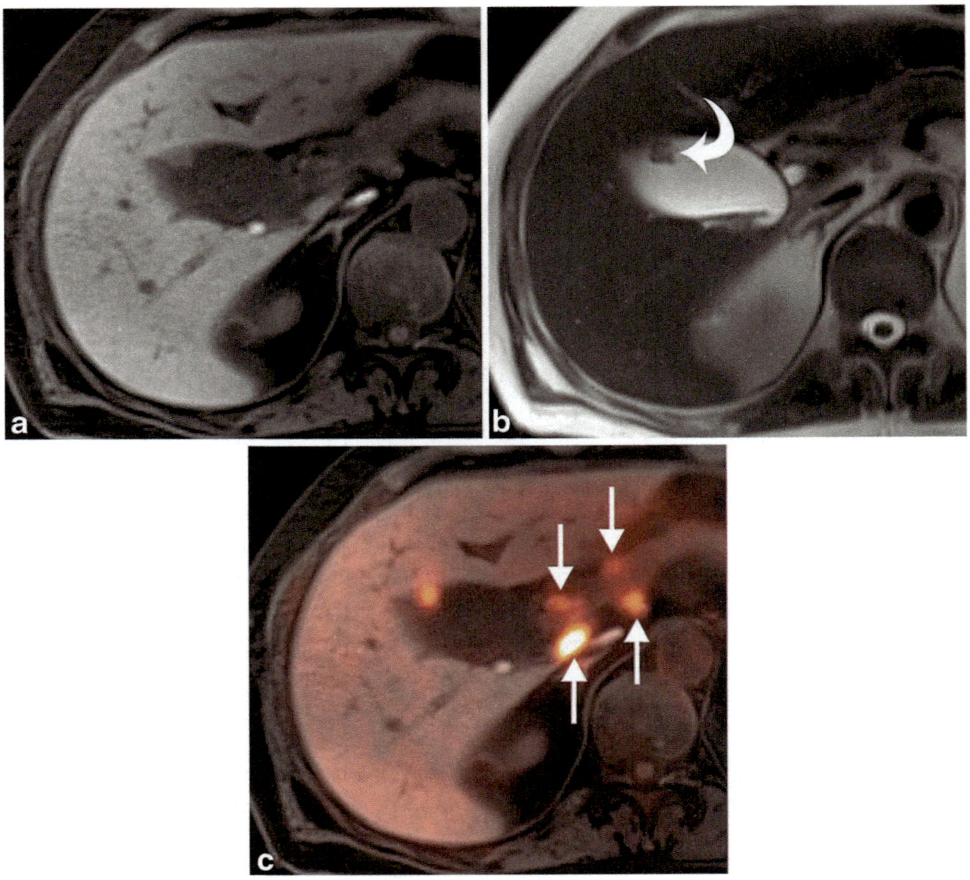

Fig. 62.1 T1 radial VIBE with fat suppression axial (**a**), T2 HASTE axial (**b**), and PET/MR T1 radial VIBE with fat suppression axial fusion (**c**)

Malignant gallbladder polyps are usually greater than 1 cm in size. They are most commonly sessile, solitary, and show interval growth on follow-up imaging. On T1-weighted images they are hypointense relative to the liver and are T2 hyperintense. Following gadolinium contrast, malignant polyps show delayed contrast enhancement that is greater than the normal gallbladder wall. Benign lesions tend to have early enhancement with delayed washout. Malignant gallbladder polyps demonstrate a higher degree of FDG uptake compared to benign polyps, although there is overlap in the SUV values.

Suggested Reading

Andren-Sandberg A. Diagnosis and management of gallbladder polyps. N Am J Med Sci. 2012;4(5):203–11.

Lee J, Yun M, Kim KS, Lee JD, Kim CK. Risk stratification of gallbladder polyps (1–2 cm) for surgical intervention with 18F-FDG PET/CT. J Nucl Med. 2012;53(3):353–8.

Case 63
Diverticulitis

Robert Matthews

History

A 49-year-old female with cervical cancer presents with abdominal pain (Fig. 63.1).

Diagnosis

Diverticulitis

Findings

- Enlarged sigmoid diverticulum that is T1 isointense and T2 hyperintense.
- T2-weighted images with fat suppression show high T2 signal in the sigmoid diverticulum characteristic of intense inflammation (curved arrow). More moderate inflammatory changes are seen in the surrounding fat with moderate T2 signal (arrowheads).
- PET/MR fusion shows intense hypermetabolic activity consistent with acute diverticulitis.

Discussion

Diverticulosis of the colon has a high prevalence in the western aging population. Diverticulosis is related to an extended low fiber diet. It can be detected by imaging in more than half of all people over the age of 65. It is characterized by outpouching of the wall of the colon, which is most commonly asymptomatic. At times, it can cause mild abdominal discomfort, bloating, and cramping. Diverticulitis occurs when the diverticulum gets inflamed or infected and that may cause fever, nausea, abdominal pain, and cramping. Many cases of diverticulitis are asymptomatic.

Multislice CT with IV and oral contrast is the preferred method in the diagnosis of acute diverticulitis. Magnetic resonance imaging can also be used to detect acute diverticulitis with a sensitivity of around 90% and a specificity of around 90%. Diverticulitis is most commonly detected in an asymptomatic patient undergoing PET/MR imaging for a cancer-related workup. MRI findings show segmental bowel wall thickening, pericolic fat stranding that is much more extensive than the wall thickening, and multiple diverticula. Active inflammation shows high T2-weighted signal, restricted diffusion, and gadolinium enhancement. MRI can also show complications of the diverticulosis such as fluid and air in the peritoneal cavity, abscess formation, and development of fistulas.

There are many causes of focal FDG uptake within the colon on PET imaging, which include normal physiological uptake, inflammation or infection, and malignancy. When there are no abnormalities detected on the accompanying MRI images, diagnosis is more difficult. In the case of diverticulitis, the abnormal FDG focus will be on the outer aspect of the colonic wall and

R. Gupta et al., *PET/MR Imaging*, https://doi.org/10.1007/978-3-319-65106-4_63

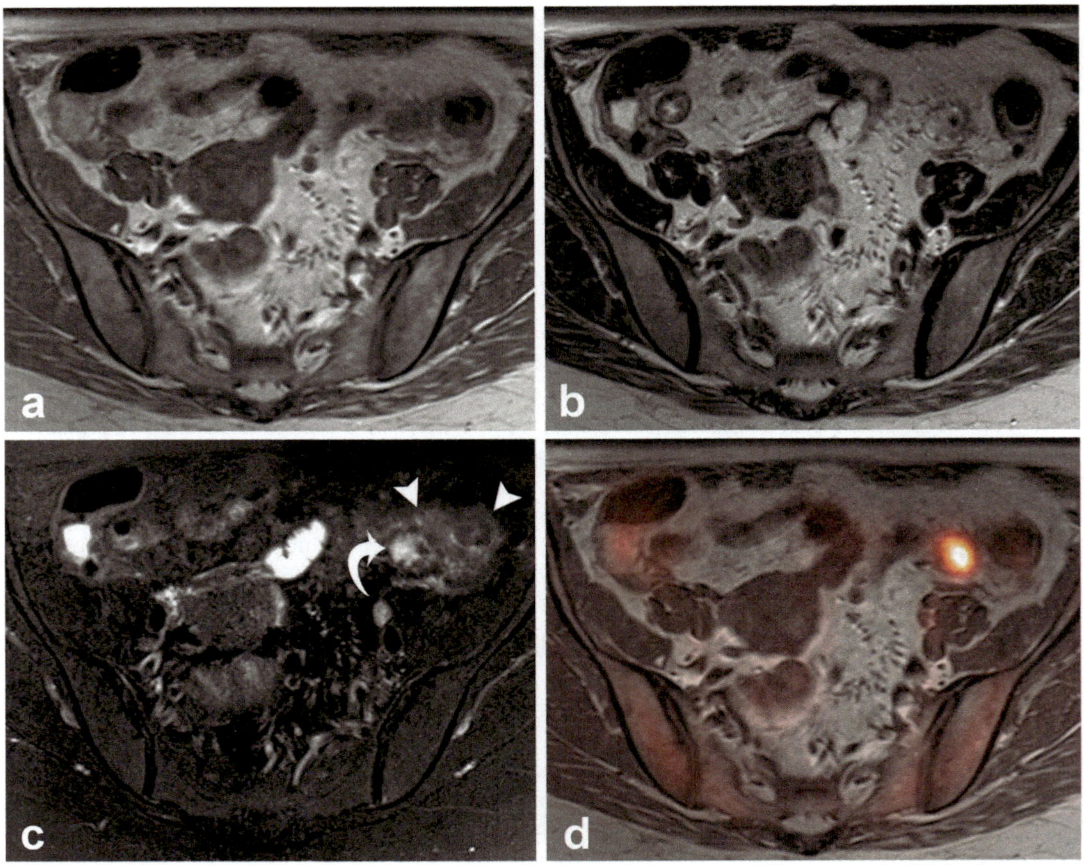

Fig. 63.1 T1 radial VIBE axial (**a**), T2 HASTE axial (**b**), T2 HASTE with fat suppression axial (**c**), and PET/MR T1 radial VIBE axial fusion (**d**)

there may be diffuse FDG uptake in the surrounding pericolic fat from inflammation. Peritoneal implants may appear similar on PET, but there will be no pericolic inflammatory response on MRI. It is not uncommon with small peritoneal implants to have very little if any abnormal MRI findings.

Suggested Reading

DeStigter KK, Keating DP. Imaging update: acute colonic diverticulitis. Clin Colon Rectal Surg. 2009;22:147–55.

Prabhakar HB, Sahani DV, Fischman AJ, Mueller PR, Blake MA. Bowel hot spots at PET-CT. Radiographics. 2007;27:145–59.

Case 64
Splenic Lymphoma

Robert Matthews

History

A 21-year-old male with newly diagnosed Hodgkin's lymphoma presents for initial staging (Fig. 64.1).

Diagnosis

Splenic lymphoma

Findings

- T1-weighted image shows multiple ill-defined hyperintense lesions (arrowheads).
- T2-weighted images demonstrate lesions to be hyperintense.
- PET/MRI and PET images show intense heterogenous FDG activity corresponding to the MRI lesions consistent with malignancy.
- Additional hypermetabolic lesion are seen in the liver consistent with metastatic disease.

Discussion

Lymphoma is the most common type of cancer involving the spleen. It may be primary splenic lymphoma or be part of a more systemic lymphomatous process. Splenic involvement may be important in deciding the correct chemotherapy regimen as well as in providing prognostic factors. Splenic involvement of lymphoma can be quite variable. Lymphomatous involvement of the spleen often presents with splenomegaly and enlarged spleen. There may be microscopic involvement, diffuse involvement, or focal lesions being either single or multiple. Both Hodgkin's and non-Hodgkin's lymphoma can have splenic lesions.

MRI imaging of the normal splenic tissue shows inhomogeneous early enhancement that becomes more uniform on delayed imaging. Typically, splenic lymphoma is best seen on the T2-weighted images showing a mild intense signal, although in some cases lymphoma can by T2 hypointense. The lesions on T1-weighted images may be either mildly hypointense or hyperintense. Following the administration of gadolinium contrast, there is usually poor enhancement with lesions being hypovascular. Microscopic diffuse lymphomatous involvement of the spleen may appear normal on MRI image or as ill-defined small hypoenhancing nodules. Following treatment of lymphoma, the lesions become less defined on T1 and T2-weighted images.

PET imaging has high sensitivity and specificity in evaluating both Hodgkin's and non-Hodgkin's lymphoma. Both primary and secondary lymphomatous involvement of the spleen may appear as solitary or multiple lesions with focally increased FDG activity. The more aggressive high-grade lymphomas would have higher SUV uptake compared to

R. Gupta et al., *PET/MR Imaging*, https://doi.org/10.1007/978-3-319-65106-4_64

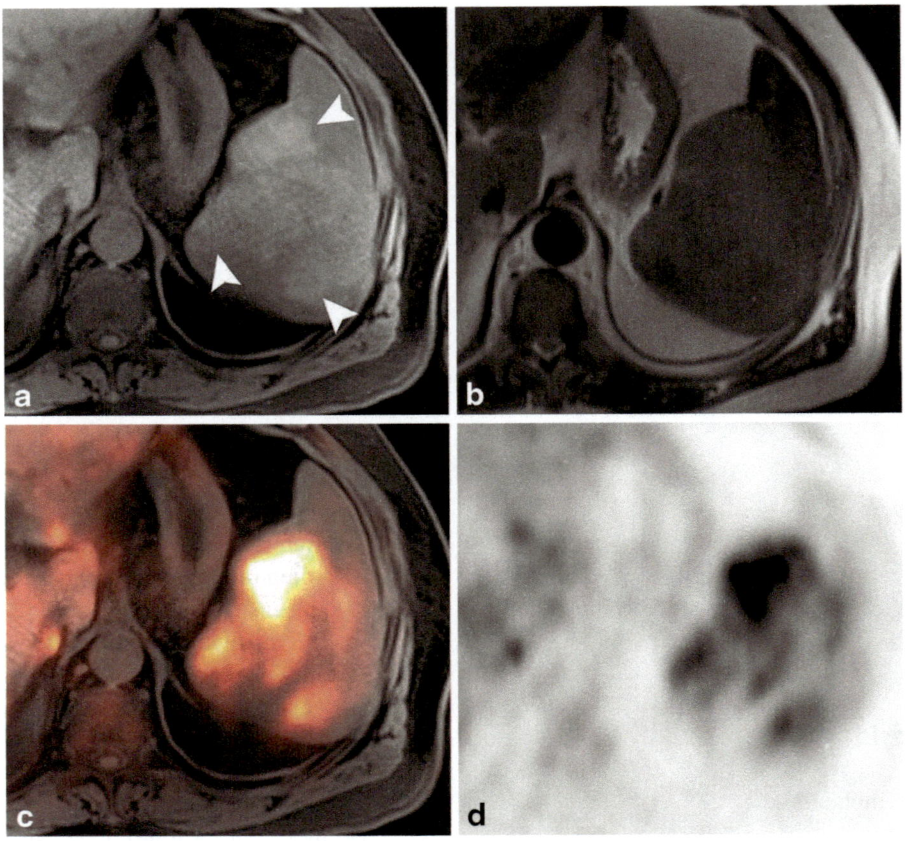

Fig. 64.1 T1 radial VIBE with fat suppression axial (**a**), T2 HASTE axial (**b**), PET/MR T1 radial VIBE with fat suppression axial fusion (**c**), and PET axial (**d**)

low-grade lymphomas. Diffuse lymphomatous involvement of the spleen can be difficult to detect with diffusely increased FDG uptake that can simulate splenic stimulation following chemotherapy.

Suggested Reading

Luna A, Ribes R, Caro P, Luna L, Aumente E, Ros PR. MRI of focal splenic lesion without and with dynamic gadolinium enhancement. AJR. 2006;186:1533–47.

Saboo SS, Krajewski KM, O'Regan KN, Giardino A, Brown JR, Ramaiya N, et al. Spleen in haematological malignancies: spectrum of imaging findings. Br J Radiol. 2012;85:81–92.

Case 65
Gastric Adenocarcinoma

Robert Matthews

History

A 64-year-old female newly diagnosed stomach mass (Fig. 65.1).

Diagnosis

Gastric adenocarcinoma with lymph node metastasis

Findings

- T2-weighted images demonstrate prominent gastric folds (arrowheads).
- T1-weighted image shows an enlarged hyperintense 1.5 cm gastrohepatic lymph node (curved arrow).
- PET/MR fusion image reveals intense FDG uptake involving the stomach as well as a hypermetabolic gastrohepatic lymph node compatible with malignancy.
- PET MIP images show hypermetabolic gastrohepatic lymph node (wide arrow) adjacent to the intensely FDG avid stomach. Note that there is mild physiological uptake in the antrum of the stomach.

Discussion

Stomach cancer is the second most common cancer in the world. It is more common in East Asia including Japan, China, and South Korea. Gastric cancer often produces nonspecific symptoms in its early stages, with abdominal pain, anorexia, and weight loss in advanced cases. In the United States gastric cancer has a poor prognosis since it is usually diagnosed at a late stage. The only proven curative therapy is complete resection of the affected portion of the stomach with adjacent lymph node removal. Traditionally, preoperative evaluation includes contrast enhanced CT scan, upper endoscopy, and endoscopic ultrasound.

MRI is very useful in evaluating tumor size, gastric wall invasion, as well as lymph node metastases. MRI allows depiction of gastric wall layers to determine the depth of tumor invasion; however, improved accuracy may require distention of the stomach by oral water contrast agents, fast breath-hold sequences, and antiperistaltic medications. The gastric cancer on MRI usually shows an abrupt transition between thickened and adjacent normal wall with thickness greater than 6 mm. Invasion of adjacent structures will show elimination of the perigastric fat plane on

R. Gupta et al., *PET/MR Imaging*, https://doi.org/10.1007/978-3-319-65106-4_65

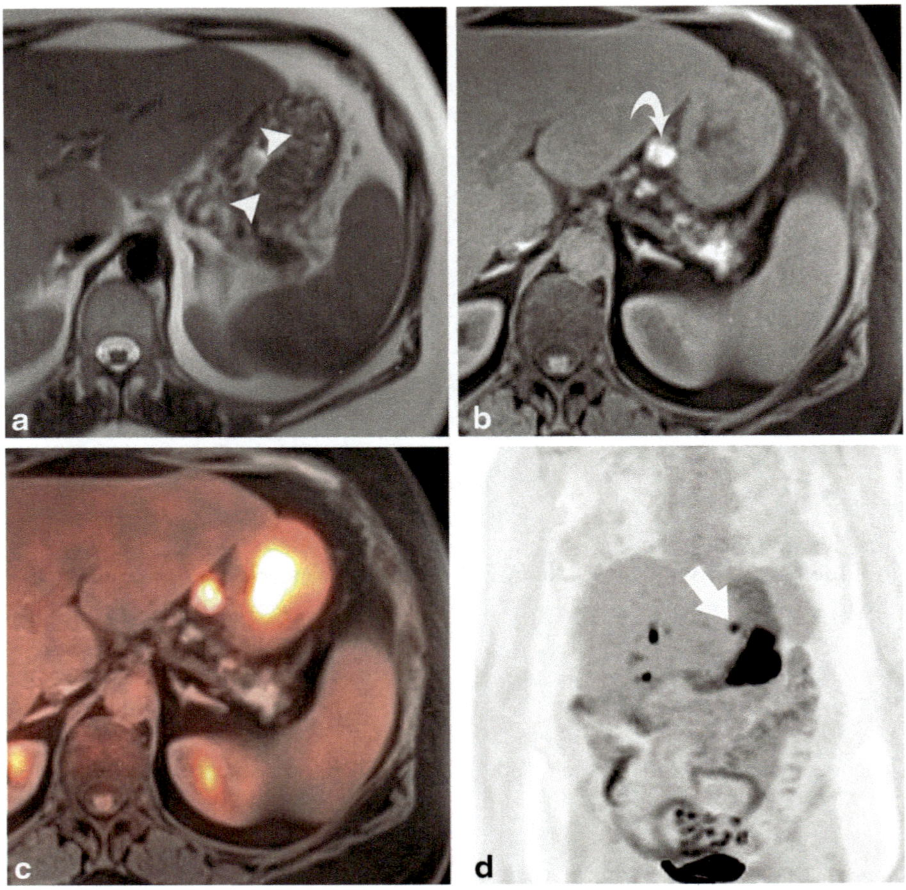

Fig. 65.1 T2 HASTE axial (**a**), T1 radial VIBE with fat suppression axial (**b**), PET/MR T1 radial VIBE with fat suppression axial fusion (**c**), and PET MIP (**d**)

T2-weighted imaging. On MRI, lymph nodes greater than 8 mm in short axis are suspicious for metastases. T1-weighted images show strong enhancement following the administration of contrast. Although MRI has 80% detection rate, omental metastases and peritoneal carcinomatosis are difficult to see on MRI.

FDG PET imaging is an alternative imaging modality demonstrating high accuracy in the initial diagnosis of disease and has the ability to detect abnormal metabolic activity in normal-sized regional lymph nodes. PET is especially useful for finding distant metastatic disease that would upstage the patient. Although there is normal physiological radiotracer uptake within the stomach, with PET/MR stomach cancer can be detected due to higher FDG uptake in areas of wall thickening. In addition to effective initial staging, PET/MR can also help to predict treatment response to chemotherapy in patients with unresectable cancer.

Suggested Reading

Huang Z, Xie DH, Guo L, Hu CH, Fang X, Meng Q, et al. The utility of MRI for pre-operative T and N staging of gastric carcinoma: a systematic review and meta-analysis. Br J Radiol. 2015;88:20140552.

Lee DH, Kim SH, Im SA, Oh DY, Kim TY, Han JK. Multiparametric fully-integrated 18-FDG PET/MRI of advanced gastric cancer for prediction of chemotherapy response: a preliminary study. Euro Radiol. 2016;26:2771–8.

Lim JS, Yun MJ, Kim MJ, Hyung WJ, Park MS, Choi JY, et al. CT and PET in stomach cancer: preoperative staging and monitoring of response to therapy. Radiographics. 2006;26:143–56.

Case 66
Rectal Cancer

Robert Matthews

History

A 47-year-old male for staging of rectal cancer (Fig. 66.1).

Diagnosis

Rectal cancer

Findings

- Hypointense T1 mass in the left rectum with moderate gadolinium contrast enhancement (arrowheads).
- T2-weighted image shows infiltration of the high signal rectal cancer into the perirectal fat consistent with a T3 tumor (thin arrows).
- PET/MR fusion image with intense hypermetabolic activity compatible with malignancy.

Discussion

More than 40,000 people in the United States are diagnosed with rectal cancer each year. Of these, 90% are adenocarcinomas with the majority beginning as adenomas. Of patients presenting with rectal cancer, 5–10% are locally advanced.

The rectum is surrounded by the high T1 and T2 mesorectal fat. This is clearly visible on non-suppressed fat sequences. This fat is in turn circumscribed by the mesorectal fascia, demonstrated by a thin low signal line on MR. Only the upper anterior parts of the rectum are covered by the peritoneum, which can be seen as a thin hypointense line on T2-weighted images.

Rectal cancer usually has low signal intensity on T1-weighted images and moderate to high signal intensity on T2-weighted images. Following the administration of gadolinium contrast, there is moderate tumor enhancement. MRI cannot reliably differentiate between the mucosa, submucosa, and muscularis propria layers of the rectum, without an endorectal coil. Usually, MRI is unable to distinguish between in situ, T1, and T2 grade tumors. However because in the rectum there is no bowel wall serosal layer, MRI can identify T3 grade tumor extension through the external muscularis that invades the mesorectum. With invasion, the high T2-weighted signal of the tumor may be noted extending into the fat. MRI can also identify T4 grade tumors that spread invading the peritoneum, adjacent organs, or the levator musculature.

FDG PET does not offer any advantages over MRI in determining the depth of rectal wall involvement. However, PET imaging has been helpful to guide radiation therapy and dose intensification during neoadjuvant treatments. PET in conjunction with MRI can determine the extent of invasive disease and involvement of other organs. MRI is limited in its ability to deter-

R. Gupta et al., *PET/MR Imaging*, https://doi.org/10.1007/978-3-319-65106-4_66

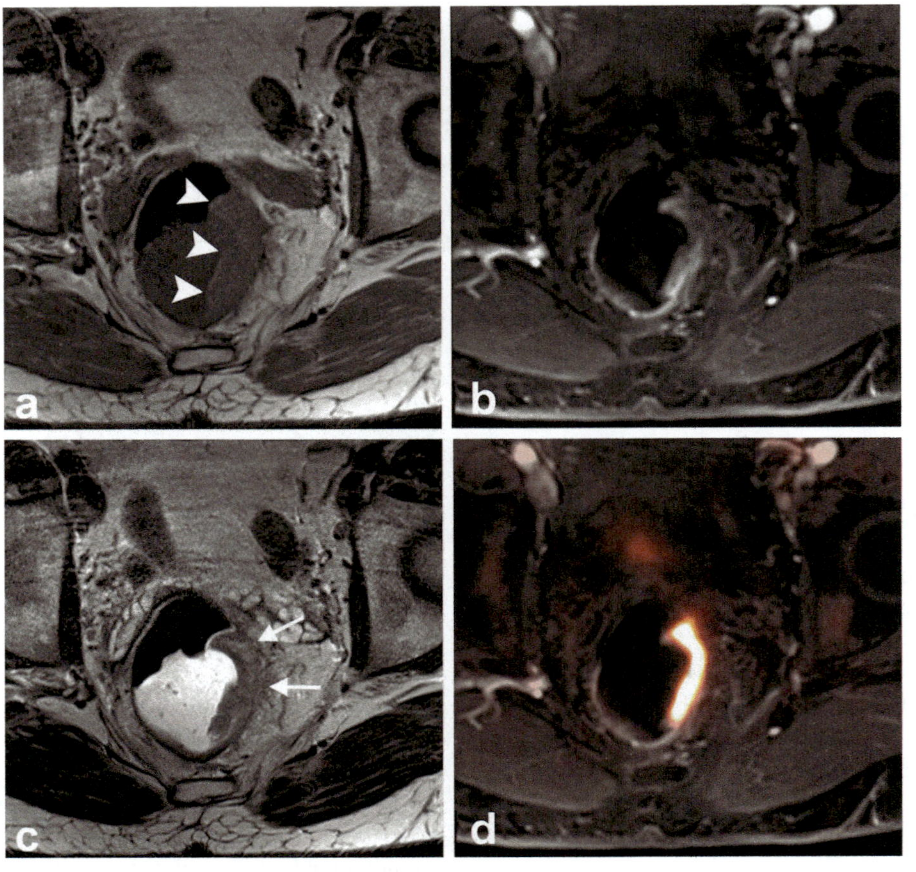

Fig. 66.1 T1 VIBE axial (**a**), T1 VIBE with fat suppression post-gadolinium contrast axial (**b**), T2 HASTE axial (**c**), and PET/MR T1 VIBE with fat suppression post-gadolinium contrast axial fusion (**d**)

mine pelvic lymph node invasion since diagnosis is based on changes in size, morphology, or enhancement. With the addition of PET imaging showing the level of metabolic activity, accurate assessment of regional lymph node involvement can be made. This information may help in treatment decisions where neoadjuvant chemotherapy, rather than surgical resection, is offered to patients with T3 tumor grade or lymph node metastases.

Suggested Reading

Chowdhury FU, Shah N, Scarsbrook AF, Bradley KM. [18F]FDG PET/CT imaging of colorectal cancer: a pictorial review. Postgrad Med J. 2010 Mar;86(1013):174–82.

Raman SP, Chen Y, Fishman EK. Evolution of imaging in rectal cancer: multimodality imaging with MDCT, MRI, and PET. J Gastrointest Oncol. 2015 Apr;6(2):172–84.

Case 67 FDG Avid Hepatocellular Carcinoma

Mark K. Youssef

History

A 71-year-old male with cirrhosis and neutropenia (Fig. 67.1).

Diagnosis

FDG avid hepatocellular carcinoma

Findings

- Heterogeneous hyperintense T2 and hypointense T1 large mass diffusely infiltrating the left hepatic lobe (white arrowheads).
- Hepatocyte-specific early and delayed contrast enhanced images show no appreciable enhancement within the large liver mass.
- PET fusion and MIP images show abnormal hypermetabolic activity within the mass (black wide arrow).
- Combination of tumor thrombus and bland thrombus within the main portal vein and both right and left portal veins (thin black arrow).

Discussion

Hepatocellular carcinoma (HCC) is the most common primary cancer of the liver. Early diagnosis has significant implications for both prognosis and treatment. Imaging in these patients therefore plays a pivotal role, both in making the initial diagnosis and for the monitoring treatment response. Ultrasound and serum alpha fetoprotein are often used as the intial surveillance test in patients with high risk for HCC. Computed tomography and MRI show higher sensitivity for diagnosing HCC, with PET as an important adjunct in patients who are found to have focal hepatic lesions.

The MRI signal characteristics of HCC generally include T1 hypointensity, T2 hyperintensity, arterial phase contrast enhancement, and rapid washout. There can be some variability particularly on the T1 and T2 sequences, depending on the macroscopic subtype and composition of the tumor, as well as the intensity of the background liver. In fact, the MR appearance is so specific that it may obviate the need for biopsy. The massive or focal subtype of HCC appears as a single large mass, while the nodular or multifocal subtype appears as multiple masses. The infiltrative subtype is diffuse, often similar in appearance to surrounding liver cirrhosis. Approximately 50–60% of cases of HCC demonstrate increased hypermetabolic activity. Hypermetabolism on PET/MR imaging, as quantified by the SUV, is directly proportional to the biological aggressiveness of the tumor.

Surgical resection or liver transplantation in the appropriate cases can often be curative, although most patients are beyond a resectable stage at the time of diagnosis of HCC. Additionally,

R. Gupta et al., *PET/MR Imaging*, https://doi.org/10.1007/978-3-319-65106-4_67

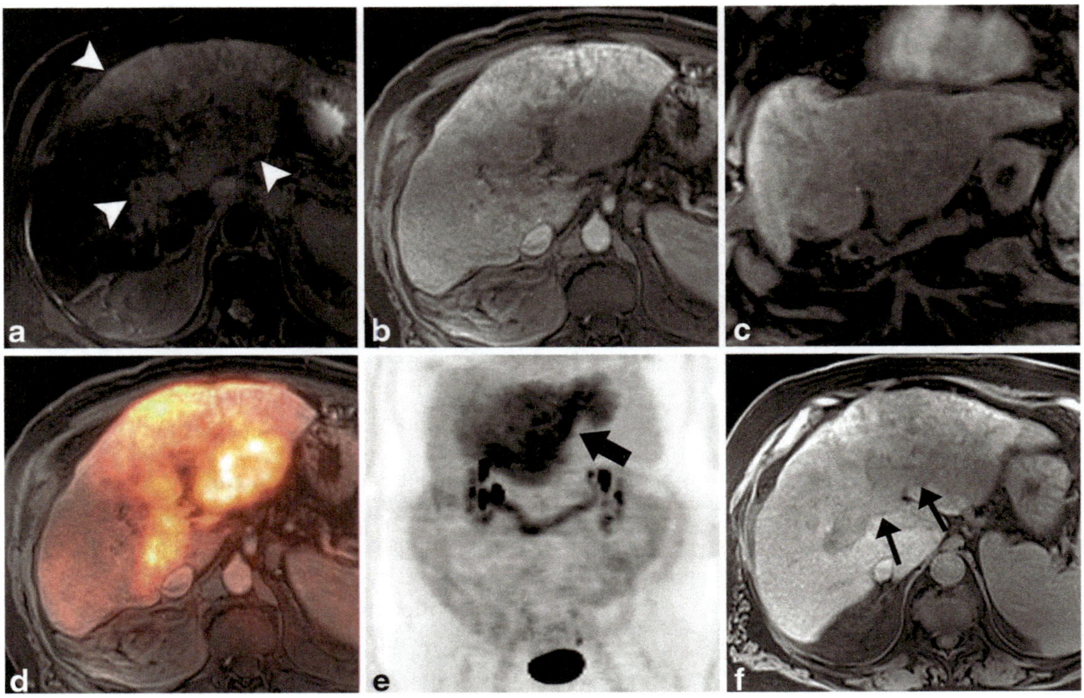

Fig. 67.1 T2 TSE with fat suppression axial (**a**), T1 VIBE with fat suppression post early hepatocyte-specific contrast axial (**b**), T1 VIBE with fat suppression 20 min delayed hepatocyte-specific contrast coronal (**c**), PET/MR T1 VIBE with fat suppression post early hepatocyte-specific contrast axial fusion (**d**), PET MIP (**e**), and T1 radial VIBE with fat suppression axial (**f**)

many patients fall outside the Milan criteria for transplantation. Non-operative treatment modalities including chemoembolization, systemic chemotherapy, and radiofrequency ablation have shown the potential to increase survival in cases of advanced HCC. A relatively newer modality, radioembolization with the intra-arterial hepatic injection of yttrium-90 microspheres spheres, delivers high dose radiation to the neoplasm, and has been shown to decrease tumor burden, sometimes allowing for surgical resection or transplantation in patients who were previously deemed inoperable. Following such treatments, the imaging characteristics of the tumor may change to reflect necrosis and the absence of arterial phase contrast enhancement.

Suggested Reading

Agnello F, Salvaggio G, Cabibbo G, Maida M, Lagalla R, Midiri M, et al. Imaging appearance of treated hepatocellular carcinoma. World J Hepatol. 2013;5(8):417–24.

El-Serag HB, Davila JA. Surveillance for hepatocellular carcinoma: in whom and how? Therap Adv Gastroenterol. 2011;4(1):5–10.

Mosconi C, Cappelli A, Pettinato C, Golfieri R. Radioembolization with yttrium-90 microspheres in hepatocellular carcinoma: role and perspectives. World J Hepatol. 2015;7(5):738–52.

Case 68 Metastatic Pancreatic Insulinoma with Gallium DOTATATE

Rajesh Gupta and Robert Matthews

History

A 54-year-old female with islet cell cancer of the pancreas who is currently on chemotherapy undergoes PET gallium DOTATATE (Fig. 68.1). Octreotide scan has been unchanged for past 3 years.

Diagnosis

Metastatic pancreatic insulinoma detected with gallium DOTATATE

Findings

- Octreotide scan shows foci of increased tracer uptake reflecting metastatic islet cell cancer in the left supraclavicular region, left upper abdomen, and right acetabulum (black arrowheads).
- In addition to the lesions above, Ga-68 DOTATATE PET image shows markedly more extensive metastatic disease in the mediastinum, liver, and abdomen.
- Fusion image of the abdomen demonstrates metastatic disease in the liver, pancreas, left paraaortic, and posterior pararenal space (thin white arrows). On MR the liver lesion and pancreatic lesions are not well visualized.
- In the pelvis the acetabular bone lesion shows intense radiotracer uptake with T1 hyperintensity compared to the surrounding bone (curved white arrow).

Discussion

Insulinomas are the most common functioning pancreatic neuroendocrine tumor (NET), accounting for 40% of all functioning pancreatic NETs. They have an incidence of 2–4 per million people, each year. Although typically sporadic, insulinomas have an association with multiple endocrine neoplasia type I (MEN I) and have also been reported in patients with neurofibromatosis type I. Patients with insulinomas can present with Whipple's triad that consists of fasting hypoglycemia (<50 mg/dL), symptoms of hypoglycemia, and immediate relief of symptoms after the administration of IV glucose. They typically present earlier than other NETs and therefore have the best prognosis. However, approximately 10% of insulinomas demonstrate malignant behavior.

Most insulinomas are intrapancreatic, with an even distribution throughout the pancreatic head, body, and tail. They are usually small at diagnosis, the majority being less than 2 cm, and are most often solitary. However, multiple lesions may be seen in up to 10% of patients, particularly in

R. Gupta et al., *PET/MR Imaging*, https://doi.org/10.1007/978-3-319-65106-4_68

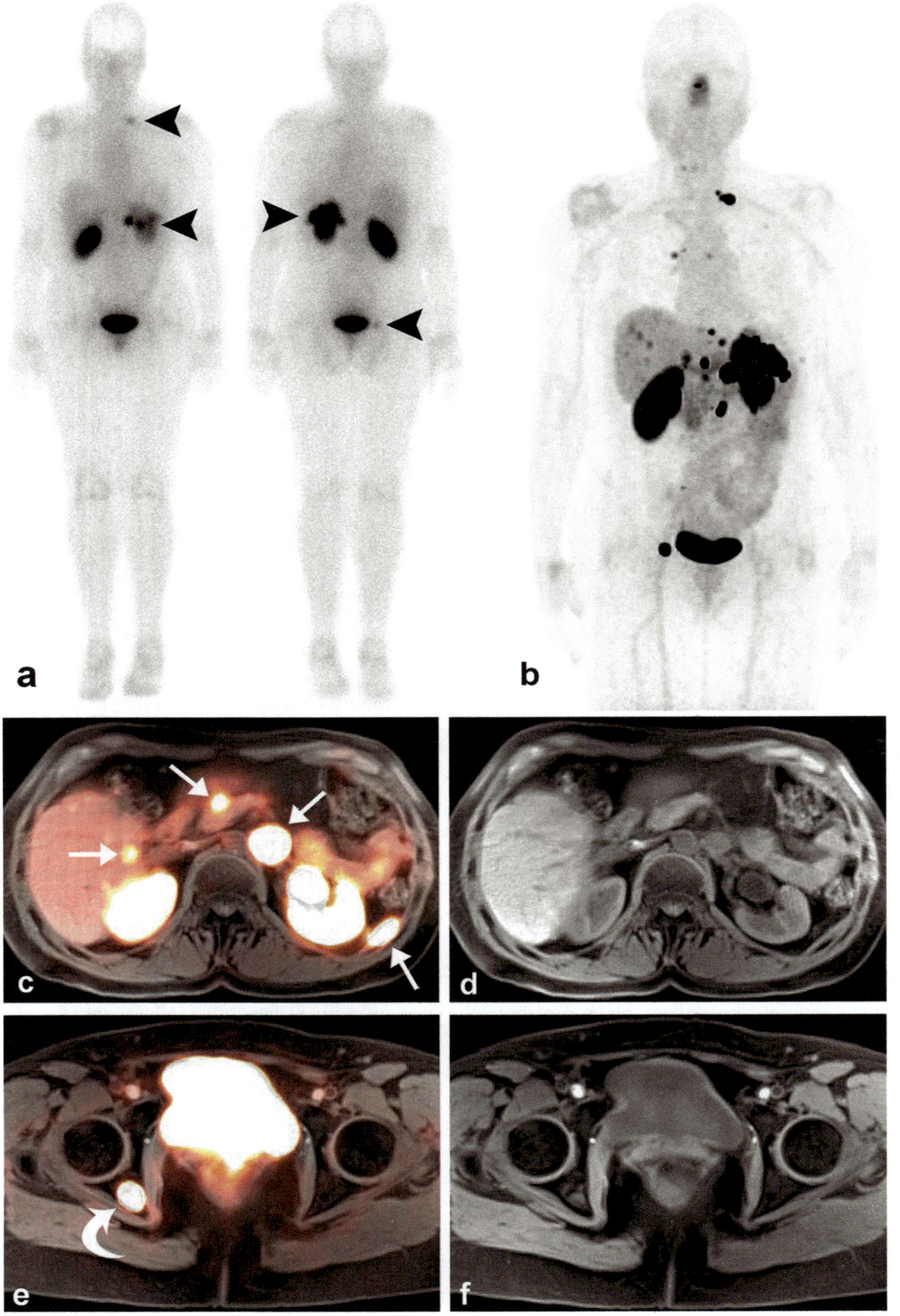

Fig. 68.1 Whole-body anterior and posterior octreotide scan (4 months prior) (**a**), Gallium-68 DOTATATE PET MIP (**b**), PET/MR T1 radial VIBE with fat suppression axial fusion (abdomen) (**c**), T1 radial VIBE with fat suppression axial (abdomen) (**d**), PET/MR T1 radial VIBE with fat suppression axial fusion (pelvis) (**e**), and T1 radial VIBE with fat suppression axial (pelvis) (**f**)

those with MEN I. On MRI, the normal pancreas demonstrates high signal intensity on T1-weighted images. Insulinomas, and other pancreatic NETs, are relatively hypointense on T1 and hyperintense on T2-weighted sequences compared to the background parenchyma. They are typically homogenous and hyperenhancing post contrast administration. Larger lesions may show ring-like and heterogeneous enhancement with cystic or necrotic areas. NET metastases also demonstrate low T1 and high T2-weighted signal intensity with early enhancement.

Nuclear imaging can be useful to detect and localize a pancreatic NET, evaluate for metastatic disease or recurrence, and assess receptor status for possible radionuclide-based treatment. The most common scintigraphic technique utilizes octreotide to bind to somatostatin type 2 receptors, which are commonly expressed by NETs. The sensitivity is highest for gastrinomas, and lowest for insulinomas as they express fewer somatostatin receptors. However, metastatic insulinomas often demonstrate increased octreotide uptake. Additionally, NETs do not usually take up FDG unless they are poorly differentiated. Research studies with Ga-68 DOTATATE PET in pancreatic NETs have shown superior lesion detection, with higher sensitivity and specificity, and change in clinical management in patients where octreotide scintigraphy demonstrated negative findings or only faint uptake. Patients with positive Ga-68 DOTATE findings may benefit from somatostatin analog radiotherapy, even when octreotide scintigraphy findings are negative. PET/MR imaging with Ga-68 DOTATATE is an excellent tool to provide detailed anatomical localization, characterization, and superior detection of pancreatic NETs as well as metastatic and recurrent disease.

Suggested Reading

Lewis RB, Lattin GE Jr, Paal E. Pancreatic endocrine tumors: radiologic-clinicopathologic correlation. Radiographics. 2010;30(6):1445–64.

Srirajaskanthan R, Kayani I, Quigley AM, Soh J, Caplin ME, Bomanji J. The role of 68Ga-DOTATATE PET in patients with neuroendocrine tumors and negative or equivocal findings on 111In-DTPA-octreotide scintigraphy. J Nucl Med. 2010;51(6):875–82.

Case 69
Focal Nodular Hyperplasia

Robert Matthews

History

A 31-year-old female for staging of Hodgkin's lymphoma (Fig. 69.1).

Diagnosis

Focal nodular hyperplasia

Findings

- T1 mildly hypointense and T2 mildly hyperintense focal hepatic lesion (arrowheads).
- Central stellate scar that is moderately T1 hypointense and moderately T2 hyperintense (thin arrow).
- Early moderate enhancement of the peripheral hyperplastic portion that persists on delayed image (curved arrows). The central scar does not enhance with hepatocyte-specific contrast.
- PET images show minimally decreased FDG uptake within the focal hepatic lesion.

Discussion

Focal nodular hyperplasia (FNH) is the second most common benign tumor of the liver, after hemangiomas. It is composed of hyperplastic elements of benign liver parenchyma including hepatocytes, bile ducts, and arteries with intercepting fibrous septa, radiating from a central stellate scar. FNH has a strong predilection for young females, ranging from adolescents to middle age, and only appears 15% of the time in males. The tumor has no malignant potential but may need to be surgically removed if rapidly increasing in size, due to potential hemorrhage or rupture.

FNH appears as a well-defined soft tissue mass that is mildly hypointense on T1-weighted images and mildly hyperintense on T2-weighted images. On MR imaging, the central stellate scar is detected in 50% of lesions. This scar shows more hypointense signal on T1-weighted images and more hyperintense signal on T2-weighted images. With the administration of gadolinium contrast, the main soft tissue lesion shows intense homogenous early enhancement that fades on the delayed images. The central stellate scar shows slow, gradual, delayed enhancement. With hepatocyte-specific contrast agents, there is moderate to intense early enhancement with delayed equilibrium of the lesion to the normal liver parenchyma due to the functioning hepatocytes. The central scar does not demonstrate uptake of these specific agents.

On FDG PET imaging, focal nodular hyperplasia has normal to decreased radiotracer uptake relative to normal liver parenchyma. If there is increased uptake, then malignancy or other space-occupying liver mass needs to be

R. Gupta et al., *PET/MR Imaging*, https://doi.org/10.1007/978-3-319-65106-4_69

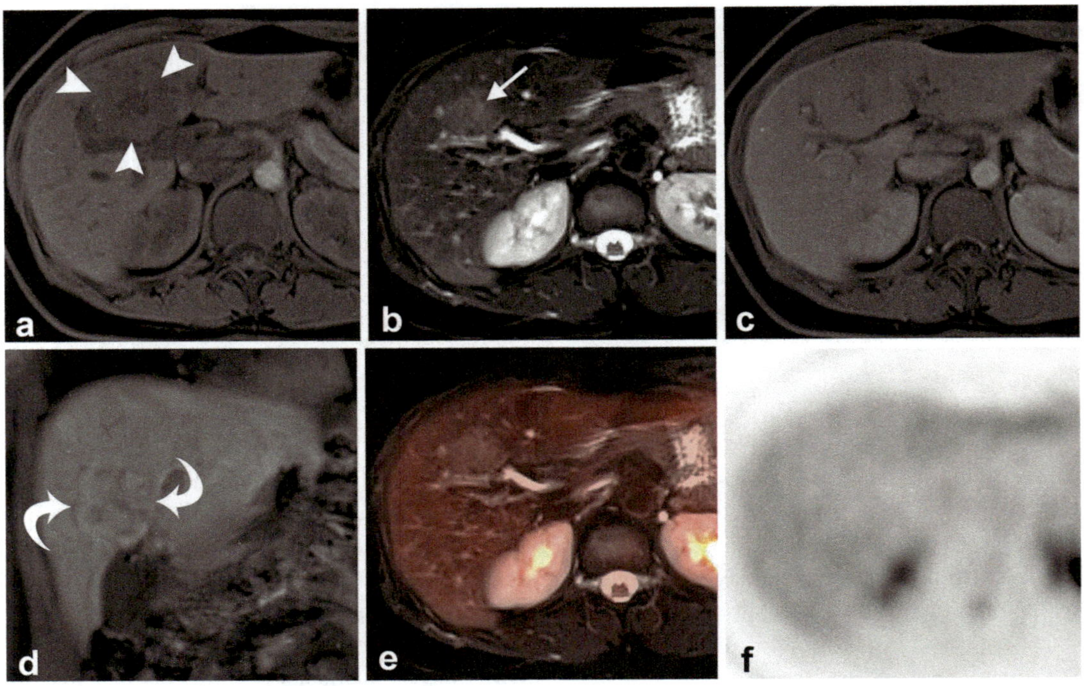

Fig. 69.1 T1 VIBE with fat suppression axial (**a**), T2 BLADE with fat suppression axial (**b**), T1 VIBE with fat suppression early post hepatocyte specific contrast axial (**c**), T1 VIBE with fat suppression post delayed hepatocyte-specific contrast coronal (**d**), PET/MRI T2 BLADE with fat suppression axial fusion (**e**), and PET axial (**f**)

strongly considered. In the past, nuclear technetium sulfur colloid SPECT imaging had been advocated for diagnosis, based on normal or increased radiotracer uptake that could be, however, also be seen in other liver neoplasms including adenoma and hepatoma. The amount of radiotracer uptake depends on the concentration of kupffer cells in the FNH lesion and it can be low in about a third of cases. Nuclear hepatobiliary agents do somewhat better with most of the lesions showing increased uptake that is diagnostic of FNH, but the lesion may be photon deficient in a number of cases.

Suggested Reading

Hussain SM, Terkivatan T, Zondervan PE, Lanjouw E, de Rave S, Ijzermans JN, et al. Focal nodular hyperplasia: findings at state-of-the-art MR imaging, US, CT, and pathologic analysis. Radiographics. 2004;24(1):3–17.

Kurtaran A, Becherer A, Pfeffel F, Müller C, Traub T, Schmaljohann J, et al. 18F-fluorodeoxyglucose (FDG)-PET features of focal nodular hyperplasia (FNH) of the liver. Liver. 2000;20(6):487–90.

Purysko AS, Remer EM, Coppa CP, Obuchowski NA, Schneider E, Veniero JC. Characteristics and distinguishing features of hepatocellular adenoma and focal nodular hyperplasia on gadoxetate disodium-enhanced MRI. AJR Am J Roentgenol. 2012;198(1):115–23.

Case 70
Acute Enteritis

Robert Matthews

History

A 55-year-old female for the evaluation of gynecological malignancy (Fig. 70.1).

Diagnosis

Acute enteritis

Findings

- Small bowel segment showing wall thickening and luminal dilatation with increased T2 signal representing bowel wall edema (black arrowheads).
- Fusion images show intense hypermetabolic activity corresponding to areas of wall thickening.
- An enlarged mesenteric lymph node is demonstrated on the T2 image (curved arrow) compatible with a reactive lymph node, having only mild FDG uptake on the fusion images.
- Metal-induced susceptibility artifact from pedicle screws in the spine (thin black arrow).

Discussion

Enteritis refers to a variety of disorders leading to inflammation of the small bowel. The etiologies are extensive and include a variety of infectious agents, ischemia, radiation, inflammatory bowel disease, scleroderma, amyloidosis, and chemotherapy induced. The main feature of enteritis is small bowel wall thickening associated with mucosal edema. There may be infiltration of the wall as well as wall hemorrhage. Chronic enteritis may lead to bowel wall dilatation, stricture, and obstruction. Fistulas and adhesions can occur, as well as abscesses.

In the acute phase of enteritis, the small bowel wall measures greater than 3 mm and there is fold thickening, which may be hard to see on MRI. Bowel that is under distended on MRI may falsely appear to have a thickened wall. Acute enteritis results in edema that is best seen on T2-weighted images with fat suppression. Mural ulceration, as seen with inflammatory bowel disease, appears as irregular T2 hyperintense signal in the wall. With enteritis there is often dilatation of intestinal loops and mesenteric fat stranding. There is also contrast enhancement of the intestinal wall. Enhancement of the bowel wall should

R. Gupta et al., *PET/MR Imaging*, https://doi.org/10.1007/978-3-319-65106-4_70

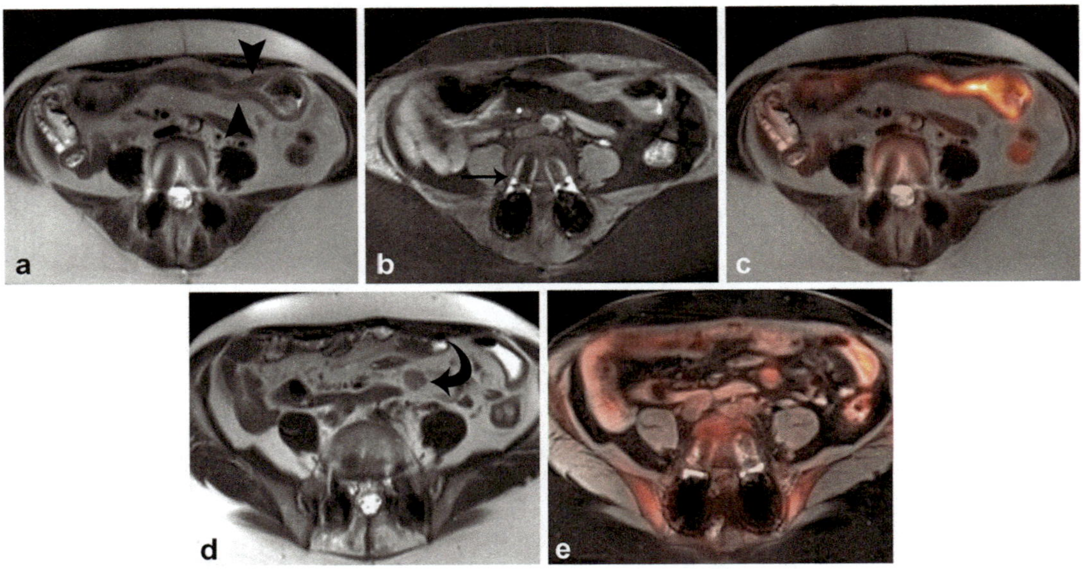

Fig. 70.1 T2 HASTE axial (**a**), T1 radial VIBE with fat suppression axial (**b**), PET/MR T2 HASTE axial fusion (**c**), T2 HASTE axial, at more inferior level (**d**), and PET/MRI T1 radial VIBE with fat suppression axial fusion, at more inferior level (**e**)

be compared to other unaffected bowel loops as an internal standard. Usually, the mucosa enhances more than the outer intestinal wall. Magnetic resonance enterography with oral contrast provides better bowel wall evaluation. When there is more extensive inflammation the mesentery may enhance as well. Enlarged reactive mesenteric lymph nodes may be seen.

On PET/MR imaging, the normal FDG uptake within the small and large bowel is quite variable. There may be segments of diffusely increased uptake, focal uptake, heterogeneous uptake, and no uptake all of which may represent physiological FDG distribution. In addition, bowel FDG uptake may be luminal. Areas of acute enteritis will demonstrate intense FDG uptake within the small bowel wall. There may be adjacent abnormal FDG uptake in the accompanying mesentery with reactive lymph nodes. There is usually good correlation of FDG uptake and abnormal signal on MRI. Care must be taken in interpreting PET/MRI studies in diabetic patients taking metformin, as bowel may characteristically show intense FDG activity without concurrent abnormal findings on MRI.

Suggested Reading

Casciani E, De Vincentiis C, Polettini E, Masselli G, Di Nardo G, Civitelli F, et al. Imaging of the small bowel: Crohn's disease in paediatric patients. World J Radiol. 2014;6(6):313–28.

Cronin CG, Scott J, Kambadakone A, Catalano OA, Sahani D, Blake MA, et al. Utility of positron emission tomography/CT in the evaluation of small bowel pathology. Br J Radiol. 2012;85(1017):1211–21.

Kavaliauskiene G, Ziech ML, Nio CY, Stoker J. Small bowel MRI in adult patients: not just Crohn's disease-a tutorial. Insights Imaging. 2011;2(5):501–13.

Case 71
Pancreatic Head Cancer

Robert Matthews

History

A 61-year-old female with abdominal pain, nausea, and vomiting presents for staging of pancreatic cancer (Fig. 71.1).

Diagnosis

Pancreastic head cancer with metastatic lymph nodes

Findings

- Pancreatic head mass that is T1 hypointense (arrowheads) and T2 hyperintense (curved arrows).
- PET/MR fusion images show intense hypermetabolic activity within this lesion compatible with pancreatic head malignancy.
- Multiple hypermetabolic retroperitoneal lymph nodes on PET/MR fusion consistent with metastatic adenopathy (thin arrows).

Discussion

Although relatively uncommon, pancreatic cancer is one of the leading causes of cancer-related deaths around the world with a one-year survival of only 24% and a five-year survival of 5%. Cancer within the head of the pancreas occurs in 65% of cases, in the body or tail in 15%, and diffusely involving the pancreas in 20%. Pancreatic head cancer presents with slowly increasing jaundice and elevated liver enzymes caused by bile duct obstruction. Other symptoms include weight loss, pain, anorexia, dark urine and light stool, nausea, and vomiting. Proper staging of pancreatic head cancer is important since resectable disease requires the Whipple surgical procedure with removal of the pancreatic head, duodenum, gallbladder, distal stomach, common bile duct, and proximal jejunum.

On MRI, the pancreatic head may be only subtly enlarged and thus it can be challenging to detect a mass. Pancreatic cancers show low signal on T1-weighted images, are hypovascular in

R. Gupta et al., *PET/MR Imaging*, https://doi.org/10.1007/978-3-319-65106-4_71

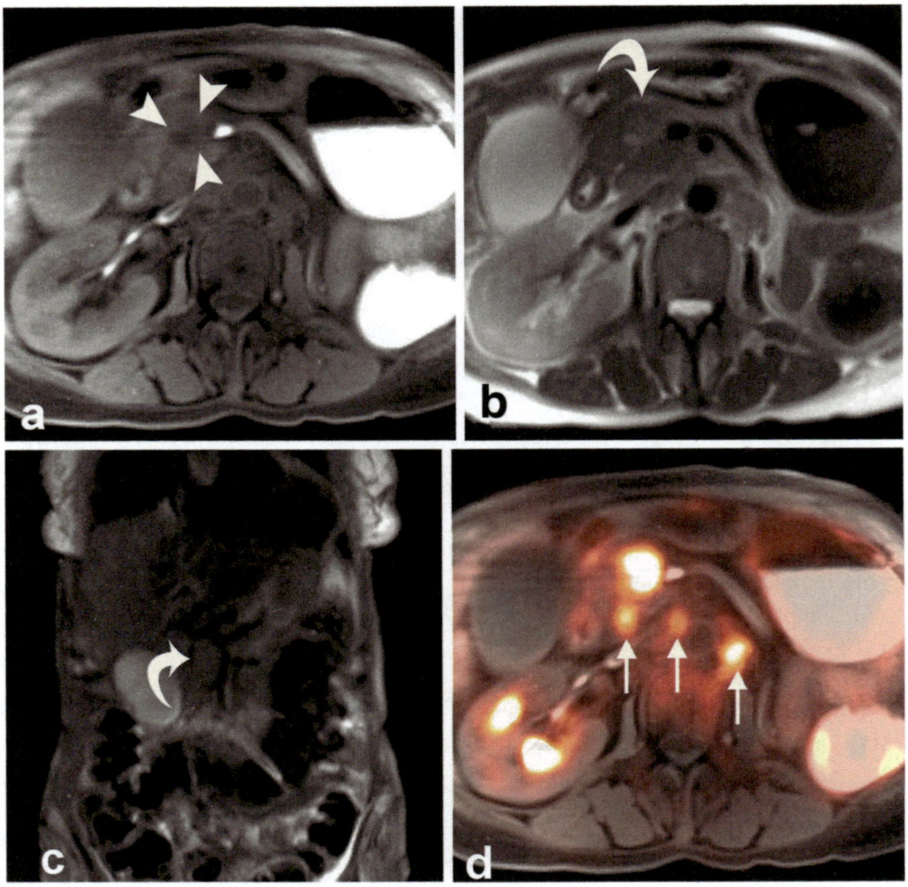

Fig. 71.1 T1 radial VIBE with fat suppression axial (**a**), T2 axial (**b**), T2 coronal (**c**), and PET/MR T1 radial VIBE with fat suppression axial fusion (**d**)

the early arterial phase of contrast administration, and demonstrate gradual delayed enhancement. Focal fat in the pancreatic head can sometimes appear to be mass-like leading to occasional confusion, but shows typical fat suppression on MRI sequences. Focal pancreatitis can also mimic pancreatic adenocarcinoma but resolves on short-term follow-up. On T2-weighted images, both the common bile duct and the pancreatic duct may be dilated leading to the double duct sign. The ductal dilation is characteristically smooth. Magnetic resonance cholangiopancreatography is a useful MR adjunct to better define the biliary tree and pancreatic ducts.

PET/MR imaging is useful in pancreatic head tumors to aid in the initial diagnosis in the jaundiced patient, since the lesions are usually FDG avid. Regional spread of cancer into surrounding structures is common and progresses rapidly, due to the absence of a pancreatic capsule. PET/MRI is an excellent tool to evaluate pancreatic and adjacent anatomy with simultaneous determination of metabolic activity. This aids in detecting local regional and metastatic spread which can help determine the most appropriate medical or surgical oncologic approach.

Suggested Reading

Shrikhande SV, Barreto SG, Goel M, Arya S. Multimodality imaging of pancreatic ductal adenocarcinoma: a review of the literature. HPB (Oxford). 2012;14(10):658–68.

Tummala P, Junaidi O, Agarwal B. Imaging of pancreatic cancer: an overview. J Gastrointest Oncol. 2011;2(3):168–74.

Case 72
GIST Hemorrhagic Metastases

Robert Matthews

History

A 48-year-old male presents following resection of gastrointestinal stromal tumor near the gastro-esophageal junction 2 years ago (Fig. 72.1). The patient recently underwent embolization of a hemorrhagic right-sided liver lesion due to new hemoperitoneum.

Diagnosis

GIST hemorrhagic liver metastases

Findings

- Large mass in the right hepatic lobe demonstrating subacute bleeding with high T1 and and heterogeneous T2 signal due to embolization (arrowheads).
- No abnormal FDG activity in the right hepatic lobe mass on fusion image indicating good treatment response.
- Left hepatic lobe mass with its peripheral solid component being T1 hypointense and T2 hyperintense.
- Fusion image demonstrates hypermetabolic activity in the solid periphery of the left hepatic lobe mass compatible with active malignancy (curved arrows).
- Layering of the central component of the left hepatic lobe mass on T1 and T2 images due to hemorrhage.
- Gallbladder shows layering sludge (thin arrow).

Discussion

Gastrointestinal stromal tumors (GIST) are an uncommon type of tumor that originate from the interstitial cells of Cajal. These cells form part of the autonomic nervous system and help to regulate digestion. The majority of the GIST occur in the stomach while the reminder occur in the small intestines. Rarely, GIST may occur in other areas of the abdomen including the peritoneum. Clinically GIST present with gastrointestinal bleeding, but other symptoms such as abdominal discomfort, pain, nausea, vomiting, and weight loss can occur. Although GIST can be benign, usually the tumor is malignant and locally aggressive. Despite their large size, these tumors rarely cause gastrointestinal obstruction.

On MRI, the solid components of GIST have a low signal on T1-weighted images and a high signal on T2-weighted images. Lesions show post contrast enhancement that is more intense and heterogeneous when the lesions are larger. In their early stage, these endoluminal tumors often appear as a smooth, well-circumscribed mass. As the tumor grows and invades the stomach or intestinal wall, there are often areas of hemor-

R. Gupta et al., *PET/MR Imaging*, https://doi.org/10.1007/978-3-319-65106-4_72

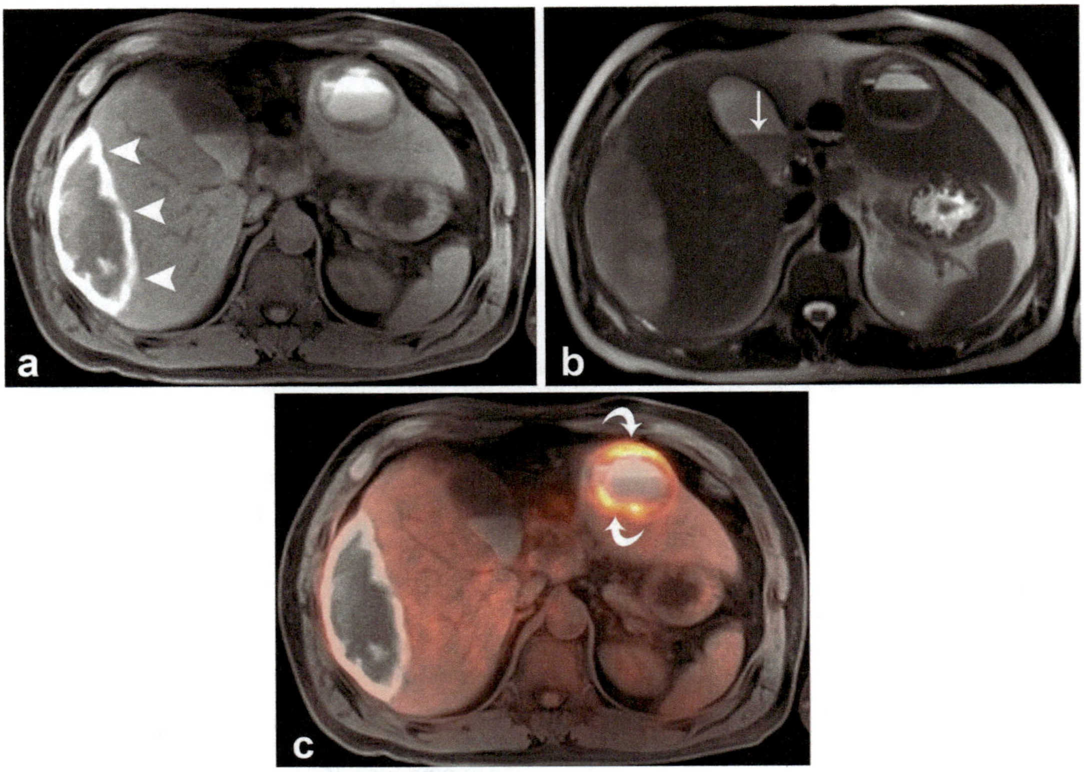

Fig. 72.1 T1 radial VIBE with fat suppression axial (**a**), T2 HASTE axial (**b**), and PET/MR T1 radial VIBE with fat suppression axial fusion (**c**)

rhage, necrosis, and cystic changes with a heterogeneous appearance that when large communicates with the lumen. When necrotic, the tumor can have variable T1 and T2 signal changes. Often when GIST is diagnosed, the tumor has become extremely large in size with extensive abdominal metastatic disease.

In patients with gastrointestinal stromal tumors, PET/MR improves the detection of the primary tumor and metastatic lesions. GIST is intensely FDG avid. PET imaging is superior in detecting local metastatic disease and can detect more lesions than a contrast-enhanced CT scan. On PET/MR imaging, GIST is most often seen as a large infiltrating mass of the stomach or intestines with intense hypermetabolic activity. There is usually extensive metastatic disease in the peritoneum and surrounding structures with abnormal increased FDG uptake. The appearance of metastatic disease on PET/MR imaging is much more extensive than patients with adenocarcinoma of the stomach or primary intestinal malignancies, although some cases of lymphoma may appear similar but without the hemorrhage, necrosis, and cystic changes. PET/MR is also excellent at assessing treatment response since the bulky lesions may not significantly change in size following a good response to therapy, however they should demonstrate decreased metabolic activity.

Suggested Reading

King DM. The radiology of gastrointestinal stromal tumours (GIST). Cancer Imaging. 2005;5:150–6.

Ulusan S, Koç Z. Radiologic findings in malignant gastrointestinal stromal tumors. Diagn Interv Radiol. 2009;15(2):121–6.

Case 73
Recurrent Colon Cancer

Robert Matthews

History

An 87-year-old female presented with colon cancer treated 5 years ago with sigmoidectomy with primary anastomosis, and chemotherapy (Fig. 73.1).

Diagnosis

Recurrent colon cancer

Findings

- Mass infiltrating the small bowel that is T1 hypointense and T2 isointense compared to the normal bowel (curved white arrow).
- PET fusion image demonstrates intense hypermetabolic activity compatible with colon cancer recurrence.
- Midline ventral hernia containing a loop of small bowel (white arrowhead).
- Artifact from right hip prostheses.

Discussion

Between 30% and 50% of patients undergoing curative surgery for colorectal cancer will eventually develop recurrent disease. Recurrence may even occur in patients with node negative Stage I and II disease. Recurrences commonly appear as nodal metastases, lung metastases, liver metastases, and local recurrence. Most local recurrences occur within the first 3 years since surgery in an asymptomatic patient. Rectal cancer tends to have more locoregional recurrence because of the confined space of the pelvis limiting the depth of surgical resection and margins. Colon cancer, on the other hand, treated with wider surgical margins usually manifests as distant metastases with recurrences in the peritoneum, retroperitoneum, and other organs.

Intraluminal recurrence at the anastomotic site can be easily detected with colonoscopic surveillance and biopsy, although granulation tissue may make it more difficult to diagnose recurrence. However, most recurrences do not occur within the lumen. Outside the bowel lumen, the determination of local recurrence is highly dependent on cross-sectional imaging. Rising tumor markers do not correlate with the extent of recurrence nor can they localize the recurrence Tumor marker measurements do not lead to significant improvements in patient survival. CT, often the first modality to look for recurrence of colorectal cancer, may miss recurrence and when noted usually underestimates the tumor burden.

FDG PET/MR imaging for recurrence of colorectal cancer has higher sensitivity and specificity than CT or MR. It has an excellent rate of detection of local recurrence including locoregional lymph nodes, peritoneal recurrence, and

R. Gupta et al., *PET/MR Imaging*, https://doi.org/10.1007/978-3-319-65106-4_73

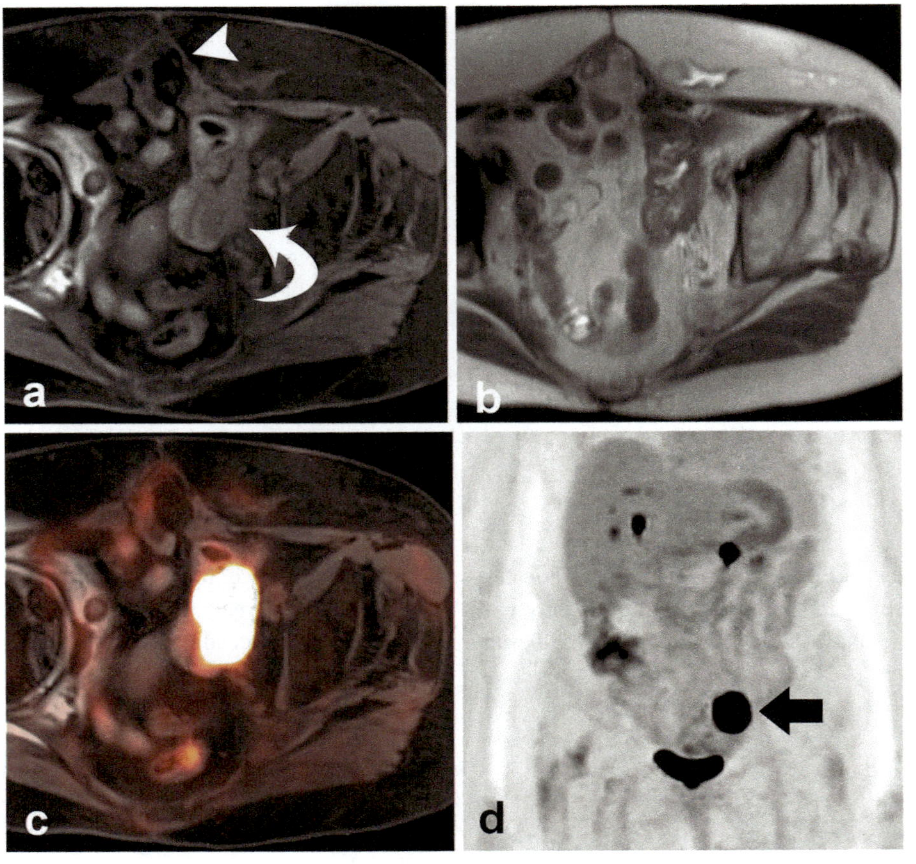

Fig. 73.1 T1 radial VIBE with fat suppression axial (**a**), T2 HASTE axial (**b**), PET/MR T1 radial VIBE with fat suppression axial fusion (**c**), and PET MIP (**d**)

hepatic metastases. PET/MR can better determine the extent and tumor burden of extrahepatic dissemination. CT and MR alone can be difficult to interpret due to distorted anatomy with scarring following surgical resection and radiation therapy. The high T2 signal on MR can be due to granulation tissue, hematoma, and radiation-induced inflammatory changes that can persist up to 2 years after therapy. A seroma can mimic a mucin-producing tumor recurrence being hyperintense on T2-weighted images, hypointense on T1-weighted images, and show peripheral enhancement. Inflammatory changes can also be seen with PET imaging with increased FDG activity leading to false-positive findings. PET is superior at detecting small metastatic lymph nodes that do not fit the size criteria as well as in detecting distant metastatic disease. PET/MR has a particular advantage when looking for local recurrence in rectal cancer where the MR component has better detection capabilities than imaging with CT.

Suggested Reading

Israel O, Kuten A. Early detection of cancer recurrence: 18F-FDG PET/CT can make a difference in diagnosis and patient care. J Nucl Med. 2007;48(Suppl 1):28S–35S.

Young PE, Womeldorph CM, Johnson EK, Maykel JA, Brucher B, Stojadinovic A, et al. Early detection of colorectal cancer recurrence in patients undergoing surgery with curative intent: current status and challenges. J Cancer. 2014;5(4):262–71.

Case 74
Neuroendocrine Tumor Gallbladder

Robert Matthews

History

A 44-year-old male presented for initial staging of a neuroendocrine tumor (Fig. 74.1).

Diagnosis

Invasive neuroendocrine tumor of the gallbladder with lymph node metastases

Findings

- Thickened gallbladder wall demonstrating hypointense T1 and hyperintense T2 signal with abnormal hypermetabolic activity on the fusion images compatible with malignancy (white arrowheads).
- Hypermetabolic retroperitoneal lymph nodes consistent with metastatic disease (thin white arrows).
- Metastatic infiltration of the liver with hypointense T1 and hyperintense T2 signal with abnormal hypermetabolic activity (wide white arrow).
- Small porta hepatis lymph nodes (curved white arrow) are seen with corresponding abnormal hypermetabolic activity on the fusion images.
- Tumor progression along the intrahepatic biliary tree with dilated bile ducts (curved black arrow) and corresponding increased FDG activity.
- Dilated bile ducts in the left hepatic lobe with increased T2 signal indicating obstruction (black arrowheads).

Discussion

Primary neuroendocrine tumors of the gallbladder comprise only a small percent (<1%) of all neuroendocrine tumors. Neuroendocrine cells are involved in visceral regulation by secreting amines and polypeptide hormones. Neuroendocrine cells can be found in a variety of tissues in the body, but most commonly occur in the lungs, pancreas, appendix, adrenal gland, and peripheral nerves. Gallbladder neuroendocrine tumors arise from intestinal or gastric metaplasia of the gallbladder wall. These tumors are commonly associated with gallstones and chronic cholecystitis. From a clinical standpoint, neuroendocrine gallbladder tumors behave similarly to gallbladder adenocarcinoma.

On imaging, it is not usually possible to differentiate between neuroendocrine tumors of the gallbladder and gallbladder adenocarcinomas. In the early stages, MRI depicts the tumor as a well-defined mass in the gallbladder fossa. The tumors

R. Gupta et al., *PET/MR Imaging*, https://doi.org/10.1007/978-3-319-65106-4_74

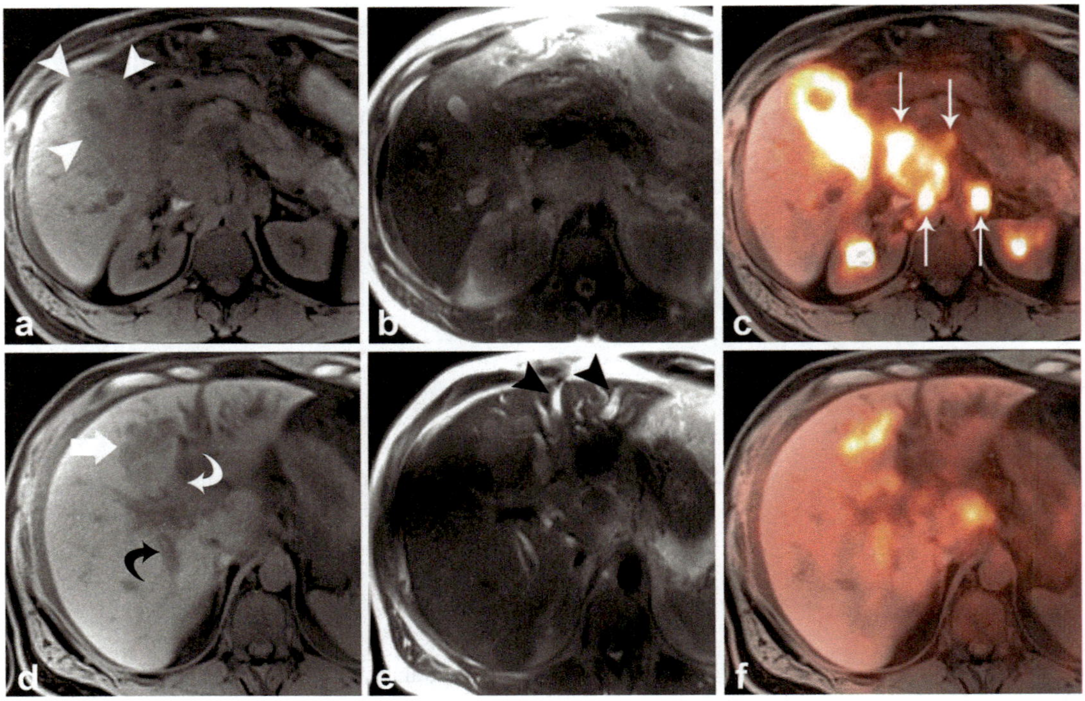

Fig. 74.1 T1 radial VIBE with fat suppression axial (**a**), T2 HASTE axial (**b**), PET/MRI T1 radial VIBE with fat suppression axial fusion (**c**), T1 radial VIBE with fat suppression axial, at more superior level (**d**), T2 HASTE axial, at more superior level (**e**), and PET/MRI T1 radial VIBE with fat suppression axial fusion, at more superior level (**f**)

show low signal on T1-weighted images and high signal on T2-weighted images. Following IV gadolinium administration, the lesions avidly enhance in the early phase due to hypervascularity. In more advanced cases, MRI can detect a large mass in the gallbladder fossa that begins to infiltrate the liver. Neuroendocrine tumors are often associated with necrotic, enlarged metastatic abdominal lymph nodes that are easily detected by MRI.

On PET/MR imaging, gallbladder neuroendocrine tumors intensely accumulate FDG radiotracer due to their aggressive nature. The combination of PET/MRI for gallbladder neuroendocrine tumors has a high detection rate and can accurately delineate the extent of spread into adjacent structures, especially the liver and bile ducts. The gallbladder wall is thickened with intense metabolic activity that is often not discernable from the liver. There may be areas of tumor necrosis with high T2 signal and an absence of metabolic activity. Neuroendocrine gallbladder tumors are often associated with intrahepatic bile duct dilatation. The tumor is often hard to distinguish from gallbladder adenocarcinoma, gallbladder lymphoma, primary liver malignancies, and gallbladder metastasis. New gallium-68-labeled somatostatin receptor PET imaging agents may play an imaging role in the future.

Suggested Reading

Eltawil KM, Gustafsson BI, Kidd M, Modlin IM. Neuroendocrine tumors of the gallbladder: an evaluation and reassessment of management strategy. J Clin Gastroenterol. 2010;44(10):687–95.

Monier A, Saloum N, Szmigielski W, Alrashid A, Napaki SM. Neuroendocrine tumor of the gallbladder. Pol J Radiol. 2015;80:228–31.

Case 75 Hepatic Chemoembolization Resulting in Chemical Cholecystitis

Christopher Shackles and Amit Gupta

History

A 54-year-old female who had chemoembolization of the right hepatic artery 1 month ago, presented for restaging of breast cancer (Fig. 75.1).

Diagnosis

Hepatic chemoembolization resulting in chemical cholecystitis

Findings

- Large masses in the right hepatic lobe that are T1 hypointense and T2 hyperintense (curved arrow).
- Masses demonstrate a necrotic photopenic center and no significant FDG uptake on fusion images consistent with treated metastases.
- Gallbladder demonstrates diffuse increased wall thickening (arrowheads) with mildly increased FDG activity that reflects chemical cholecystitis from chemoembolization.

Discussion

Transarterial chemoembolization therapy (TACE) is a method of administrating localized chemotherapy directly to a liver tumor via a transarterial catheter. TACE is most commonly used for the treatment of hepatocellular carcinoma (HCC). However, TACE has also been used in the treatment of colorectal metastases as well as primary cholangiocarcinoma. HCC after TACE typically demonstrates variable signal intensity on T1- and T2-weighted sequences. Hypointensity within a lesion on T2-weighted sequences typically corresponds to areas of coagulation necrosis, while conversely, hyperintensity corresponds to hemorrhage or residual tumor. It can be difficult to ascertain viable tumor from necrotic areas on non-contrast sequences. On post contrast images, viable tumor will demonstrate post gadolinium enhancement while necrotic tissue will not. Iodized oil results in beam hardening artifact on CT, which may hinder assessment of post contrast enhancement on CT. Lipiodol does not alter signal intensity on MRI, thus making it easier to identify residual tumor on gadolinium-enhanced MR images. However, it may be difficult to

R. Gupta et al., *PET/MR Imaging*, https://doi.org/10.1007/978-3-319-65106-4_75

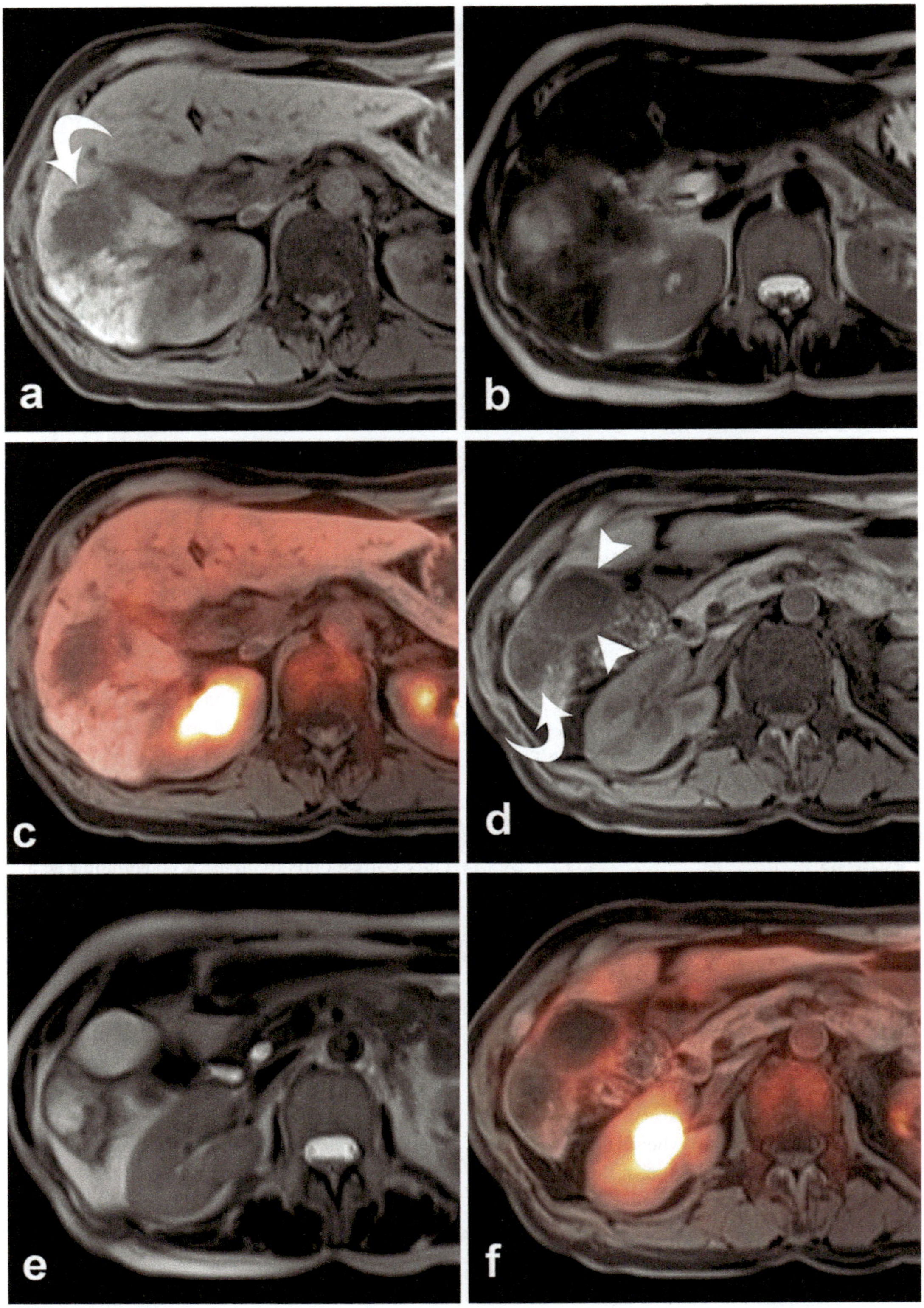

Fig. 75.1 T1 radial VIBE with fat suppression axial (mid liver) (**a**), T2 HASTE axial (mid liver) (**b**), PET/MR T1 radial VIBE with fat suppression axial fusion (mid liver) (**c**), T1 radial VIBE with fat suppression axial (lower liver) (**d**), T2 HASTE axial (lower liver) (**e**), and PET/MR T1 radial VIBE with fat suppression axial fusion (lower liver) (**f**)

appreciate small areas of residual tumor as the tumor capsule typically appears as a hyperintense ring on both early and delayed post contrast sequences. In these equivocal cases, subtraction images may provide additional value. In addition, metabolic information provided by PET can prove helpful.

As we know, FDG is a glucose analog and becomes trapped within highly active tumor cells after being metabolized into FDG-6-phosphate. The normal liver is typically concentrated in glucose-6-phototase activity causing rapid dephosphorylation resulting in lower background activity. Together, these differences may result in visible increased FDG uptake in viable HCC. However, some HCCs can demonstrate relatively low FDG uptake, despite viability, secondary to dephosphorylation. Decreased or absent FDG uptake after TACE in a previously FDG avid HCC lesion has been associated with tumor necrosis. Studies have demonstrated that decreased FDG uptake is not only more sensitive than CT findings, but often may occur earlier than CT changes. Limited resolution of PET scanners and respiratory motion during acquisition may limit the utility of PET in the evaluation of smaller tumors (<1 cm in size). Overall, PET and MRI can play a complimentary role and help in better assessment of liver lesions in these otherwise challenging post TACE cases.

Typically for right hepatic lobe chemoembolization, the catheter is placed in the right hepatic artery beyond the cystic artery origin. However, this is sometimes not possible, as the extent of disease in the right hepatic lobe requires placement of a catheter before the origin of the cystic artery. This can lead to embolization of the cystic artery and can result in chemical cholecystitis. This appears as thickened gallbladder wall on MR images. Most cases of chemical cholecystitis can be managed conservatively.

Suggested Reading

Clark TW. Complications of hepatic chemoembolization. Semin Interv Radiol. 2006;23(2):119–25.

Lim HS, Jeong YY, Kang HK, Kim JK, Park JG. Imaging features of hepatocellular carcinoma after transcatheter arterial chemoembolization and radiofrequency ablation. AJR Am J Roentgenol. 2006;187(4):W341–9.

Torizuka T, Tamaki N, Inokuma T, Magata Y, Yonekura Y, Tanaka A, et al. Value of fluorine-18-FDG-PET to monitor hepatocellular carcinoma after interventional therapy. J Nucl Med. 1994;35(12):1965–9.

Part IV

Genitourinary

Case 76
Cervical Cancer

Rajesh Gupta

History

A 76-year-old female presents with postmenopausal bleeding (Fig. 76.1).

Diagnosis

Cervical cancer (invasive squamous cell carcinoma) with lymph node metastases

Findings

- Sagittal MRI images show an irregular cervical mass which extends superiorly into the uterine fundus, inferiorly into the vagina, and anteriorly to invade the bladder wall. It displays relatively high signal on T2-weighted images, isointense on T1-weighted images, and enhances avidly following contrast administration.
- PET and fusion images show prominent FDG uptake within the cervical mass consistent with malignancy.
- The endometrial canal is dilated with fluid and debris due to obstruction from the cervical mass (asterisk).
- Low T2-weighted round submucosa fibroma is seen below the asterisk.
- Axial images show parametrial tumor extension with hypermetabolic lymph nodes (arrows).

Discussion

Carcinoma of the cervix is the third most common gynecological malignancy. It typically occurs in younger women with an average age of onset at around 45 years. The most common histologic subtype is squamous cell. The human papillomavirus (HPV) is central to the development of cervical neoplasia and is sexually transmitted. The most common presenting symptoms include vaginal bleeding and discharge. Mortality from cervical cancer has decreased significantly with the advent of the Papanicolau screening test.

Presurgical evaluation of cervical cancer is crucial in determining early stage versus advanced disease for treatment considerations. MRI can accurately determine tumor size and location, depth of stromal invasion, extension into the lower uterine segment, and evaluate regional lymph node metastases. Cervical tumors are best seen on T2-weighted images as a relatively hyperintense mass compared to the lower signal intensity stroma. Axial oblique T2-weighted FSE images are important to assess for parametrial invasion. The addition of fat saturation

R. Gupta et al., *PET/MR Imaging*, https://doi.org/10.1007/978-3-319-65106-4_76

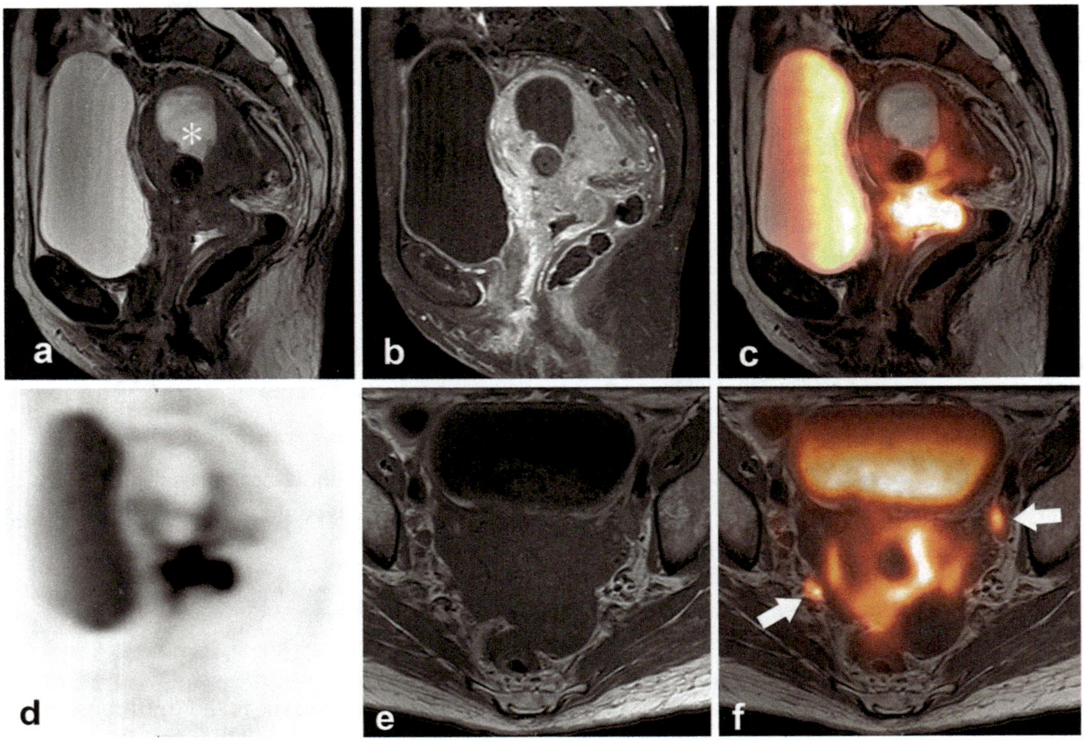

Fig. 76.1 T2-weighted sagittal pelvis (**a**), T1 VIBE with fat suppression post-gadolinium contrast sagittal pelvis (**b**), PET/MR T2-weighted sagittal pelvis fusion (**c**), PET sagittal (**d**), T1-weighted axial pelvis (**e**), and PET/MR T1-weighted axial fusion (**f**)

sequences can improve evaluation for parametrial extension. On T1-weighted images, cervical tumors are usually isointense to the normal cervix and may not be visible. However, T1-weighted images are important to identify enlarged abdominopelvic lymph nodes, and assess for the nodal morphology. The use of contrast in cervical cancer is usually not necessary as it does not improve staging accuracy compared to unenhanced images. Dynamic contrast-enhanced MRI can, however, be helpful to determine tumor recurrence from postsurgical changes.

The role of PET in cervical cancer is increasing, especially with improved spatial resolution from hybrid PET/MR systems. Prior reports have shown PET to have a sensitivity of 85–92% for detecting primary lesions in patients with FIGO stage IB disease or higher in tumors greater than 2 cm. Several reports have shown PET to be useful in the evaluation of lymph node metastases and is essential for detection of distant metastases and accurate initial staging. PET/MR can detect small early metastatic pelvic lymph nodes. PET is particularly helpful in identifying recurrent malignant lesions, especially after surgery where the anatomy has become distorted. Several studies have investigated the accumulation of FDG in the primary tumor, lymph nodes and uterine body and found that SUV was the only significant variable that can correlate with overall survival and prediction of poor prognosis.

Suggested Reading

Nogami Y, Iida M, Banno K, Kisu I, Adachi M, Nakamura K, et al. Application of FDG PET in cervical cancer and endometrial cancer: utility and future prospects. Anticancer Res. 2014;34(2):585–92.

Sala E, Wakely S, Senior E, Lomas D. MRI of malignant neoplasms of the uterine corpus and cervix. AJR Am J Roentgenol. 2007;188(6):1577–87.

Case 77
Simple Renal Cysts

Rajesh Gupta

History

A 75-year-old female presented with incidental bilateral renal lesions (Fig. 77.1).

Diagnosis

Simple renal cysts

Findings

- T1 hypointense and T2 hyperintense exophytic right renal lesion.
- PET/MR fusion axial image shows absence of FDG activity within the renal cyst (arrow).
- PET/MR fusion coronal image demonstrates two adjacent thin-walled renal cysts without FDG uptake.

Discussion

Renal cysts are common incidental lesions found in the kidneys on various imaging modalities with an overall population prevalence of 41% as determined by CT-based studies. Their incidence increases with patient age and renal dysfunction. The vast majority of these lesions are benign, meeting the criteria of a simple cyst with thin, well-defined walls and no enhancement following gadolinium contrast on MRI. The Bosniak classification is based on the morphological appearance and enhancement of renal cysts on CT and defines a simple cyst as one with a hairline thin wall, no internal septa, no calcifications, and no enhancement with no need for follow-up. MRI T2-weighted images are the most helpful in distinguishing a simple cyst from other renal lesions, as they show a homogenous fluid filled lesion that is hyperintense due to its water content with a thin surrounding wall. Intralesional septa and solid nodules are also readily visualized on T2-weighted images. Simple cysts will have low signal intensity on T1-weighted and no post contrast enhancement. On FDG PET, simple cysts will appear photopenic compared to the background renal parenchyma with no wall FDG uptake.

Complicated renal cysts with hemorrhagic or proteinaceous components may have a mildly increased T1-weighted signal and decreased T2-weighted signal. The presence of enhancement within a renal lesion is the most reliable criteria to distinguish a solid mass from a cyst on MR imaging. Renal cell carcinoma, renal metastases, and lymphomatous kidney involvement will have increased FDG uptake

R. Gupta et al., *PET/MR Imaging*, https://doi.org/10.1007/978-3-319-65106-4_77

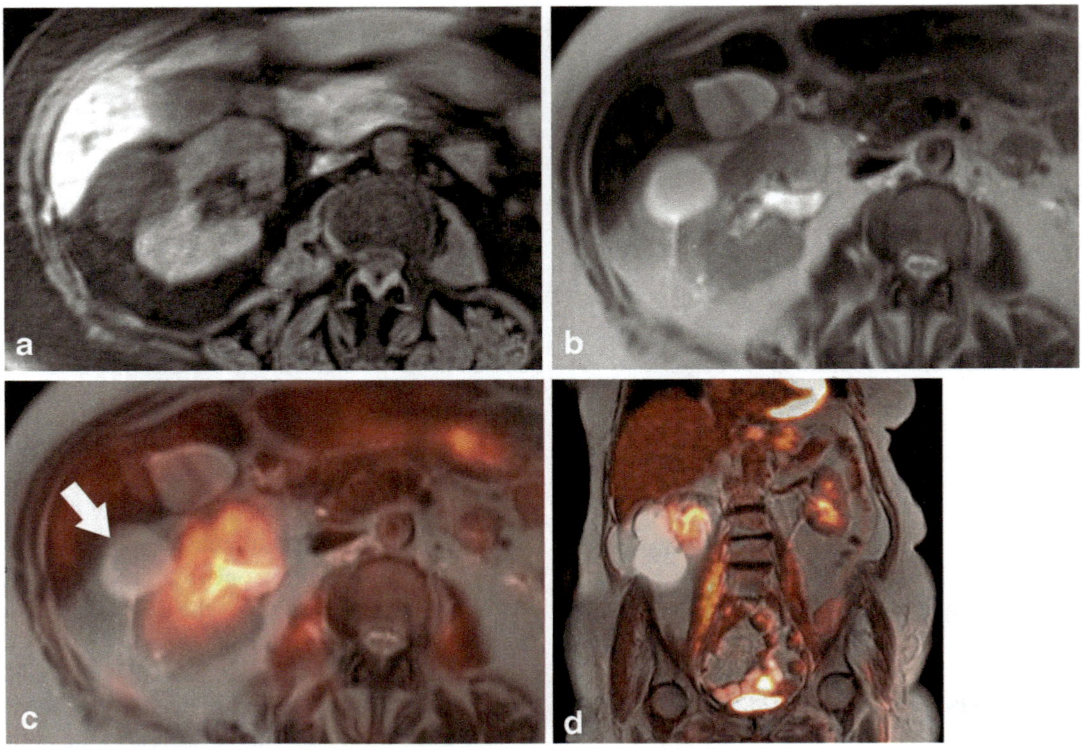

Fig. 77.1 T1 radial VIBE axial (**a**), T2 HASTE axial (**b**), PET/MR T2 HASTE axial fusion (**c**), and PET/MR T2 TSE coronal fusion (**d**)

on PET imaging. Evaluation of renal lesion may be difficult with PET due to physiological excretion of FDG through the kidneys which can interfere with image interpretation. Combined PET/MR systems allow for better PET evaluation of renal lesions as high-resolution anatomical information can be correlated with PET data. Mild or subtle FDG uptake would be better seen on PET/MR images allowing to identify more suspicious lesions.

Suggested Reading

Kochhar R, Brown RK, Wong CO, Dunnick NR, Frey KA, Manoharan P. Role of FDG PET/CT in imaging of renal lesions. J Med Imaging Radiat Oncol. 2010;54(4):347–57.

Pedrosa I, Sun MR, Spencer M, Genega EM, Olumi AF, Dewolf WC, et al. MR imaging of renal masses: correlation with findings at surgery and pathologic analysis. Radiographics. 2008;28(4):985–1003.

Simms RJ, Ong ACM. How simple are "simple renal cysts"? Nephrol Dial Transplant. 2014;29(Suppl 4):iv106–12.

Case 78
Mature Cystic Ovarian Teratoma

Rajesh Gupta

History

A 19-year-old female presents with pelvic pain (Fig. 78.1).

Diagnosis

Mature cystic ovarian teratoma (dermoid cyst)

Findings

- Large complex ovarian cystic lesion in the left adnexa that is predominantly T1 hypointense and T2 hyperintense (wide arrow).
- Within this cystic lesion there is a round protuberance with foci of T1 and T2-weighted hyperintensities representing a Rokitansky nodule (arrowhead).
- Dixon fat image confirms the presence of adipose tissue (curved arrow).
- This lesion has minimal FDG uptake confirming a benign mature cystic teratoma.
- Mild physiological FDG uptake is noted in the endometrium (thin arrow).

Discussion

Ovarian teratomas are common germ cell neoplasms comprised of mature or immature tissues of germ cell origin. The most common histologic type is the mature cystic teratoma, also known as a dermoid cyst, which typically contains mature tissue from at least two of the three germ cell layers (ectoderm, mesoderm, or endoderm). Skin derivatives and neural tissue are usually present. Fat, bone, cartilage, and muscle manifest in over 90% of cases. A portion of endodermal tissue including gastrointestinal epithelium, bronchial epithelium, and thyroid tissue is present in the majority of cases. The solid protuberance in the ovarian cyst, also termed Rokitansky nodule or dermoid plug, contains the calcification, teeth, adipose, hair, and sebaceous components. Ovarian teratomas usually affect young women, with a mean patient age of 30 years. They tend to be asymptomatic but can present with abdominal or pelvic pain. Complications of mature cystic teratomas include rupture, malignant degeneration, and torsion which can sometimes be detected on imaging.

The majority of mature cystic teratomas can be diagnosed with ultrasound, however it can some-

R. Gupta et al., *PET/MR Imaging*, https://doi.org/10.1007/978-3-319-65106-4_78

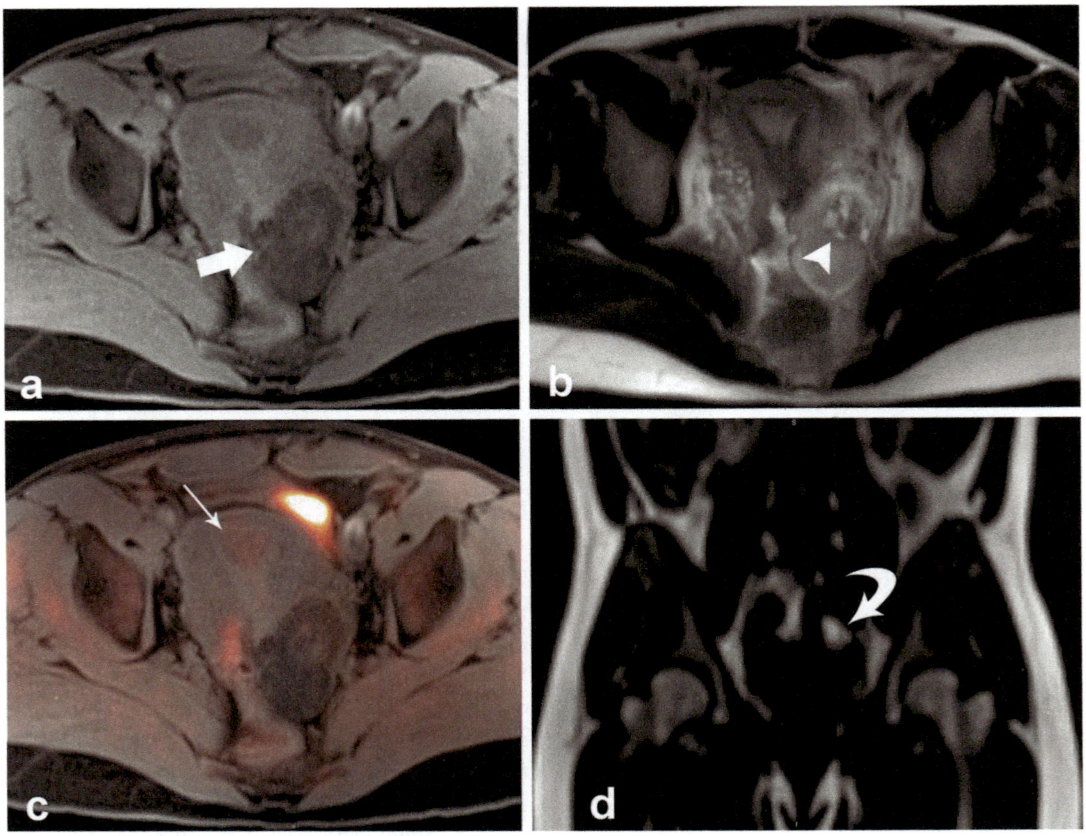

Fig. 78.1 T1 radial VIBE with fat suppression axial (**a**), T2 HASTE axial (**b**), PET/MR T1 radial VIBE with fat suppression axial fusion (**c**), and Dixon T1-weighted fat sequence coronal (**d**)

times be difficult as they can have a variety of appearances. Ultrasound can detect the characteristic Rokitansky nodule including strands of hair and teeth with varying degrees of echogenicity. On CT, the detection of fat density with or without calcification of the wall is diagnostic for mature cystic teratoma. On MR imaging, the sebaceous fat component will demonstrate high T1-weighted signal, however the T2-weighted signal can be variable. It can also be difficult to discern adipose tissue from hemorrhage on the basis of T1-weighted and T2-weighted signal intensities. Therefore, on MRI fat suppression techniques, chemical-shift in and out-of-phase imaging, and Dixon fat sequences are more advantageous in confirming a mature cystic teratoma.

Mature cystic teratomas are usually benign but can rarely undergo malignant degeneration. On the other hand, immature teratomas are generally malignant. FDG PET/CT has been found to have a high diagnostic accuracy in distinguishing between benign and malignant lesions in ovarian teratomas. Mature cystic teratomas with malignant degeneration and immature teratomas were determined to have a higher SUV than the benign teratomas. Additionally, FDG PET is useful in detecting metastases or peritoneal dissemination. Combining PET with MR provides even greater soft tissue characterization to distinguish benign from malignant pelvic lesions.

Suggested Reading

Outwater EK, Siegelman ES, Hunt JL. Ovarian teratomas: tumor types and imaging characteristics. Radiographics. 2001;21(2):475–90.

Yokoyama T, Takehara K, Yamamoto Y, Okame S, Shiroyama Y, Yokoyama T, et al. The usefulness of 18F-FDG PET/CT in discriminating benign from malignant ovarian teratomas. Int J Clin Oncol. 2015;20(5):960–6.

Case 79 Papillary Urothelial Neoplasm of the Bladder, Low Malignant Potential

Rajesh Gupta

History

A 75-year-old female presents with painless hematuria (Fig. 79.1).

Diagnosis

Papillary urothelial neoplasm of the bladder, low malignant potential (PUNLMP)

Findings

- Papillary mass is seen within the posterior bladder at the left uterovesicle junction which is isointense on T1, and hyperintense on T2 images (arrows).
- No abnormal focal hypermetabolism associated with this bladder lesion because of its low-grade malignant potential. The lesion is seen on PET as a "defect" with surrounding FDG urinary activity.
- No evidence of muscular invasion since T2 hypointense line of the detrusor muscle is intact.

Discussion

There are various subtypes of bladder cancer, with the most recognized type being invasive urothelial carcinoma, also referred to as transitional cell carcinoma. Non-invasive urothelial neoplasms are divided into flat and papillary subgroups. Papillary lesions of the bladder can be benign, have malignant potential, or contain low- or high-grade urothelial carcinoma identified within the lesion on histopathological analysis. The typical presenting symptom for bladder cancer is painless hematuria. Papillary urothelial neoplasm of low malignant potential (PUNLMP) occurs predominantly in the lateral and posterior walls of the bladder, close to the ureteral orifices. PUNLMPs recur in up to 30–40% of patients; however, disease progression and mortality are exceedingly rare.

On T2-weighted MR images, superficial or papillary bladder cancer lesions are hypo to isointense filling defects relative to the high signal intensity of urine. The detrusor muscle of the bladder wall appears as a hypointense line on T2-weighted images. Lesions that invade the muscularis propria of the bladder interrupt this

R. Gupta et al., *PET/MR Imaging*, https://doi.org/10.1007/978-3-319-65106-4_79

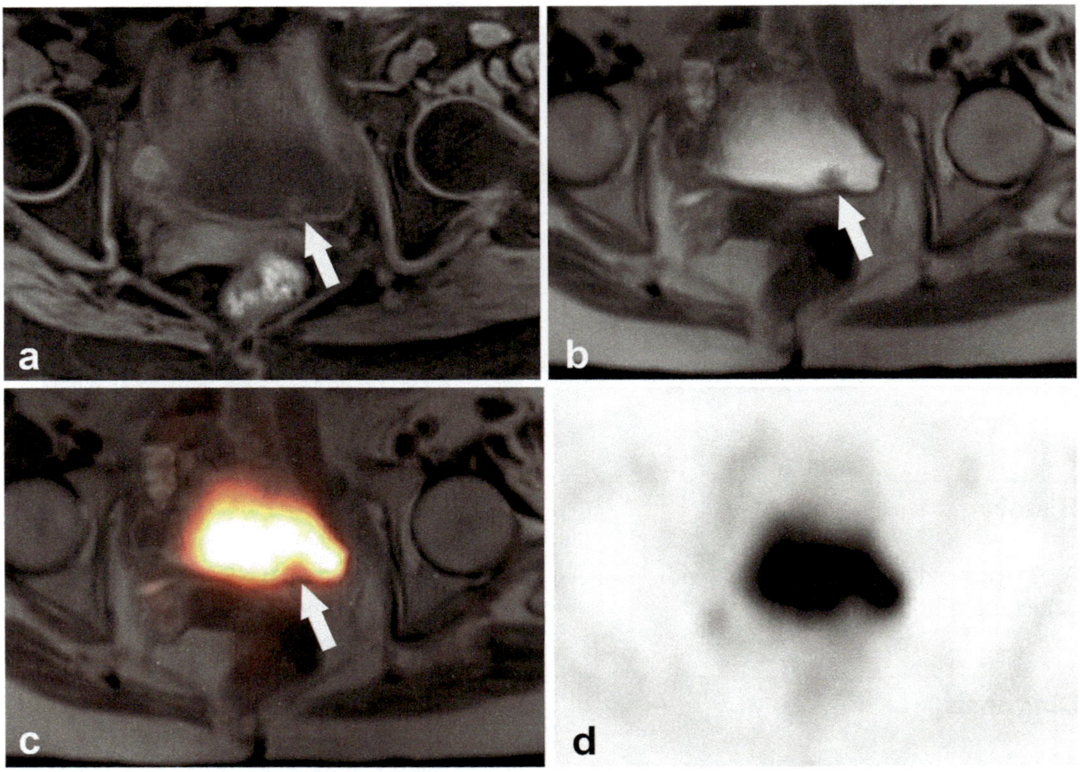

Fig. 79.1 T1 radial VIBE axial with fat saturation (**a**), T2 HASTE axial (**b**), PET/MR T2 HASTE axial fusion (**c**), and PET axial (**d**)

hypointense line on T2-weighted images. Bladder cancers are usually isointense on T1-weighted images. The bladder wall enhances slightly on dynamic contrast-enhanced MRI; however, bladder cancer lesions enhance earlier and more intensely. Extravesical disease that spreads to adjacent organs can be readily seen on both T1 and T2-weighted images on MRI. Evaluation of lymph nodes and bone marrow is best done through fat-saturated T1-weighted sequences.

Use of FDG PET is limited in the evaluation of primary bladder cancer due to interference of intensely radioactive luminal urine with assessment of the bladder wall lesions. PET in combination with MR is more useful in evaluating high-grade lesions, extravesical extension, and in particular nodal and distant metastases.

Suggested Reading

Bouchelouche K, Turkbey B, Choyke PL. PET/CT and MRI in bladder cancer. J Cancer Sci Ther. 2012;S14(1). pii: 7692.

Verma S, Rajesh A, Prasad SR, Gaitonde K, Lall CG, Mouraviev V, et al. Urinary bladder cancer: role of MR imaging. Radiographics. 2012;32(2):371–87.

Case 80
Adrenal Adenoma

Rajesh Gupta

History

An 85-year-old female with stage II sigmoid colon cancer presents for restaging 2 years after surgical resection (Fig. 80.1).

Diagnosis

Adrenal adenoma

Findings

- Left adrenal nodule that is isointense to muscle on both T1 and T2-weighted images (wide arrow).
- PET/MR fusion image demonstrates moderate increased FDG uptake in the left adrenal nodule greater than the liver.
- In-phase image shows isointense uptake (thin arrow) that drops in signal on the out-of-phase image (curved arrow) consistent with microscopic fat.
- Small hemorrhagic cyst in the left kidney that is hyperintense on T1-weighted image (arrowhead), hypointense on T2-weighted image, and demonstrates no FDG uptake.

Discussion

Adrenal adenomas are the most common adrenal mass lesion, found in 3% of patients at autopsy. They are benign fat-containing lesions that are usually incidentally found on abdominal imaging. The frequency of adrenal adenomas increases with age. The majority are non-functioning and therefore asymptomatic. Hyperfunctioning adrenal gland adenomas can manifest with symptoms corresponding to excess hormone secretion. Small, non-functioning adrenal adenomas do not require treatment.

Imaging plays a role in confirming the likely benignity of adrenal adenomas, and excluding malignancies and myelolipomas, another fat-containing adrenal lesion. Chemical shift imaging, with in and out-of-phased sequences, is sensitive to intravoxel fat, characteristic of adre-

R. Gupta et al., *PET/MR Imaging*, https://doi.org/10.1007/978-3-319-65106-4_80

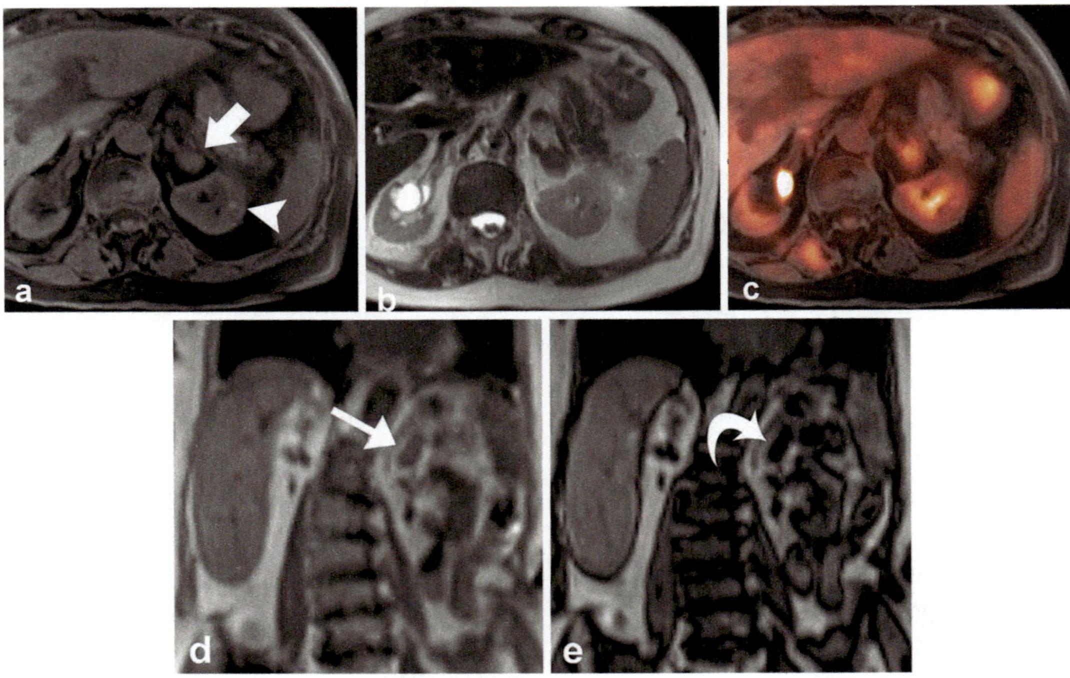

Fig. 80.1 T1 radial VIBE with fat suppression axial (**a**), T2 HASTE axial (**b**), PET/MR T1 radial VIBE with fat suppression axial fusion (**c**), Dixon T1-weighted in-phase coronal (**d**), and Dixon T1-weighted out-of-phase coronal (**e**)

nal adenomas. Lesions with intravoxel fat will drop in signal on out-of-phase sequences, where a drop greater than 20% is considered diagnostic for a benign adrenal adenoma. This lesion will not suppress on fat-saturated images, while on the other hand, myelolipoma contains macroscopic fat, and will suppress. Rarely, adrenal adenomas can contain foci of hemorrhage which will have varying T1 and T2 signal depending on its age. Adenomas typically demonstrate homogenous enhancement after contrast administration and do not exhibit restricted diffusion, whereas malignant adrenal lesions typically do. Adrenal adenomas are bilateral in 10–15% of the cases.

On FDG PET, adrenal adenomas usually have less uptake than the liver, with most demonstrating uptake less than maximum SUV of about 3.0. A maximum SUV in an adrenal nodule greater than 3.1 has a specificity for malignancy of 75.9% while SUV ratio of liver to nodule greater than 1.0 has a specificity for malignancy of 65.5%. Functional adenomas can have a higher degree of uptake compared to non-functioning ones. Malignant primary adrenal masses and metastases will usually have markedly increased FDG uptake and are typically larger in size than benign lesions. Because it may be difficult to differentiate benign from malignant adrenal lesions on FDG PET alone, PET/MR imaging can be very effective as it simultaneously includes MR characterization with chemical shift imaging. Importantly, the Dixon-based sequence is currently routinely used in PET/MR imaging for attenuation correction.

Suggested Reading

Blake MA, Holalkere NS, Boland GW. Imaging techniques for adrenal lesion characterization. Radiol Clin N Am. 2008;46(1):65–78. vi.

Dong A, Cui Y, Wang Y, Zuo C, Bai Y. (18)F-FDG PET/CT of adrenal lesions. AJR Am J Roentgenol. 2014;203(2):245–52.

Elsayes KM, Mukundan G, Narra VR, Lewis JS Jr, Shirkhoda A, Farooki A, et al. Adrenal masses: MR imaging features with pathologic correlation. Radiographics. 2004;24(Suppl 1):S73–86.

Case 81
Invasive Cancer of the Vulva

Rajesh Gupta

History

An 85-year-old woman with a history of hysterectomy presents with cancer of the vulvus (Fig. 81.1).

Diagnosis

Invasive cancer of the vulva

Findings

- T1-weighted images of the perineum show an isointense signal corresponding to an ovoid lesion of the vaginal introitus (wide arrow).
- T2-weighted sagittal images show a hyperintense signal of the vulvar lesion (curved arrow) that enhances following gadolinium contrast.
- PET/MR fusion demonstrates intense hypermetabolic activity in the lesion of the vaginal introitus.
- No uterus is visualized due to a prior hysterectomy.

Discussion

Vulvar cancer is an uncommon type of gynecologic cancer involving the external female genitalia, representing only 5–8% of all gynecological malignancies. Although the rate of invasive vulvar cancer has remained steady over the past two decades, the incidence of in situ disease has more than doubled. The most prevalent histologic subtype is squamous cell carcinoma, usually through HPV infection. Patients with vulvar cancer may present with pruritus, bleeding pain, and burning sensations. Lesions may be flat, raised, ulcerated, or plaque-like. Modes of spread include direct extension to adjacent organs, lymphatic spread to superficial inguinal nodes, and hematogenous dissemination late in the disease.

Imaging evaluation of vulvar cancer is performed to assess tumor size, local extension, pelvic lymph node involvement, and distant metastases. MRI is excellent at identifying soft tissue, vaginal, and rectal invasion that allows for accurate local staging of vulvar cancer. Both high-resolution T2-weighted sequence and T1-weighted images in the sagittal plane area are useful in determining the extent of tumor involvement.

R. Gupta et al., *PET/MR Imaging*, https://doi.org/10.1007/978-3-319-65106-4_81

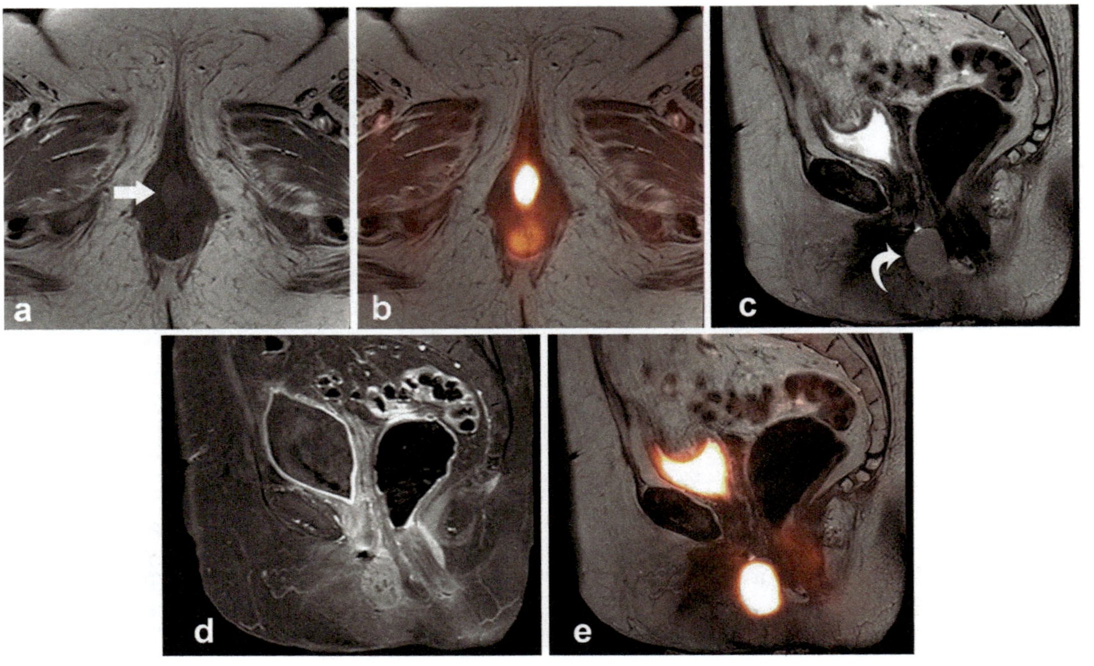

Fig. 81.1 T1-weighted axial perineum (**a**), PET/MR T1-weighted fusion axial perineum (**b**), T2-weighted sagittal pelvis (**c**), T1 TSE with fat suppression post-gadolinium contrast sagittal pelvis (**d**), and PET/MR T2-weighted sagittal pelvis fusion (**e**)

Vulvar cancer shows low signal or isointense signal on T1-weighted images and intermediate to high signal on T2-weighted images. Additionally, vulvar cancer shows contrast enhancement that adds to the detection of small tumors and helps determine involvement of adjacent structures. Axial T1-weighted pelvic images with a large field of view are used to identify metastatic regional lymph node including the inguinal lymph nodes as well as osseous involvement. The most commonly accepted size criteria for suspicious lymph node involvement is a short-axis diameter > 10 mm. Other features include irregular contour and necrotic changes within the node.

FDG PET/MR is useful in detecting nodal involvement and distant metastasis as well as soft tissue delineation of local extension. While normal size metastatic lymph node can be detected by PET, PET/MR helps to see necrotic nodes with less FDG avidity. Whole-body PET/MR imaging can detect retroperitoneal lymph nodes and other more distant lesions.

Suggested Reading

Cohn DE, Dehdashti F, Gibb RK, Mutch DG, Rader JS, Siegel BA, et al. Prospective evaluation of positron emission tomography for the detection of groin node metastases from vulvar cancer. Gynecol Oncol. 2002;85(1):179–84.

Kataoka MY, Sala E, Baldwin P, Reinhold C, Farhadi A, Hudolin T, et al. The accuracy of magnetic resonance imaging in staging of vulvar cancer: a retrospective multi-centre study. Gynecol Oncol. 2010;117(1):82–7.

Viswanathan C, Kirschner K, Truong M, Balachandran A, Devine C, Bhosale P. Multimodality imaging of vulvar cancer: staging, therapeutic response, and complications. AJR Am J Roentgenol. 2013;200(6):1387–400.

Case 82
Physiological FDG Uptake in the Uterus and Ovary

Jerrin Varghese and Amit Gupta

History

An 18-year-old female presents with lymphoma for staging (Fig. 82.1).

Diagnosis

Physiological FDG uptake in the uterus and ovary

Findings

- Physiological FDG uptake in the endometrium cavity with normal endometrial fluid on the T2 sequence (thin arrow).
- Physiological FDG uptake in the bilateral ovaries that contain small cysts in this premenopausal female (arrowheads).

Discussion

The uterus is a female reproductive organ and consists of an outer epithelial lining (serosa), an inner muscular layer (myometrium), and an inner epithelial layer (endometrium). The normal FDG uptake for the uterus depends upon many factors, including whether the patient is pre- or post-menopausal and at what point in the menstrual cycle imaging takes place. In postmenopausal women, the endometrium demonstrates lower FDG uptake, with an SUV <2. In premenopausal patients, the endometrium demonstrates the most increase uptake during the menstrual and ovulatory phases, with an SUV of about 5.0 and 3.7, respectively. The FDG uptake in premenopausal women on oral contraceptives is lower, and is similar to FDG uptake during proliferative and secretory phases on women not on oral contraceptives. The presence of intrauterine contraceptive devices does not significantly increase FDG uptake in the uterus.

Hormonal replacement therapy has been shown to increase the thickness of the endometrium. However, it does not significantly increase endometrial FDG uptake. Menstrual cycle abnormalities can create changes in uterine FDG uptake; for example, in oligomenorrhea FDG uptake can increase and resemble that of ovulatory phase, and amenorrhea decreases normal FDG uptake, resembling that of postmenopausal women. Knowledge of these normal physiological FDG uptake patterns is important to differentiate a benign process from endometrial cancer, which significantly increases uterine FDG uptake.

MRI of the uterus offers significant advantages over CT in its ability to differentiate the aforementioned layers of the uterus. In fact, it was the first technology capable of elucidating the "junctional zone," or the distinct inner myometrium, even ahead of its demonstration on light microscopy. On the T2-weighted image, the endometrium demonstrates high signal, the myome-

R. Gupta et al., *PET/MR Imaging*, https://doi.org/10.1007/978-3-319-65106-4_82

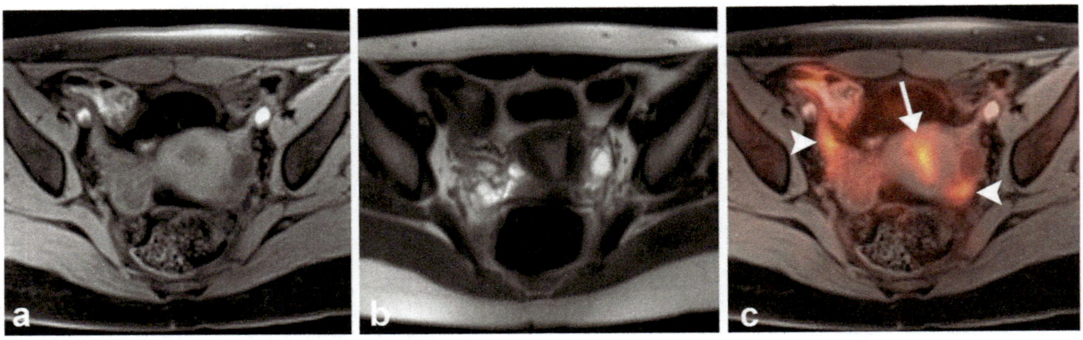

Fig. 82.1 T1 radial VIBE with fat suppression axial (**a**), T2 HASTE axial (**b**), and FDG PET/MR T1 radial VIBE with fat suppression axial (**c**)

trium demonstrates intermediate signal, and the junctional zone demonstrates relatively low signal. On T1 post-contrast images, the endometrium and myometrium enhance more avidly than the junctional zone. In adenomyosis, the low T2 signal junctional zone thickens over 12 mm, representing smooth muscle hypertrophy. Leiomyomas demonstrate low T2 signal, but can demonstrate high T1 signal if hemorrhagic. They enhance relatively less than surrounding myometrium. Endometrial cancer is isointense to surrounding endometrial tissue on T1 and mixed in signal on T2. On post-contrast imaging, it demonstrates avid enhancement with early washout. MRI is usually reserved for the staging of endometrial cancer.

The ovaries are the female reproductive organs responsible for ovulation and sex hormone production. In premenopausal women, increased FDG uptake can be seen in the ovulatory phase, and is therefore not very specific for malignancy. In postmenopausal women, however, increased ovarian uptake is fairly specific for malignancy, as the ovulatory phase no longer occurs.

Although ultrasound is the most common imaging modality for evaluation of ovarian and adnexal lesions, MRI boasts of superior specificity and its ability to differentiate benign from malignant adnexal lesions. On T1-weighted images, the normal ovaries demonstrate low to intermediate signal. On T2-weighted images, the ovarian follicles demonstrate relative increased signal. Ovarian cysts demonstrate expected high T2 signal and low T1 signal. Lesions containing fat such as teratomas demonstrate high signal on T1 and drop signal on T1 fat-saturated sequences. Lesions containing blood products such as endometriosis or hemorrhagic cysts will maintain high signal on T1 and T1 fat-saturated sequences. Lesions concerning for malignancy will demonstrate nodular enhancement and thick septations.

Suggested Reading

Iyer VR, Lee SI. MRI, CT, and PET/CT for ovarian cancer detection and adnexal lesion characterization. AJR Am J Roentgenol. 2010;194(2):311–21.

Lerman H, Metser U, Grisaru D, Fishman A, Lievshitz G, Even-Sapir E. Normal and abnormal 18F-FDG endometrial and ovarian uptake in pre- and postmenopausal patients: assessment by PET/CT. J Nucl Med. 2004;45(2):266–71.

Novellas S, Chassang M, Delotte J, Toullalan O, Chevallier A, Bouaziz J, et al. MRI characteristics of the uterine junctional zone: from normal to the diagnosis of adenomyosis. AJR Am J Roentgenol. 2011;196(5):1206–13.

Case 83
Renal Cell Carcinoma

Robert Matthews

History

A 53-year-old male presents with laryngeal cancer for restaging after surgical excision (Fig. 83.1).

Diagnosis

Renal cell carcinoma (chromophobe)

Findings

- Large mass in the right kidney which is heterogenous but predominantly hypointense on a T1-weighted image, as compared to the renal parenchyma (wide arrow) and mildly hyperintense on T2-weighted images.
- Central stellate scar is hyperintense on T2-weighted images (arrowhead).
- PET/MR fusion image shows abnormal heterogenous FDG uptake within the renal mass with abnormal uptake in the stellate scar.
- CT scan shows lack of enhancement in the central stellate scar (thin arrow).
- Overall findings may be seen in both chromophobe renal cell carcinoma and renal oncocytoma.

Discussion

Chromophobe renal cell carcinoma (CRCC) is the third most common type of renal cell carcinoma comprising between 4 and 10% of all renal cell carcinomas (RCC). It usually appears as a solitary, non-capsulated mass that is larger than most RCC and often presents in the sixth decade of life. In general, CRCC has a better prognosis than more typical RCC. CRCC has two types, eosinophilic and mixed type, where the eosinophilic variant has many histological and macroscopic features that are similar to RCC.

Renal oncocytoma is the second most common benign renal tumor comprising 3–7% of all renal neoplasms. These are most commonly detected between 40 and 69 years of age and have an average size of 6 cm at presentation. Most cases are asymptomatic and are discovered incidentally. There are usually unilateral, but may be bilateral in 5% of cases, and can occur at the same time as renal cell carcinoma.

On MRI, both chromophobe renal cell carcinoma and renal oncocytoma have overlapping features. The most common of these features is a central stellate fibrous scar that does not enhance following gadolinium contrast. This appears in 45% of renal oncocytomas. CRCC often also has

R. Gupta et al., *PET/MR Imaging*, https://doi.org/10.1007/978-3-319-65106-4_83

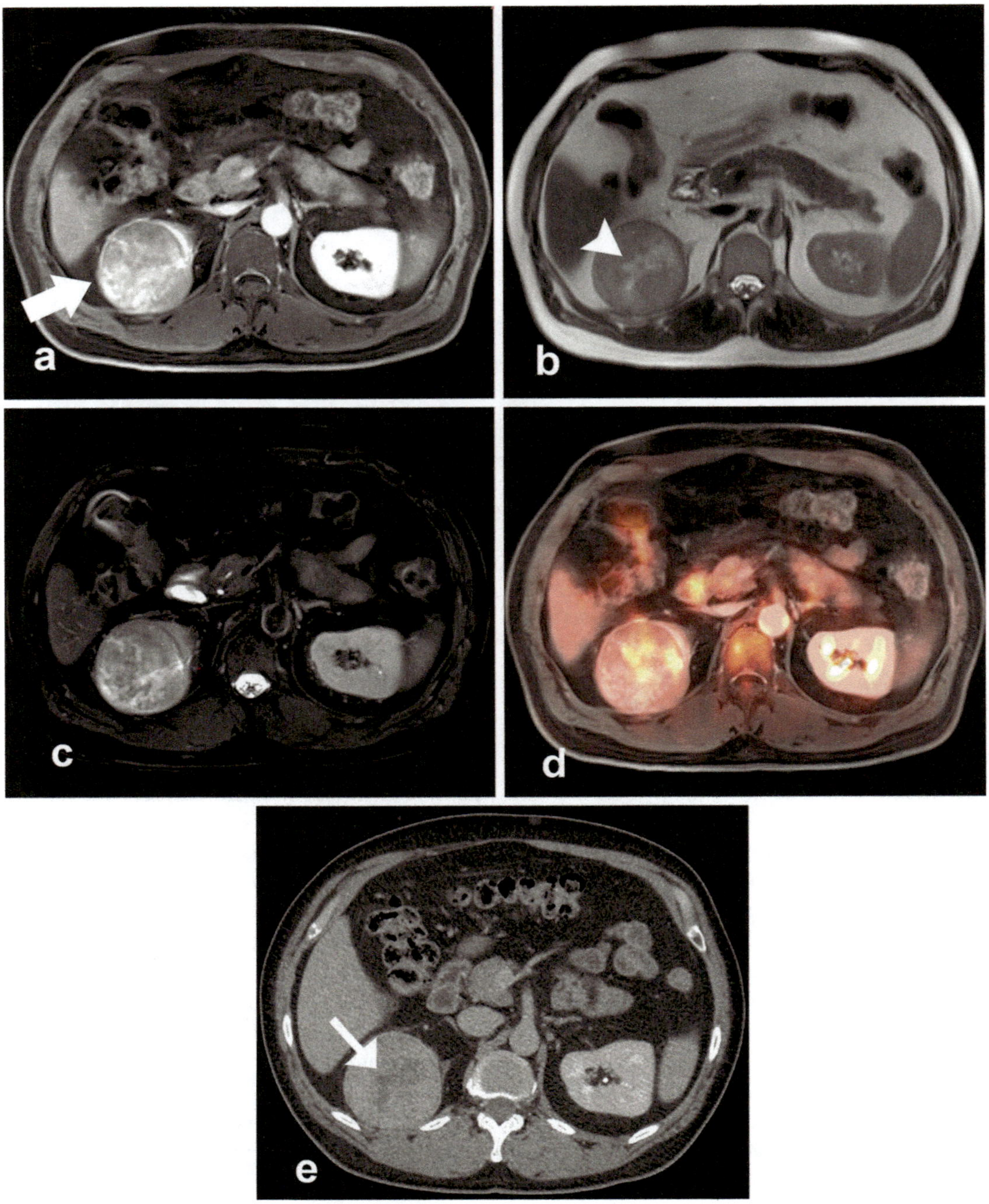

Fig. 83.1 T1 radial VIBE with fat suppression axial (**a**), T2 HASTE axial (**b**), T2 BLADE with fat suppression axial (**c**), PET/MR T1 radial VIBE with fat suppression axial fusion (**d**), and CT scan with delayed contrast enhancement axial (**e**)

a central stellate fibrous scar in 23% of cases and may also display central necrosis that can simulate appearance of a scar. Both CRCC and renal oncocytomas are typically located in the periphery of the kidney, and may demonstrate areas of hemorrhage, T2 hyperintensity with a quarter being homogenous, and both may enhance following contrast. Both tumors are usually well-circumscribed lesions but uncommonly may show perinephric fat invasion.

On FDG PET/MR imaging, uptake of FDG in renal oncocytoma ranges from very intense to background level uptake which is usually in a heterogeneous pattern. FDG uptake in RCC may also range from very intense to no appreciable uptake. FDG PET in detection of primary RCC has a sensitivity of 60–75% and a specificity of 80–100%. RCC that have a higher grade tend to have higher FDG uptake. Part of the difficulty in detecting RCC with PET is the physiological excretion of FDG through the urinary system. Giving a diuretic such as furosemide to allow the kidneys to wash out the tracer may improve detection. PET/MR does play an important role in the detection of recurrent RCC as well as metastatic disease especially since higher grade lesions are more like to recur and metastasize.

Suggested Reading

Kochhar R, Brown RK, Wong CO, Dunnick NR, Frey KA, Manoharan P. Role of FDG PET/CT in imaging of renal lesions. J Med Imaging Radiat Oncol. 2010;54(4):347–57.

Rosenkrantz AB, Hindman N, Fitzgerald EF, Niver BE, Melamed J, Babb JS. MRI features of renal oncocytoma and chromophobe renal cell carcinoma. AJR Am J Roentgenol. 2010;195(6):W421–7.

Case 84
Urinoma: Urinary Fistula

Rajesh Gupta

History

A 50-year-old male with metastatic rectal cancer presents for restaging following coloproctectomy, bladder repair, and chemoradiotherapy (Fig. 84.1).

Diagnosis

Urinoma—urinary fistula

Findings

- T2-weighted image shows a hyperintense fluid collection posterior to the bladder with a Foley catheter. The fluid collection is layered indicating debris (arrow).
- T1 image show contrast enhancement between the bladder and fluid collection indicating inflammation (arrowheads).
- PET/MR fusion demonstrates intense FDG activity within the hyperintense portion of the fluid collection with SUV 74 indicating the presence of radioactive urine.
- A fistula tract containing radioactive urine is identified connecting the urinoma with the inferior aspect of the bladder (curved arrow).

Discussion

Urinomas contain collections of urine, usually found in the retroperitoneum, outside of the normal pathway that urine travels. Within the retroperitoneum, they most commonly occur in the perirenal space secondary to urinary obstruction. Other causes include surgery, trauma, or diagnostic instrumentation. Damage to the kidneys, ureter, or bladder during abdominal or pelvic surgery can result in a urinoma as a leakage from a technically inadequate or dehisced anastomosis of the urinary system. In renal transplants, urinary leak occurs in 1–5% of cases, with technical error of the anastomosis occurring usually in the first week and ischemia of the ureter as a cause of the leak after the first week.

Typical clinical presentations of a urinoma include sensations of pressure and pain due to mass effect on adjacent structures. They may be asymptomatic and found incidentally on imaging. Urinomas may be secondarily infected leading to fever and elevated white blood cell count. Ultrasound and CT can readily identify a fluid collection; however, the delineation between a urinoma from seroma or abscess may be difficult. Contrast-enhanced CT is more effective at determining a urinoma as it can detect the flow of urine into the collection on delayed images.

R. Gupta et al., *PET/MR Imaging*, https://doi.org/10.1007/978-3-319-65106-4_84

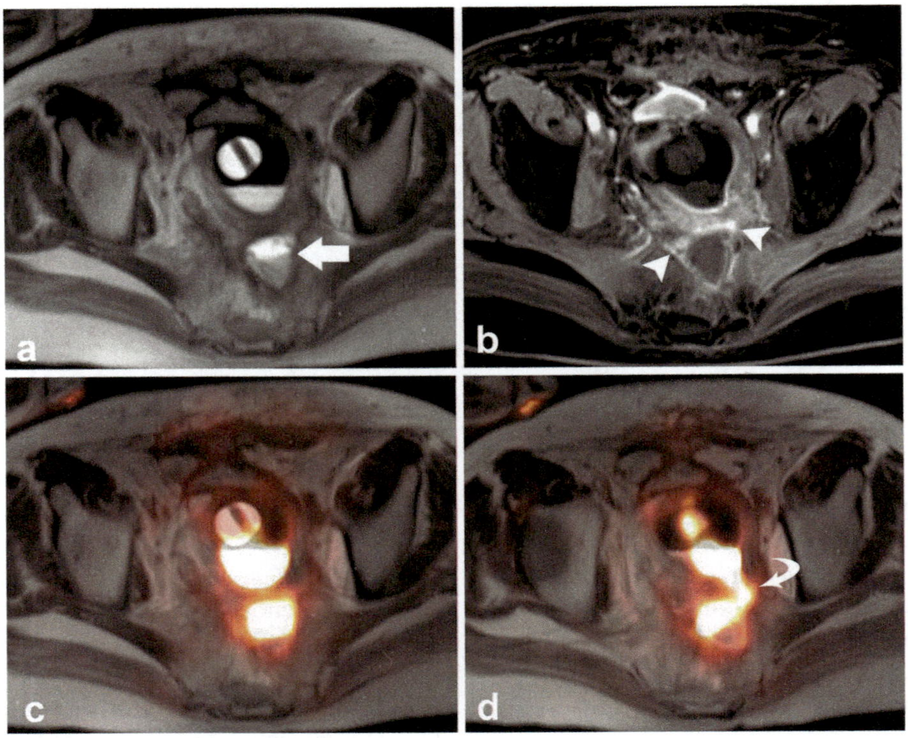

Fig. 84.1 T2-weighted images of the axial pelvis (**a**), T1 VIBE with fat suppression post-gadolinium contrast axial pelvis (**b**), PET/MR T2-weighted axial pelvis fusion (**c**), and PET/MR T2-weighted axial pelvis fusion at a more superior level (**d**)

Although MRI is rarely used to diagnose urinomas, its increased contrast resolution can identify a fistulous connection to the bladder and suggest infected fluid collections with contrast enhancement and surrounding inflammation. Direct tests such as cystography, CT cystograms, or ureterograms may be required to identify leaks with direct contrast injection.

PET imaging may be useful in confirming a urinoma by assessing the degree of radioactivity of the fluid collection in comparison to the radioactive urine within the bladder. A PET/MR system can better determine precise anatomical location, enhancement characteristics, and potential fistulous connections or leaks. Otherwise, the PET avid collection could be mistaken for hypermetabolic lymphadenopathy or mass. PET studies may also prove to be useful in follow-up to evaluate for resolution of the urinoma.

Suggested Reading

Lee J, Darcy M. Renal cysts and urinomas. Semin Interv Radiol. 2011;28(4):380–91.

Sanchez MJ, Caride VJ. Incidental, early diagnosis of urinoma by F-18 FDG PET/CT. Clin Nucl Med. 2005;30(2):102–4.

Yu NC, Raman SS, Patel M, Barbaric Z. Fistulas of the genitourinary tract: a radiologic review. Radiographics. 2004;24(5):1331–52.

Case 85
Endometrial Polyps and Tamoxifen-Associated Changes

Rajesh Gupta

History

A 67-year-old female with breast cancer, treated with surgery and radiation therapy, and on tamoxifen treatment (Fig. 85.1).

Diagnosis

Endometrial polyps and tamoxifen-associated changes

Findings

- T1-weighted image shows a low signal dilated endometrial canal.
- T2-weighted image demonstrates heterogeneous signal intensity within the endometrial canal representing endometrial thickening and polyps (arrow).
- PET/MR fusion demonstrates no abnormal FDG activity. Intense physiological bladder activity is seen in the left pelvis.
- Incidental note is made of multiple small T2-weighted hyperintense nabothian cysts in the cervix (curved arrow).

Discussion

Tamoxifen is a SERM (Selective Estrogen Receptor Modulator) used for antiestrogen hormonal therapy in patients with breast cancer that have estrogen-positive receptors. As a side effect tamoxifen has pro-estrogenic effects on the endometrium, causing increased prevalence of endometrial changes including hyperplasia, polyps, and carcinoma. As many as 50% of breast cancer patients treated with this medication develop an endometrial lesion within the first 3 years.

One of the main concerns with tamoxifen use is the propensity to cause endometrial dysplasia and carcinoma, which can be easily assessed by pelvic MRI. The normal endometrium appearance and thickness varies greatly depending on the patient's reproductive age and menses timing. On MRI, tamoxifen may cause the endometrium to appear thickened, irregular, and cystic. However, another MR imaging pattern that has been described represents endometrial atrophy or proliferative changes. This is characterized by homogenous high T2-weighted signal, contrast enhancement of the endometrium–myometrium junction, and T1-weighted

R. Gupta et al., *PET/MR Imaging*, https://doi.org/10.1007/978-3-319-65106-4_85

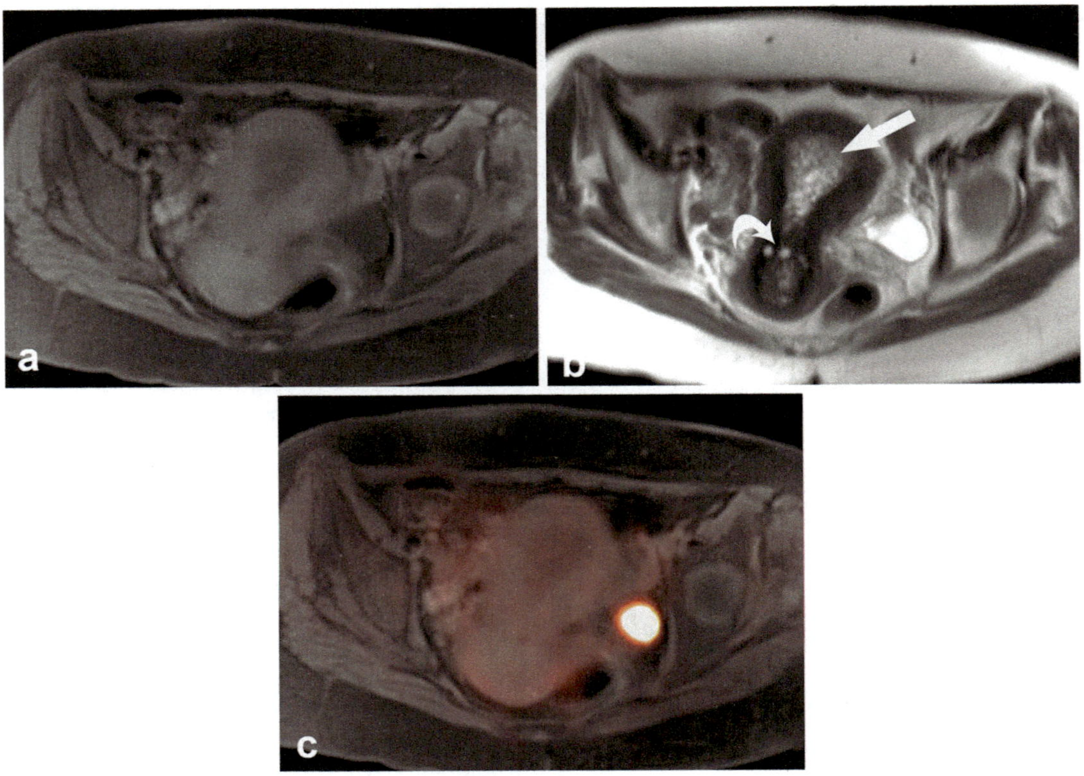

Fig. 85.1 T1 radial VIBE with fat suppression axial pelvis (**a**), T2 HASTE axial pelvis (**b**), and PET/MR T1 radial VIBE axial pelvis fusion (**c**)

signal void in the endometrial lumen. Alternatively, heterogeneous endometrial T2-weighted signal and lattice-like enhancement throughout the endometrial canal has been found to be associated with polyps.

FDG PET can be useful to avoid a false-positive interpretation of endometrial malignancy, especially when fused with MR to provide a more precise anatomic localization. Endometrial FDG uptake varies throughout the menstrual cycle, being increased at the ovulatory and menstrual phases and decreased following menopause. Hormonal therapy has not been found to influence endometrial FDG uptake.

Suggested Reading

Lerman H, Metser U, Grisaru D, Fishman A, Lievshitz G, Even-Sapir E. Normal and abnormal 18F-FDG endometrial and ovarian uptake in pre- and postmenopausal patients: assessment by PET/CT. J Nucl Med. 2004;45(2):266–71.

Nalaboff KM, Pellerito JS, Ben-Levi E. Imaging the endometrium: disease and normal variants. Radiographics. 2001;21(6):1409–24.

Case 86
Prostate Cancer

Rajesh Gupta

History

A 76-year-old male presents with gross hematuria and urinary incontinence with brachytherapy for prostate cancer 14 years ago (Fig. 86.1).

Diagnosis

Recurrent prostate cancer

Findings

- Bulky soft tissue mass involves the prostate gland and surrounds the base of the bladder with high T2-weighted signal and post contrast enhancement.
- Mass extends posteriorly to invade the anterior wall of the rectum (arrow).
- Susceptibility artifacts within the prostate gland on the T1 image represent brachytherapy seeds (arrowheads).
- PET/MR fusion images show avid FDG uptake compatible with recurrent malignancy.

Discussion

Prostate cancer is the second most common cancer in men worldwide. The use of PSA screening has increased the frequency of prostate biopsies and the diagnosis of prostate of cancer. Symptoms are nonspecific and include urinary frequency, urgency, nocturia, and hesitancy. The primary indication to perform an MRI after a biopsy-proven diagnosis of cancer is to evaluate for extracapsular extension. It may also identify suspicious areas for biopsy in a patient with an elevated PSA.

The prostate gland is comprised of the peripheral zone, central zone, and the transitional zone. The peripheral zone accounts for 70% of the prostate volume and is the most common site where adenocarcinoma arises. On T1-weighted images, the prostate gland appears homogenously medium signal intensity in all zones. With an endorectal coil, T2-weighted images of the prostate zones are well delineated but are more difficult to see with body or pelvic coils. T1-weighted images are acquired to depict post biopsy hemorrhage, tumor infiltration of the peri-prostatic fat, and metastatic disease in the pelvic lymph nodes. T2-weighted images of prostate cancer show an area of decreased signal intensity relative to the normally high signal intensity in the peripheral zone. Detection of small prostate cancer tumors is more difficult in the transitional and central zones because of normal heterogenous T2 signal. Prostate cancer may have early nodular enhancement and early washout on dynamic contrast-enhanced MR imaging. Diffusion-weighted imaging is usually useful since prostate cancer often shows restricted diffusion.

R. Gupta et al., *PET/MR Imaging*, https://doi.org/10.1007/978-3-319-65106-4_86

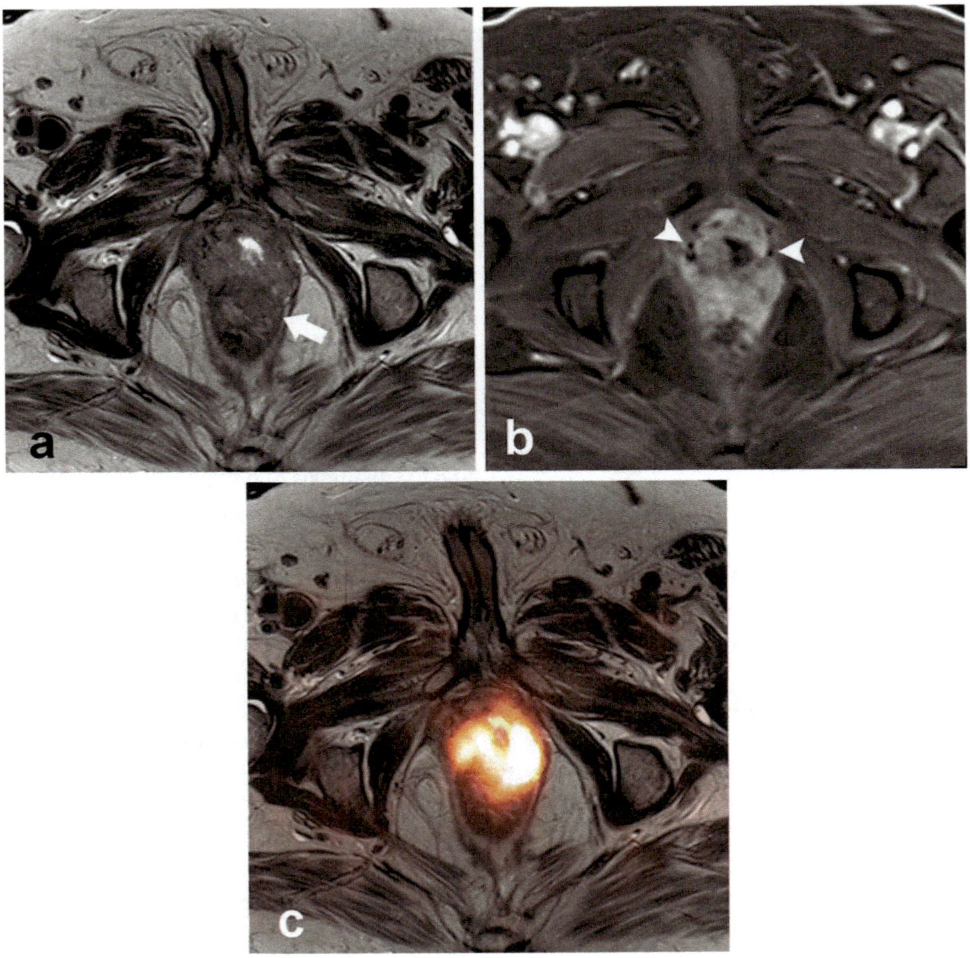

Fig. 86.1 T2-weighted axial perineum (**a**), T1 VIBE with fat suppression post gadolinium contrast axial perineum (**b**), and PET/MR T2-weighted axial perineum fusion (**c**)

FDG PET imaging has limited value in the assessment of low grade or early prostate cancer. The degree of uptake in the prostate gland can vary both by age and individually. Early prostate cancer may have only mild relative increased uptake and false-positive findings include benign prostatic hyperplasia and prostatitis. FDG PET imaging is very useful at detecting pelvic lymph node involvement and distant metastases in more aggressive forms of cancer. Accurate registration of PET/MR would allow better detection of invasive prostatic cancer. The use of newer PET agents such as C-11 and F-18 labeled amino acids, and Ga-68 and F-18 labeled PSMA (prostate-specific membrane antigen) ligands offers superior prostate cancer evaluation including initial staging and detection of recurrent disease.

Suggested Reading

Hricak H, Choyke PL, Eberhardt SC, Leibel SA, Scardino PT. Imaging prostate cancer: a multidisciplinary perspective. Radiology. 2007;243(1):28–53.

de Perrot T, Rager O, Scheffler M. Potential of hybrid ^{18}F-fluorocholine PET/MRI for prostate cancer imaging. Eur J Nucl Med Mol Imaging. 2014;41(9):1744–55.

Case 87
Colovaginal Fistula

Rajesh Gupta

History

A 54-year-old female with cervical cancer presents for restaging having history of left psoas abscess (Fig. 87.1).

Diagnosis

Colovaginal fistula

Findings

- T2-weighted images with fat suppression show a fluid collection in the left pelvic sidewall, which demonstrates low signal on T1-weighted images wide arrows. This fluid collection communicates with the sigmoid colon and vaginal lumen through the left fornix.
- T2-weighted images also show a moderately hyperintense signal adjacent to the fluid collection representing inflammation (curved arrows).
- PET/MR fusion images demonstrate moderate hypermetabolism in the area of inflammation.

Discussion

Colovaginal fistula refers to a communication between the colon and the vagina. It is most commonly associated with complicated diverticular disease, but can also be caused by gynecologic malignancy, inflammatory bowel disease, trauma, or following pelvic radiotherapy. Radiation-related fistulas most commonly involve the sigmoid colon or rectum, and in these cases recurrent cancer must be ruled out. Women may present with feces, flatus, or mucus per the vagina, as well as, abdominal pain, fever, and systemic toxicity.

MRI is ideal for demonstrating genitourinary fistulas as it can distinguish between the fistula's fluid contents and its wall. Thin fluid-weighted images in all three planes are needed and must be carefully assessed. MRI can demonstrate the fistula's location and morphology guiding surgical management. It has the important ability to detect areas of abscesses and secondary fistula extension. Fat-suppressed T2-weighted MRI sequences are essential to identify fluid containing tracts and sites of infection. T1-weighted images are excellent for anatomic overview. Active infection

R. Gupta et al , *PET/MR Imaging*, https://doi org/10.1007/978-3-319-65106-4_87

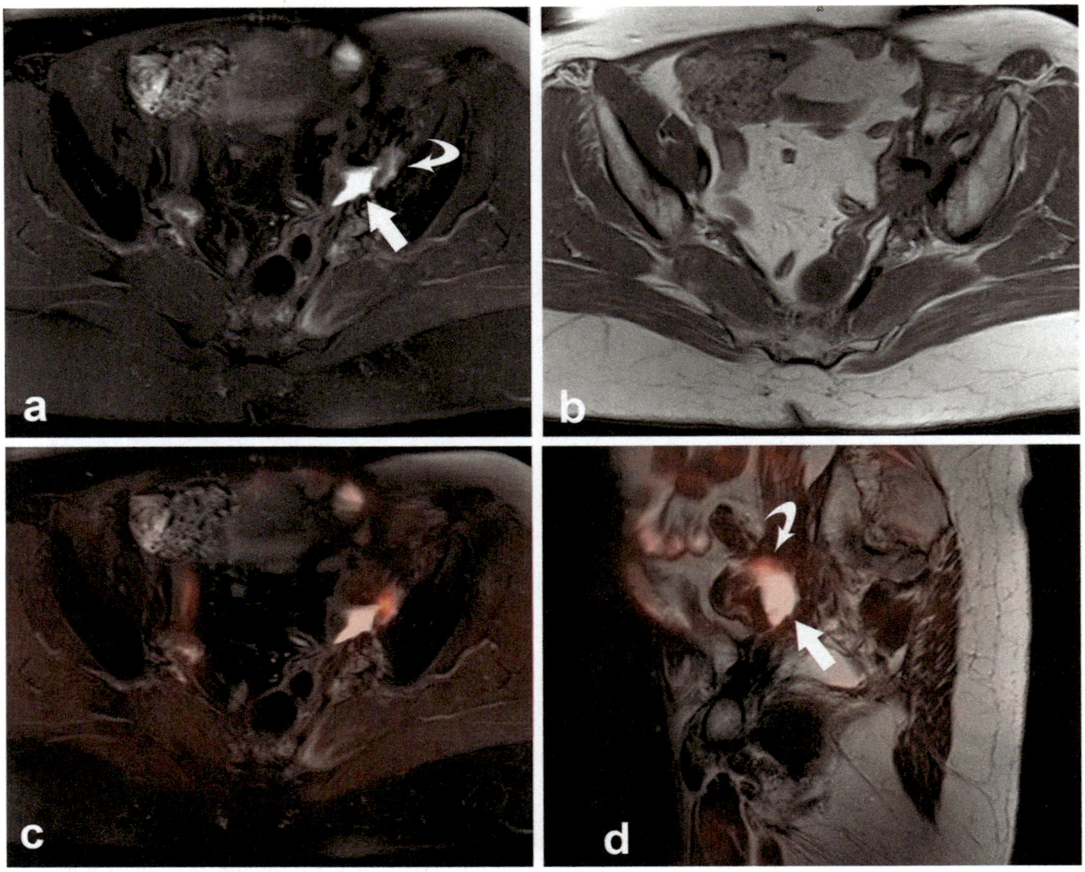

Fig. 87.1 T2-weighted with fat suppression axial pelvis (**a**), T1-weighted axial pelvis (**b**), PET/MR T2-weighted with fat suppression axial pelvis fusion (**c**), and PET/MR T2-weighted sagittal pelvis fusion (**d**)

and granulation tissue demonstrate intense contrast enhancement.

FDG PET imaging is a valuable tool in assessing for active inflammation or infection at the site of fistulation, and can reliably exclude negative cases. PET imaging can elucidate causes of fistulas including recurrent neoplasm and active infection. The combined benefit of PET/MR provides an early detection of fistulas, provide an accurate and precise assessment of the fistula tract, and identify secondary complications of fistulas.

Suggested Reading

Tang YZ, Booth TC, Swallow D, Shahabuddin K, Thomas M, Hanbury D, et al. Imaging features of colovesical fistulae on MRI. Br J Radiol. 2012;85(1018):1371–5.

Vaidyanathan S, Patel CN, Scarsbrook AF, Chowdhury FU. FDG PET/CT in infection and inflammation—current and emerging clinical applications. Clin Radiol. 2015;70(7):787–800.

Yu NC, Raman SS, Patel M, Barbaric Z. Fistulas of the genitourinary tract: a radiologic review. Radiographics. 2004;24(5):1331–52.

Case 88
Seroma: Post-Operative

Rajesh Gupta

History

A 36-year-old female with cervical cancer treated by surgical resection (Fig. 88.1).

Diagnosis

Seroma: post-operative

Findings

- Fluid collection (curved arrow) within the right subcutaneous gluteal tissues, which is hypointense on T1-weighted image and hyperintense on the T2-weighted image. The rim of the collection is hyperintense on T1.
- PET/MR fusion image shows mild hypermetabolism consistent with inflammation.
- Within this seroma, there are globular areas of low T1 and T2 signals, which represent an organized hematoma.

Discussion

Seromas are collections of serous fluid that may accumulate as a complication of surgery or after trauma. Identifying distinct imaging characteristics for seromas can be useful when attempting to differentiate it from soft tissue sarcomas or abscesses. Post-operative seromas are relatively well-defined lesions of low to intermediate T1-weighted signal intensity and high signal intensity on T2-weighted images. Often times, globular areas of low T2-weighted signal can be identified which usually represents organized hematomas or granulation tissue. An abscess will also demonstrate low T1-weighted and high T2-weighted signal on MRI. However, other differentiating characteristics include intense ring enhancement post contrast administration and diffusion restriction. It has been reported that follow-up imaging for seromas should not be performed in less than 3-month intervals to allow adequate time for resolution.

R. Gupta et al., *PET/MR Imaging*, https://doi.org/10.1007/978-3-319-65106-4_88

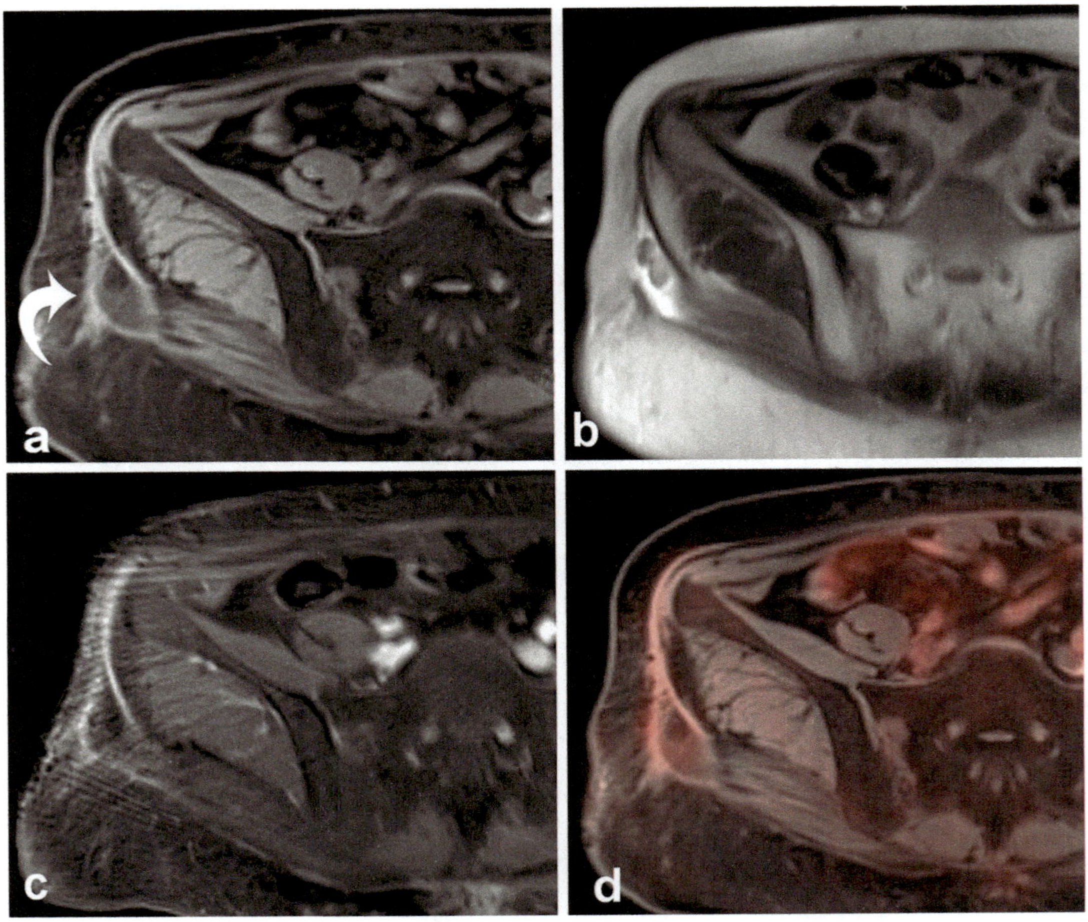

Fig. 88.1 T1 radial VIBE with fat suppression axial pelvis (**a**), T2 HASTE axial pelvis (**b**), T1 radial with fat suppression post gadolinium contrast axial pelvis (**c**), and PET/MR T1 radial VIBE with fat suppression axial pelvis fusion (**d**)

FDG PET/MR is an excellent modality to distinguish between a benign seroma versus a malignant soft tissue sarcoma or abscess as it provides precise anatomic localization and can quantify hypermetabolic activity. While benign or noninfected seromas may have mild hypermetabolic activity due to inflammation, the activity should regress over time. On the other hand, an abscess or malignant lesion will show intense FDG uptake. Previous studies have shown FDG PET/CT to have a sensitivity of 93% in differentiating benign fluid collections from soft tissue sarcomas. Statistically significant differences have been found in the maximum SUV of soft tissue sarcomas and benign fluid collections on PET.

Suggested Reading

Amini B, Madewell JE, Chuang HH, Haygood TM, Hobbs BP, Fox PS, et al. Differentiation of benign fluid collections from soft-tissue sarcomas on FDG PET/CT. J Cancer. 2014;5(5):328–35.

Poon-Chue A, Menendez L, Gerstner MM, Colletti P, Terk M. MRI evaluation of post-operative seromas in extremity soft tissue sarcomas. Skelet Radiol. 1999;28(5):279–82.

Case 89
Uterine Leiomyomas

Rajesh Gupta

History

A 71-year-old female with postmenopausal bleeding and cervical cancer (Fig. 89.1).

Diagnosis

Uterine leiomyomas

Findings

- The uterus is enlarged and contains multiple leiomyomas.
- Largest fibroid is isointense on T1-weighted images with low signal peripherally, low signal on T2-weighted images, and shows no contrast enhancement compatible with a hyaline-degenerated fibroid (wide arrow).
- More superior fibroid is isointense on the T1-weighted image, low signal on the T2-weighted image, and enhances homogenously following contrast (curved arrow).
- PET/MR fusion image shows absence of FDG uptake in the necrotic fibroid while the more superior fibroid has uptake equal to the surrounding normal uterine tissue.

Discussion

Uterine leiomyomas, also called fibroids, are the most common benign uterine neoplasm. Leiomyomas are composed of smooth muscle. They are usually incidental findings on imaging, but can sometimes cause diagnostic difficulties. Fibroids typically occur in women of reproductive age. They are responsive to hormones and commonly grow during pregnancy and involute with menopause. Presenting symptoms may include abnormal uterine bleeding, pain, and infertility but they are most often asymptomatic. Within the uterus, fibroids most commonly have an intramural location, but may be subserosal or submucosal in location. They often undergo hyaline degeneration with other types of cystic, hemorrhagic, or myxoid changes. Malignant transformation into leiomyosarcoma is rare.

The most accurate imaging technique to detect, localize, and characterize fibroids is MRI. Typically, non-degenerated leiomyomas are well-circumscribed homogenous masses with decreased T2 signal intensity compared to the outer myometrium and low to intermediate signal on T1-weighted images. They have variable contrast enhancement. Fibroids that have undergone hyaline degeneration have low T2 signal

R. Gupta et al., *PET/MR Imaging*, https://doi.org/10.1007/978-3-319-65106-4_89

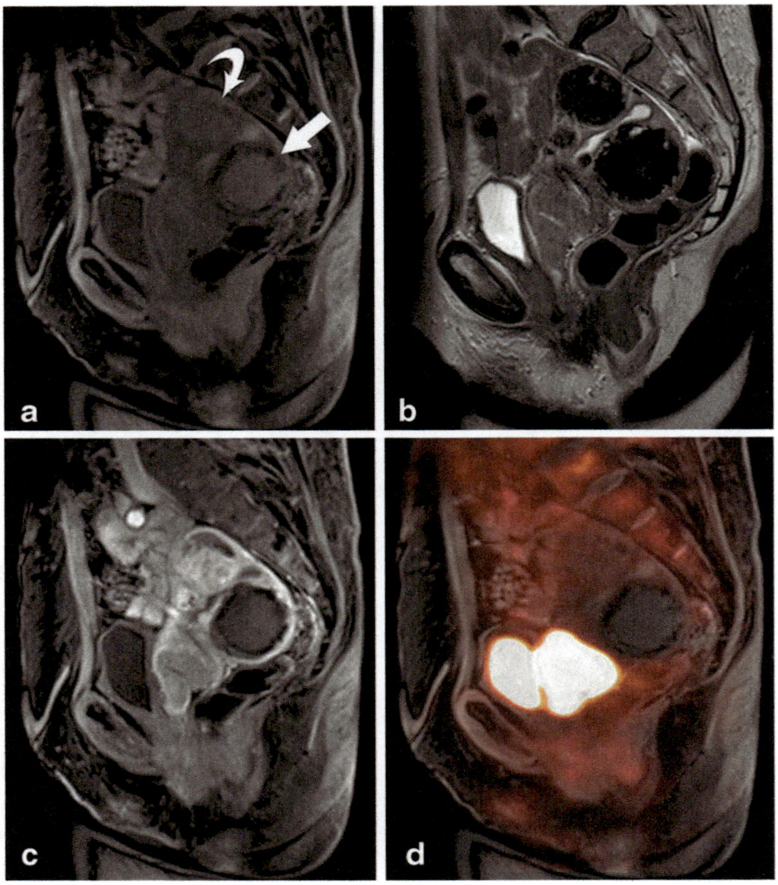

Fig. 89.1 T1 VIBE with fat saturation sagittal pelvis (**a**), T2-weighted sagittal pelvis (**b**), T1 VIBE with fat suppression post-gadolinium contrast sagittal pelvis (**c**), and PET/MR T1-weighted with fat saturation sagittal fusion (**d**)

similar to non-degenerated ones. Those that have undergone cystic degeneration usually have high signal on T2 sequences, although their appearance can be variable. Hemorrhagic degeneration is characteristically identified through peripheral or diffuse high signal intensity on T1-weighted images. Leiomyomas with myxoid degeneration show mild gradual contrast enhancement and markedly high signal on T2-weighted images.

Leiomyomas usually have mild to absent FDG PET uptake, but can infrequently show moderate to intense uptake. The exact mechanism for FDG accumulation in benign lesions such as fibroids is unclear but likely related to multiple factors including hormonal control, cellularity, vascularity, as well as variability in growth factor and receptor expression. FDG uptake within fibroids is more common in premenopausal women and also higher in the luteal phase of the menstrual cycle. FDG PET alone cannot reliably distinguish between leiomyomas and leiomyosarcomas as both can have mild to high uptake, however combined PET/MR allows for more reliable characterization.

Suggested Reading

Kitajima K, Murakami K, Kaji Y, Sugimura K. Spectrum of FDG PET/CT findings of uterine tumors. AJR Am J Roentgenol. 2010;195(3):737–43.

Murase E, Siegelman ES, Outwater EK, Perez-Jaffe LA, Tureck RW. Uterine leiomyomas: histopathologic features, MR imaging findings, differential diagnosis, and treatment. Radiographics. 1999;19(5):1179–97.

Case 90
Invasive Small Cell Bladder Cancer

Robert Matthews and Rajesh Gupta

History

A 61-year-old female presents for restaging following resection of left renal cell cancer (Fig. 90.1). Recent ultrasound showed severe right hydronephrosis and a bladder mass.

Diagnosis

Invasive small cell bladder cancer with lymph node metastasis

Findings

- T2-weighted images show a large heterogeneous hyperintense pelvic mass (asterisks) invading the detrusor muscle of the bladder with disruption of the T2 hypointense line (black arrowheads).
- T1 radial VIBE images show the mass involving the uterus with indistinct margins (white arrowheads) as well as invasion of the rectum (arrow). There is an enlarged right external iliac lymph node (curved arrow).
- Corresponding PET/MR fusion image shows intense hypermetabolic activity in the mass and lymph node with an additional small metastatic focus in the displaced uterus.
- STIR images show the large size of the right-sided pelvis mass with hyperintense signal and increased FDG activity.

Discussion

Bladder cancer is the most common malignancy arising from the urinary tract, the fourth most common cancer in males and the tenth most common cancer in females, with the average age at the time of diagnosis being 73. Risk factors for developing bladder cancer include tobacco smoke, occupational exposure to certain chemicals, arsenic in drinking water, and chronic bladder inflammation. The major type of bladder cancer is transitional cell carcinoma comprising 9 out of 10 cases. Use of cyclophosphamide as a chemotherapy agent increases the risk for transitional cell carcinoma. Small cell carcinoma of the bladder is a very rare, poorly differentiated neuroendocrine epithelial type of cancer estimated at 0.7% of all bladder cancers. It carries a poor prognosis usually being diagnosed at an advanced stage, and less than 10% 5-year survival rate. The most common presenting symptoms of small cell bladder cancer is gross hematuria, dysuria, and occasionally urinary obstruction.

MRI is excellent at localizing and assessing intramural tumor invasion and adjacent organ

R. Gupta et al., *PET/MR Imaging*, https://doi.org/10.1007/978-3-319-65106-4_90

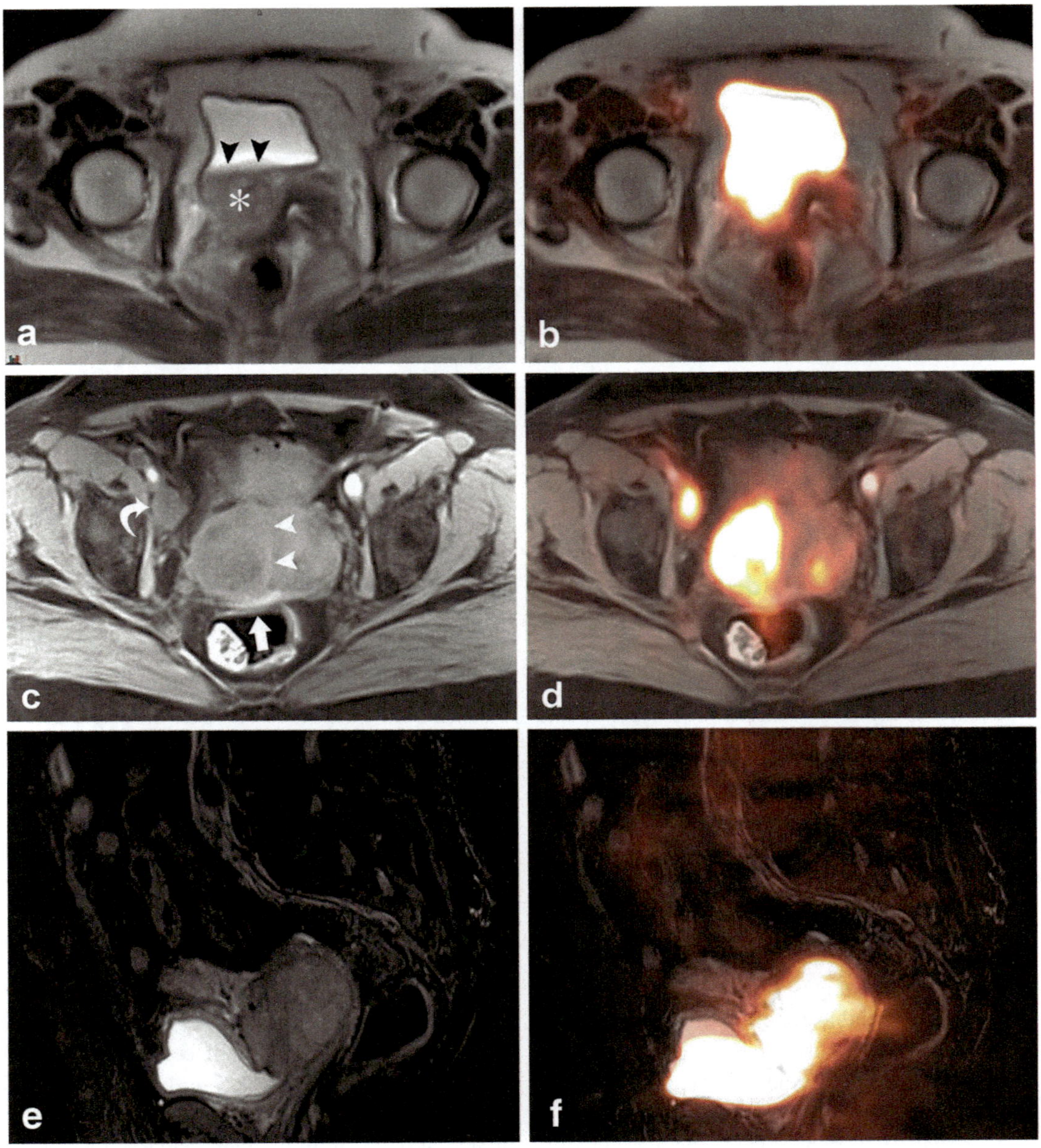

Fig. 90.1 T2-weighted axial pelvis (**a**), PET/MR T2-weighted axial pelvis fusion (**b**), T1 radial VIBE fat-suppressed axial pelvis (**c**), PET/MR T1 radial VIBE fat-suppressed axial pelvis fusion (**d**), STIR sagittal pelvis (**e**), and PET/MR STIR sagittal pelvis fusion (**f**)

involvement. For best results on MRI imaging, the bladder should be moderately full as under distension or over distension of the bladder may hide lesions. When there is invasive bladder cancer on MRI, the normal T2-weighted hypointense detrusor muscle of the bladder wall appears interrupted by tumor. On extravesical spread of bladder cancer, the mass would be seen outside the bladder on the T2-weighted images. For extravesical fat infiltration, T1-weighted images are better suited for early invasion. T1 is also valuable for intraluminal detection of tumor which may be causing urinary obstruction. With contrast-enhanced T1 sequences invasive bladder would show early focal wall enhancement due to its increased vascularity, although normal mucosa and submucosa also enhance early. T2-weighted and STIR images better depicts tumor invasion of the prostate gland, uterus, and vagina because of the high signal of the cancer making it easier to be seen.

Although FDG PET is limited in the evaluation of non-invasive bladder cancer because of the difficulty-discerning uptake from the adjacent bladder activity, PET is useful when assessing aggressive tumors with local extension and metastatic spread. PET/MR in particular can help to identify small metastatic lymph nodes, pelvic sidewall metastases, recurrence around wounds and interventional tracks, and distant metastatic spread to liver, lung, bone, adrenal gland, and intestine. It is also helpful following surgical and radiation treatment where interpretation by MRI alone can be difficult.

Suggested Reading

Bouchelouche K, Turkbey B, Choyke PL. PET/CT and MRI in bladder cancer. J Cancer Sci Ther. 2012;S14(1). pii: 7692.

Lohrisch C, Murray N, Pickles T, Sullivan L. Small cell carcinoma of the bladder: long term outcome with integrated chemoradiation. Cancer. 1999;86(11):2346–52.

Verma S, Rajesh A, Prasad SR, Gaitonde K, Lall CG, Mouraviev V, et al. Urinary bladder cancer: role of MR imaging. Radiographics. 2012;32(2):371–87.

Case 91
Bladder Cancer Causing Hydronephrosis in Patient with Duplicated Collecting System

Rajesh Gupta

History

A 61-year-old female with severe right hydronephrosis on recent ultrasound and resection of left renal cell cancer (Fig. 91.1).

Diagnosis

Bladder cancer causing hydronephrosis in patient with duplicated collecting system

Findings

- T1 image shows hydronephrosis with parenchymal thinning and dilation of the proximal right ureter. The right renal collecting system has increased signal compared to low signal on the normal left side indicating hemorrhagic and proteinaceous debris.
- PET/MR fusion image shows lack of radiotracer activity in the right collecting system due to renal obstruction.
- T2-weighted and PET/MR fusion images in the coronal view show a dilated duplicated collecting system (arrowheads). A hypermetabolic bladder mass is seen in the bladder causing the renal obstruction consistent with cancer (curved arrow). The normal left renal collecting system shows physiological FDG excretion.
- Hypermetabolic right paraaortic metastatic lymph node is seen on the PET/MR axial image.

Discussion

Obstructive uropathy can be caused by a variety of pathologies including kidney stones, bladder cancer, pelvic malignancies, blood clots, papillary necrosis, and others. Symptoms include abnormal urine flow, hematuria, renal dysfunction, and flank pain. Obstruction may not be completely apparent on CT or renal ultrasound. However, the kidney may experience progressive damage if the urinary flow is not reestablished by stent, tumor removal, or other appropriate treatment.

Renal obstruction may be detected incidentally on PET/MR while evaluating malignancy involving the pelvis. T2-weighted images may demonstrate a dilated urinary collecting system with the hydroureter or hydronephrosis leading to the site of renal obstruction. Dilatation must be distinguished from T2 bright cysts and perinephric fat on non-fat-suppressed images. If there is longstanding obstruction then the T1 signal may become bright as in this case. T1- and T2-weighted images are also used to assess renal parenchymal changes including thinning of the cortex.

R. Gupta et al., *PET/MR Imaging*, https://doi.org/10.1007/978-3-319-65106-4_91

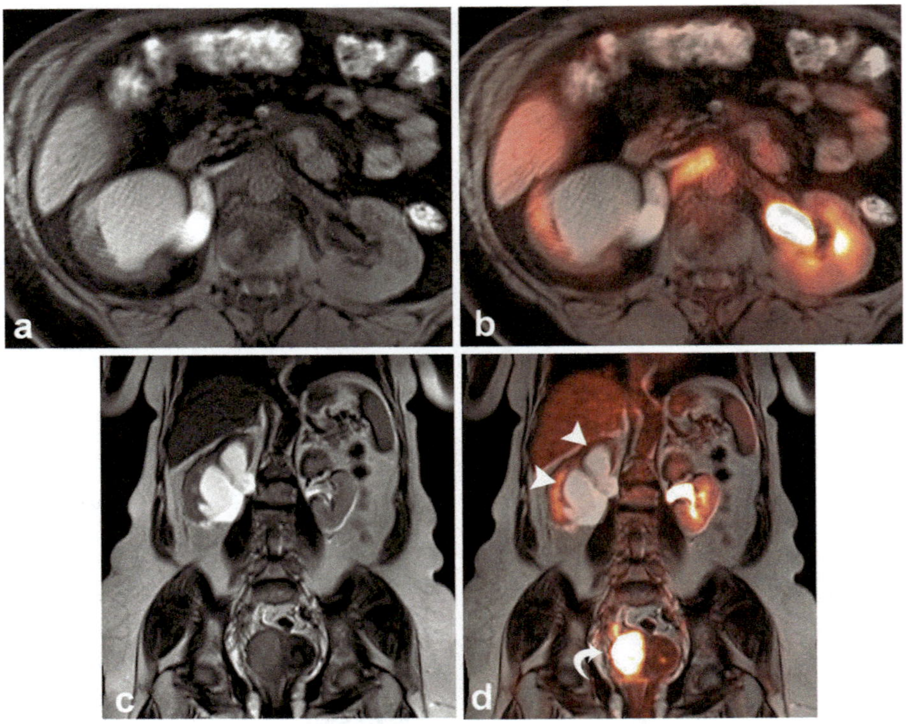

Fig. 91.1 T1 radial VIBE axial with fat suppression (**a**), PET/MR T1 radial VIBE with fat suppression axial fusion (**b**), T2 TSE coronal (**c**), and PET/MR T2 TSE fusion coronal (**d**).

Duplicated renal collecting systems characterized by incomplete fusion of the upper and lower renal pole moieties are usually asymptomatic but can be prone to infection, reflux, or obstruction. Dedicated magnetic resonance urography with gadolinium contrast provides more definite evaluation of urinary tract obstruction and duplicated renal collecting system.

In FDG PET examinations, the radiotracer is physiologically excreted by the kidneys through the urinary system resulting in radioactive urine within the renal collecting system, ureters, and bladder. This can provide information on both renal function and excretory state. In this case, the right duplicated collecting system and ureters are dilated and show no significant FDG activity compared to the left side. This finding is consistent with obstruction of the distal right ureter, related to a large right-sided bladder cancer. Lasix can be given for confirmation of the renal obstruction with delayed PET imaging.

Suggested Reading

Adeb M, Darge K, Dillman JR, Carr M, Epelman M. Magnetic resonance urography in evaluation of duplicated renal collecting systems. Magn Reson Imaging Clin N Am. 2013;21:717–30.

Nikken JJ, Krestin GP. MRI of the kidney- state of the art. Eur Radiol. 2007;17:2780–93.

Case 92
Recurrent Prostate Cancer with Fluciclovine

Ana M. Franceschi and Robert Matthews

History

A 56-year-old male referred for restaging with rising PSA and Gleason score 4 + 5 prostate diagnosed 2 years ago. He has received CyberKnife treatment and is currently on hormonal therapy hormonal therapy (Fig. 92.1).

Diagnosis

Recurrent prostate cancer detected by fluciclovine

Findings

- T1 mildly hypointense enlarged right pelvic side wall lymph node (wide white arrow) that shows homogenous contrast enhancement.
- PET/MR fusion image shows increased radiotracer uptake in the pelvic side wall lymph node compatible with metastasis.
- More superior level image shows an additional metastatic right internal iliac lymph node with increased activity (curved white arrow).
- PET MIP shows increased radiotracer in the pelvic side wall lymph node (thin black arrow) and right internal iliac lymph node (black arrowhead).

Discussion

Fluciclovine is a radiotracer recently approved by the FDA which is indicated for PET imaging in men with suspected prostate cancer recurrence based on elevated blood prostate-specific antigen (PSA) levels, and treated by hormone therapy or castrate-resistant prostate cancer. Two amino acid transporter systems located on the plasma membrane that are overexpressed by prostate cancer are L amino acid transporters (LAT) and alanine-cysteine transporters (ASCT). LAT is associated with higher Gleason score and poor survival, and ASCT with more aggressive tumor behavior. Fluciclovine is a F-18 tagged analog of the amino acid L-leucine that is taken up by through LAT and ASCT.

Fluciclovine is utilized as part of a whole-body PET/MR imaging protocol and aids in the detection of local, lymph node, and bone relapse of metastatic prostate cancer. The low uptake in the kidneys and urinary tract aids in detecting

R. Gupta et al., *PET/MR Imaging*, https://doi.org/10.1007/978-3-319-65106-4_92

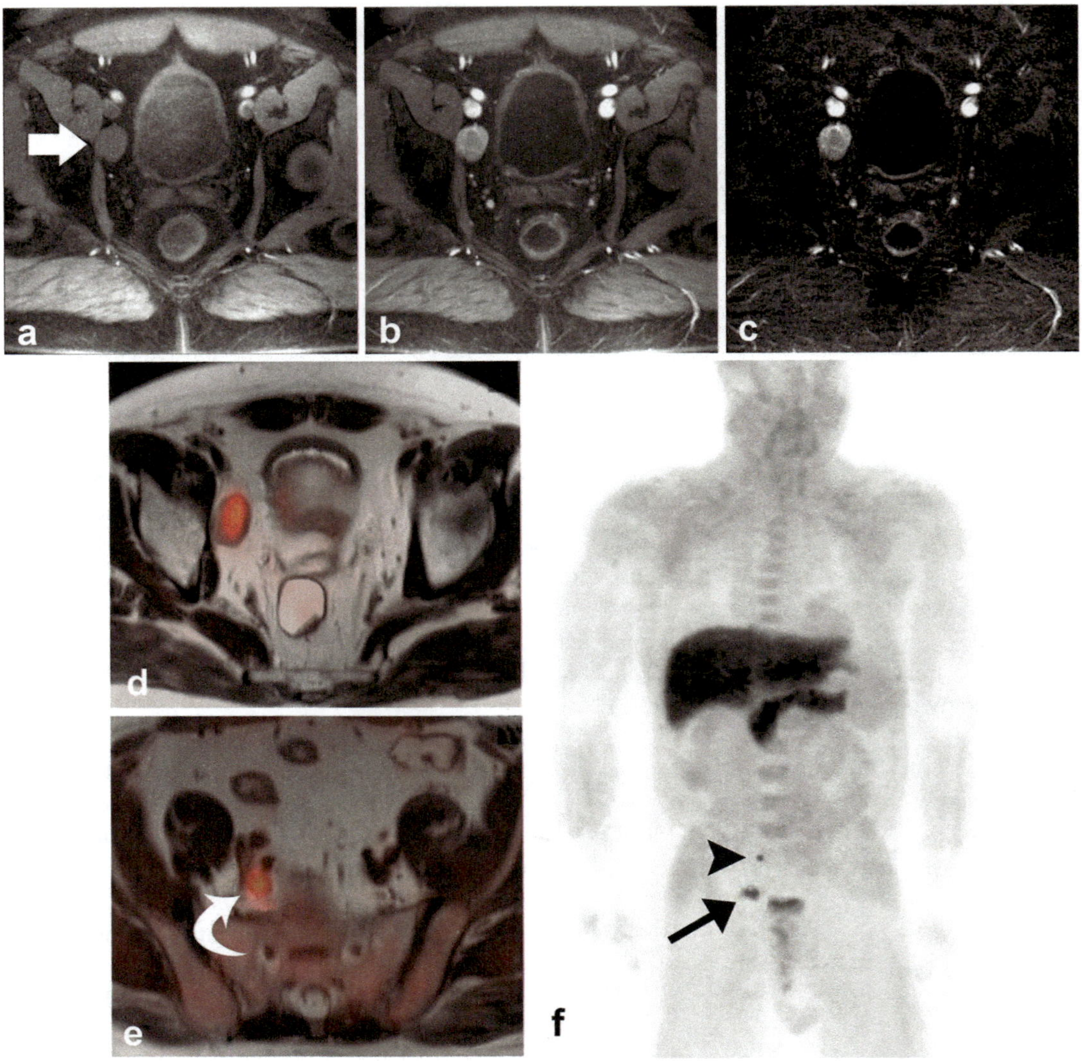

Fig. 92.1 T1 radial VIBE with fat suppression axial (**a**), T1 radial VIBE with fat suppression post-gadolinium contrast axial (**b**), Digital subtraction of gadolinium contrast axial (**c**), PET/MR T2 axial fusion (**d**), PET/MR T2 axial fusion, more superiorly (**e**), and PET MIP (**f**)

prostate bed recurrences. There is also low uptake in the brain which may be useful for the detection of brain metastases. The intense liver and pancreatic uptake might hinder detection in these organs. Though recurrent prostate cancer is typically a slowly progressive, relatively indolent disease process, it is important to identify those patients with rapid disease progression who are in need of more aggressive treatment measures. Abnormal fluciclovine scans revealing metastatic lesions, positively correlate with the PSA levels in the blood, although the exact PSA level on when to perform a scan has yet to be determined. Even with a negative nuclear bone scan, osseous metastatic lesions can be detected by fluciclovine scans. Therefore, fluciclovine is useful in patients who are in need of a systemic imaging tool which can detect metastatic disease with a high degree of sensitivity and specificity.

Several recent publications have determined that fluciclovine is an alternative radiotracer with superior results when compared to C-11 choline in the setting of patients with biochemical relapse after radical prostatectomy. In animal models, fluciclovine demonstrated higher radiotracer uptake in the lesions compared to other radiolabeled amino acids such as C-11 choline, C-11 methionine, and C-11 acetate. Furthermore, it has been shown that the results of fluciclovine PET imaging studies influenced radiotherapy management decisions in patients with recurrent prostate cancer. Clinical trials aiming to assess for differences in PSA-free survival are currently underway.

Suggested Reading

Nanni C, Schiavina R, Brunocilla E, Boschi S, Borghesi M, Zanoni L, Pettinato C, Martorana G, Fanti S. 18F-fluciclovine PET/CT for the detection of prostate cancer relapse: a comparison to 11C-choline PET/CT. Clin Nucl Med. 2015;40(8):e386–91.

Schuster DM, Nanni C, Fanti S. Evaluation of prostate cancer with radiolabeled amino acid analogs. J Nucl Med. 2016;57(Suppl 3):61S–6S.

Schuster DM, Nanni C, Fanti S. PET tracers beyond FDG in prostate cancer. Semin Nucl Med. 2016;46(6):507–21.

Testa C, Pultrone C, Manners DN, Schiavina R, Lodi R. Metabolic imaging in prostate cancer: where we are. Front Oncol. 2016;6:225.

Case 93
Endometrial Cancer

Rajesh Gupta and Apar Gupta

History

A 49-year-old female with abnormal vaginal bleeding found to have a uterine mass on ultrasound (Fig. 93.1).

Diagnosis

Endometrial cancer (undifferentiated adenocarcinoma) with metastatic lymph node

Findings

- A large, ill-defined mass is seen infiltrating the endometrium and myometrium with extension into the cervix. It is hyperintense on T2-weighted images, isointense on T1-weighted images, and demonstrates heterogeneous enhancement.
- Post contrast image demonstrates a dilated endometrial canal with non-enhancing heterogeneous material representing debris and blood (asterisk).
- PET/MR fusion and PET images show this mass to be hypermetabolic consistent with endometrial cancer. An FDG avid metastatic lymph node, without MR characteristics of malignancy, is seen (arrow).

Discussion

Endometrial cancer emanates from the inner lining of the uterus. It is the most common type of uterine cancer. Adenocarcinoma is the most common histological type of endometrial cancer. Patients may present with abnormal frequency and quantity of menstrual bleeding, abdominal pain, or vaginal discharge after menses.

On T1-weighted MRI, endometrial carcinoma is isointense to the normal endometrium. Endometrial carcinoma is hyperintense or heterogeneous on T2-weighted images. Dynamic contrast-enhanced MRI imaging improves accuracy for detecting myometrial invasion. The normal inner myometrium shows avid enhancement earlier than the outer myometrium. Endometrial cancer generally enhances earlier than normal endometrium but later than the adjacent myometrium. T1-weighted imaging is useful for evaluation of local pelvic lymph nodes and retroperitoneal involvement, as in all pelvic malignancies.

Because normal endometrium can have significant FDG activity especially during menses, use of PET is limited in evaluating the primary endometrial lesion. On PET/MR imaging, seeing structural MRI changes in the uterus in conjunction with PET findings allows for better lesion characterization. PET is helpful in identifying

R. Gupta et al., *PET/MR Imaging*, https://doi.org/10.1007/978-3-319-65106-4_93

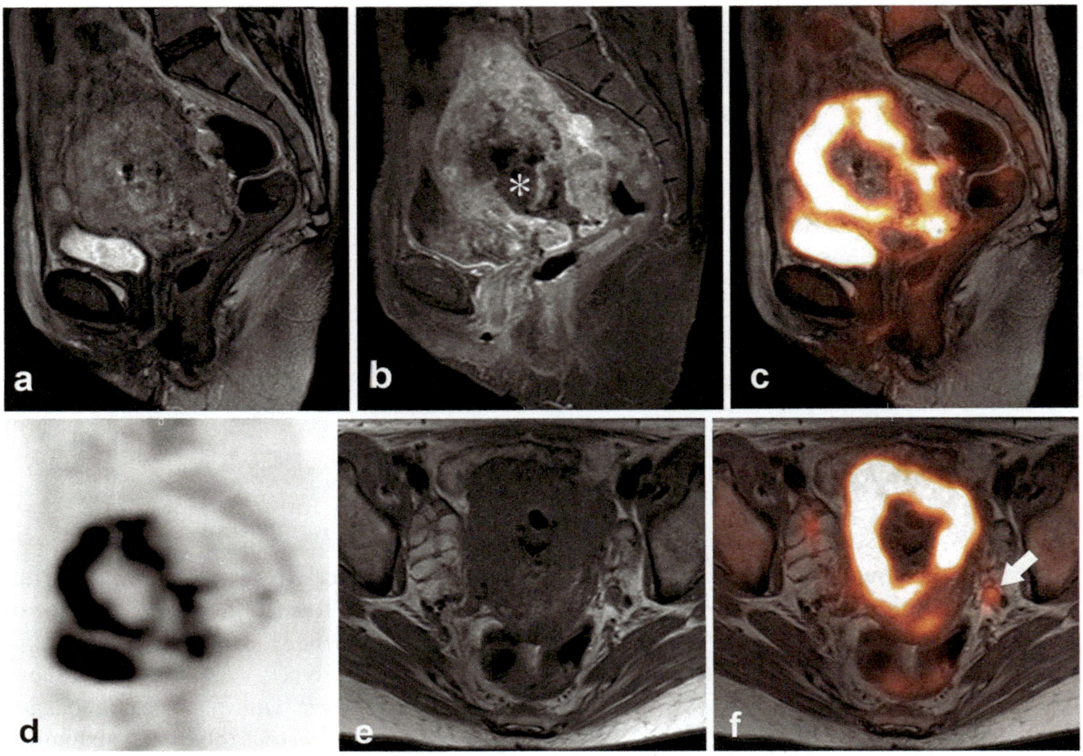

Fig. 93.1 T2-weighted sagittal pelvis (**a**), T1 TSE with fat suppression post-gadolinium contrast sagittal pelvis (**b**), PET/MR T2-weighted sagittal pelvis fusion (**c**), PET sagittal pelvis (**d**), T1 VIBE axial pelvis (**e**), and PET/MR T1 VIBE axial fusion (**f**)

lymph node metastases with higher sensitivity and specificity than MRI alone, especially in normal size lymph nodes. PET/MR has increased diagnostic accuracy when the primary tumor or enlarged lymph nodes measure at least 10–12 mm. PET/MR allows also for assessment of distant metastatic lesion localization, especially at unusual sites, such as the supraclavicular region, mediastinum, bone, and intramuscular spaces which contributes to overall tumor staging. PET is also useful in detecting recurrent lesions when post therapy changes may confound MRI findings.

Suggested Reading

Nogami Y, Iida M, Banno K, Kisu I, Adachi M, Nakamura K, et al. Application of FDG PET in cervical cancer and endometrial cancer: utility and future prospects. Anticancer Res. 2014;34(2):585–92.

Sala E, Wakely S, Senior E, Lomas D. MRI of malignant neoplasms of the uterine corpus and cervix. AJR Am J Roentgenol. 2007;188(6):1577–87.

Part V

Head and Neck

Case 94
Orbital Rhabdomyosarcoma

James Bai and Lev Bangiyev

History

A 14-year-old female developed swelling of left eyelid 2 weeks ago (Fig. 94.1).

Diagnosis

Orbital rhabdomyosarcoma

Findings

- MRI shows a predominantly extraconal, left well-defined left orbital mass that is T1 hypointense, T2 hyperintense (wide white arrow), and exhibits homogeneous enhancement
- There is mass effect with medial and superior displacement of the inferior rectus muscle (black arrowhead)
- The mass demonstrates increased signal on DWI with corresponding decreased signal on ADC maps indicating increased cellularity (curved arrows)
- PET/MRI fusion shows increased FDG uptake consistent with malignancy

Discussion

Rhabdomyosarcoma is the most common pediatric soft tissue sarcoma, and has a predilection for the head and neck area. The majority of tumors occur in children younger than 10 years of age. The tumor originates from striated muscle and is considered a high-grade malignancy. The clinical presentation largely depends on the location of the tumor as well as presence or absence of metastases. Histologically, rhabdomyosarcomas can be divided into three major groups: embryonal, alveolar, and pleomorphic. The most aggressive of the three types is alveolar, which affects older children and accounts for approximately 15% of cases. The embryonal type has the best prognosis. It occurs in younger children and accounts for 70% of cases.

There are three major locations of head and neck rhabdomyosarcoma: parameningeal, non-parameningeal, and orbital. Given the deep-seated location and proximity to vital structures of skull base, the parameningeal tumors have the worst prognosis with 5-year survival ranging between 64% and 73%. Imaging is essential for the initial evaluation to establish tumor location and extent, and guiding tissue biopsy. Imaging also plays a

R. Gupta et al., *PET/MR Imaging*, https://doi.org/10.1007/978-3-319-65106-4_94

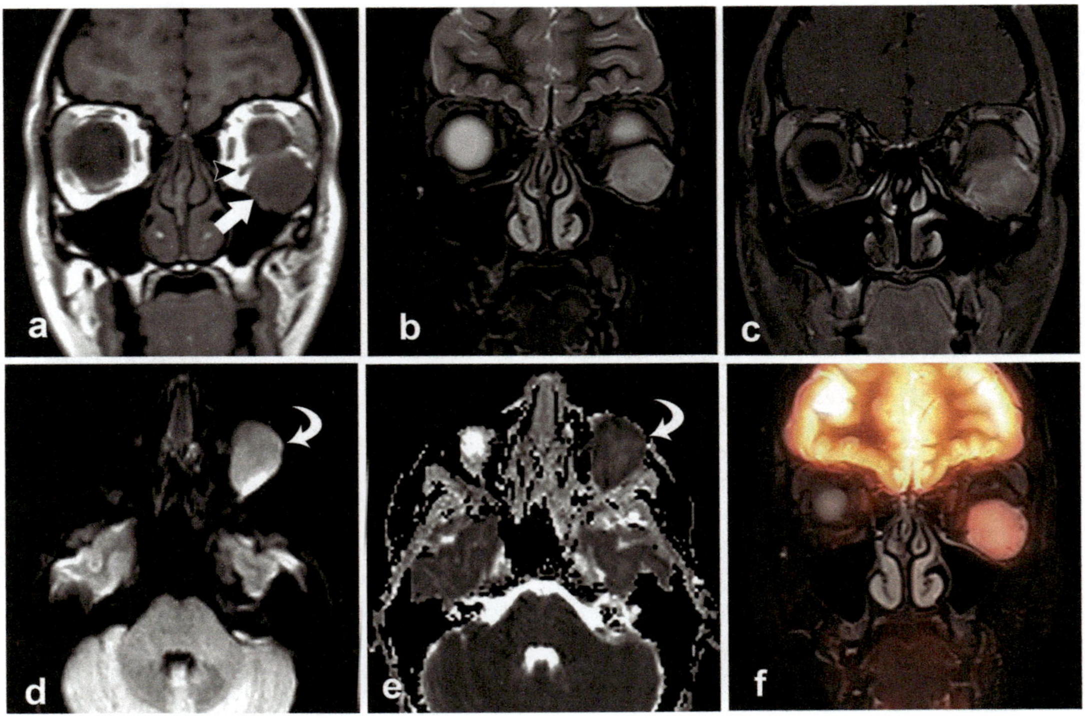

Fig. 94.1 T1 coronal (**a**), STIR coronal (**b**), T1 with fat suppression post-gadolinium contrast coronal (**c**), diffusion-weighted imaging axial (**d**), apparent diffusion coefficient axial (**e**), and PET/MRI STIR coronal fusion (**f**).

major role in assessing treatment response and tumor recurrence. Rhabdomyosarcoma is a highly cellular tumor that shows increased diffusion restriction with hyperintense signal on DWI and low ADC values. DWI also provides additional valuable assessment to differentiate postoperative changes or necrosis from a residual recurrent tumor.

FDG PET/MR imaging has advantages over conventional modalities for staging of patients with rhabdomyosarcoma due to high sensitivity for lymph node involvement and detection of distant metastases. Furthermore, PET/MRI is a great tool for assessment of treatment response combining high negative predictive value from PET, ability of MRI sequences to characterize and delineate residual tumor, and avoiding excessive radiation exposure from CT on frequent follow-ups of pediatric patients.

Suggested Readings

Freling NJM, Merks JHM, Saeed P, Balm AJM, Bras J, Pieters BR, et al. Imaging findings in craniofacial childhood rhabdomyosarcoma. Pediatr Radiol. 2010;40(11):1723–38.

Purz S, Sabri O, Viehweger A, Barthel H, Kluge R, Sorge I, et al. Potential pediatric applications of PET/MR. J Nucl Med. 2014;55:32S–9S.

Vandecaveye V, De Keyzer F, Vander Poorten V, Dirix P, Verbeken E, Nuyts S, et al. Head and neck squamous cell carcinoma: value of diffusion-weighted MR imaging for nodal staging. Radiology. 2009;251(1):134–46.

Case 95
Chronic Thyroiditis

Frank Papik and Robert Matthews

History

A 57-year-old female presents for restaging of breast cancer (Fig. 95.1). The patient is on thyroid replacement hormone.

Diagnosis

Chronic thyroiditis

Findings

- PET images show intense, diffusely increased FDG uptake within the thyroid gland most consistent with chronic thyroiditis.
- Mildly enlarged thyroid gland that is slightly hyperintense on T1-weighted image and isointense signal on T2-weighted image.
- No thyroid nodules identified.

Discussion

Thyroiditis is a general term that refers to inflammation of the thyroid gland. There are many different forms of this disorder, and they can be grouped into acute, subacute, and chronic thyroiditis depending on the time-course of their presentation. Acute thyroiditis is a rare disease, usually caused by a bacterial infection. Rarely, it may result from thyroid trauma. Although early on these patients may have a transient hyperthyroidism, their thyroid hormone levels are usually normal. Symptoms include acute onset of fever and anterior neck pain. Antibiotics are the typical treatment and surgical intervention is rarely required.

Subacute thyroiditis is more common, typically affecting women aged 20–60 years old. This disorder usually appears after an upper respiratory viral infection and symptoms could include weakness, fever, dysphagia, or unilateral anterior neck pain that can radiate to chest, mandible, or ear. Early on these patients have a temporary hyperthyroidism but later on they can end up with a hypothyroidism that can last for months or in rare cases be permanent. Chronic thyroiditis can be caused by autoimmune disorders including Hashimoto's thyroiditis, Graves' disease, and postpartum thyroiditis. It can result in hypo- or hyperthyroidism depending on the disorder.

Normal thyroid tissue on MRI scans should be slightly hyperintense on T1 and isointense to slightly hyperintense on T2-weighted images compared to surrounding neck muscles and enhance homogenously. On MR imaging in patients with subacute thyroiditis, the thyroid glands would appear with irregular, indistinct margins and increased signal intensity on T1- and especially T2-weighted images. On MR images of chronic thyroiditis, the thyroid may appear blurred on the edges, normal or hyperin-

R. Gupta et al., *PET/MR Imaging*, https://doi.org/10.1007/978-3-319-65106-4_95

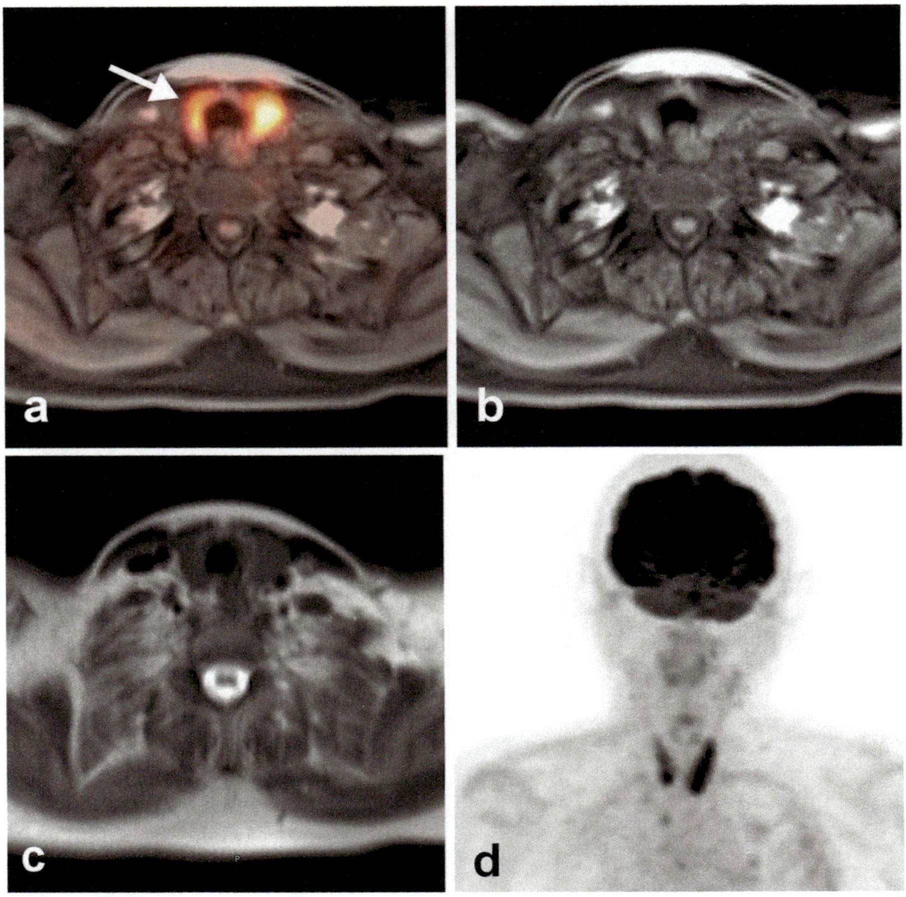

Fig. 95.1 FDG PET/MR T1 radial VIBE with fat suppression axial fusion (**a**), T1 radial VIBE with fat suppression axial (**b**), T2 HASTE axial (**c**), and PET MIP coronal (**d**)

tense on T1 and T2-weighted imaging. There are often spots of focally increased intensity on T2-weighted images.

FDG does not usually accumulate in normal thyroid tissue to a significant amount, so the gland may not be visible on the PET part of a PET/MR imaging. With thyroiditis, the thyroid gland shows mild to intense, homogenous activity often detected as an incidental finding generally more intense with subacute thyroiditis. Patients with incidentally often detected mild or intense diffuse FDG uptake in the thyroid gland should undergo thyroid function tests and antibody profiling if there is no clinical history of thyroid disease. Focal FDG thyroid uptake on PET imaging is typically associated with a benign or malignant tumor, with higher SUVs more likely found in malignancy. Focal thyroid uptake should always be correlated with ultrasound and often biopsy of underlying nodules to distinguish between benign and malignant nodules.

Suggested Reading

Agrawal K, Weaver J, Ngu R, Krishnamurthy MH. Clinical significance of patterns of incidental thyroid uptake at (18)F-FDG PET/CT. Clin Radiol. 2015;70(5):536–43.

Karantanis D, Bogsrud TV, Wiseman GA, Mullan BP, Subramaniam RM, Nathan MA, et al. Clinical significance of diffusely increased 18F-FDG uptake in the thyroid gland. J Nucl Med. 2007;48:896–901.

Jhaveri K, Shroff MM, Fatterpekar GM, Som PM. CT and MR imaging findings associated with subacute thyroiditis. AJNR Am J Neuroradiol. 2003;24(1):143–6.

Case 96
Base of the Tongue Squamous Cell Carcinoma

James Bai and Lev Bangiyev

History

A 62-year-old male with a history of tobacco smoking presents with a base of tongue lesion. Biopsy revealed squamous cell carcinoma of the tongue (Fig. 96.1).

Diagnosis

Base of the tongue squamous cell carcinoma

Findings

- MRI shows a T1 isointense, STIR hyperintense soft tissue mass in the right base of the tongue that extends across the midline to involve the contralateral side (arrowheads).
- Heterogeneous enhancement of the base of tongue lesion following gadolinium contrast.
- PET fusion images show markedly increased FDG uptake within the base of tongue lesion consistent with malignancy (thin arrows).

Discussion

The base of the tongue is an anatomic subset of the oropharynx that extends from the circumvallate papillae to the valleculae. The vast majority of malignant tumors occurring in the oropharynx, including the base of the tongue, are squamous cell carcinoma (SCC). SCC accounts for over 90% of tongue neoplastic cases. The rest of the malignant lesions in this anatomic location include minor salivary gland tumors, lymphoma, and mesenchymal tumors. Imaging of SCC should include evaluation for submucosal extent, involvement of the intrinsic muscles of the tongue, crossing the midline, pre-epiglottic invasion, bone involvement, and spread to the cervical lymph nodes.

FDG PET/MR imaging has recently gained interest in imaging of head and neck cancer. MRI provides excellent soft tissue contrast to delineate the complex anatomy of the head and neck region, and is considered the modality of choice for imaging tumors of the oral cavity and pharynx. In evaluating metastatic lymph nodes, conventional MRI relies on morphological criteria, with relatively low sensitivity and specificity. Combining superior MRI anatomic and morphologic delineation of the soft tissues with metabolic characterization of tissues with PET may significantly increase sensitivity and specificity. In addition, MRI can offer physiologic imaging utilizing advanced techniques such as diffusion-weighted imaging and dynamic contrast-enhanced (DCE) imaging, which can further aid in characterization of the tumor and lymph nodes. DCE MR imaging allows evaluation of tumor vascularity, permeability, and blood flow, which are important features of malignant tumors.

R. Gupta et al., *PET/MR Imaging*, https://doi.org/10.1007/978-3-319-65106-4_96

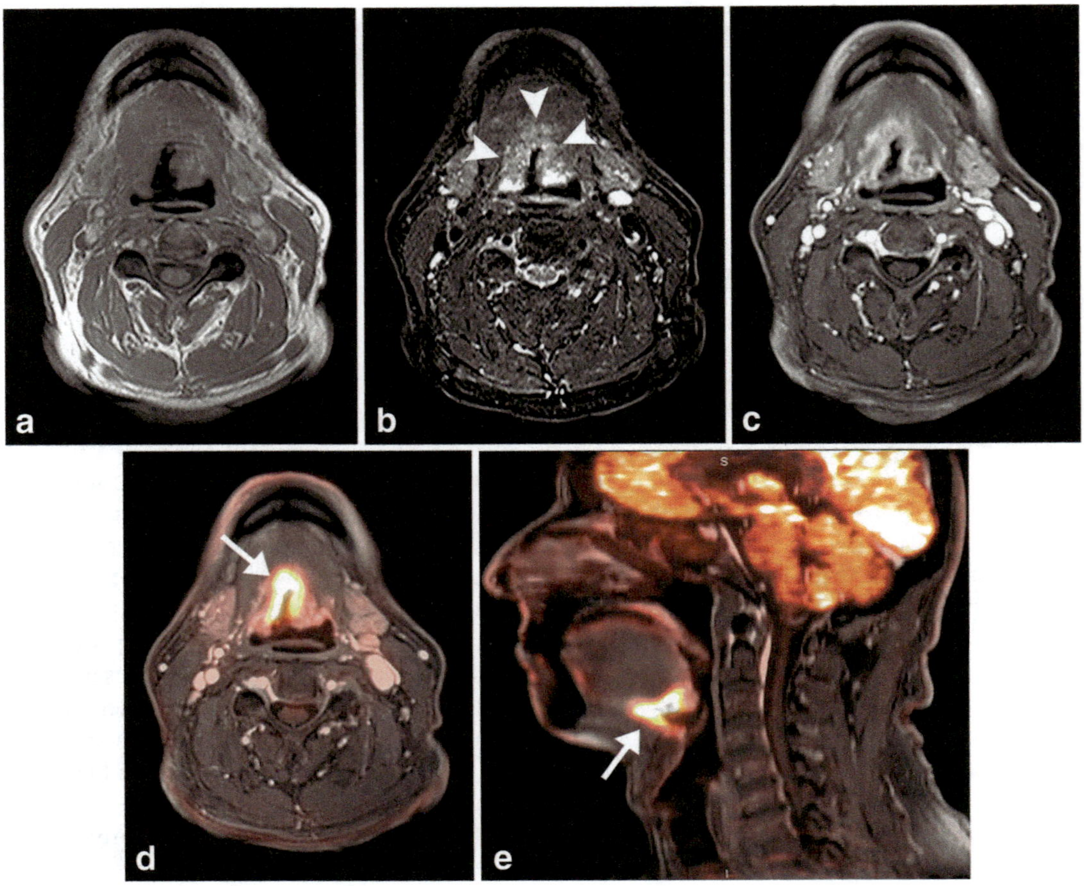

Fig. 96.1 T1 axial (**a**), STIR axial (**b**), T1 VIBE post-gadolinium contrast axial (**c**), PET/MR T1 VIBE post-gadolinium contrast axial fusion (**d**), and PET/MR T1 VIBE post-gadolinium contrast sagittal fusion (**e**)

When compared to PET/CT, advantages of PET/MRI are the minimization of ionizing radiation, superior soft tissue contrast resolution, and wider range of acquisition. An additional advantage of PET/MRI is lower susceptibility to dental filling artifacts in the head and neck region. Although PET/MRI is a relatively new oncologic imaging modality, it has already shown promising results for staging of head and neck cancer in several clinical studies.

Suggested Reading

Bashir U, Mallia A, Stirling J, Joemon J, MacKewn J, Charles-Edwards G, et al. PET/MRI in oncological imaging: state of the art. Diagnostics (Basel). 2015;5(3):333–57.

Kosling S, Knipping S, Hofmockel T. Imaging of nasopharyngeal diseases. Radiologe. 2009;49(1):17–26.

Ong CK, Chong VF. Imaging of tongue carcinoma. Cancer Imaging. 2006;6:186–93.

Case 97
Brown Adipose Tissue

Amit Gupta

History

A 14-year-old male presents for restaging Hodgkin's lymphoma (Fig. 97.1).

Diagnosis

Brown adipose tissue

Findings

- Intense hypermetabolic activity corresponding to fat within the lateral aspects of the neck (thin arrows). Milder FDG uptake is seen in the fat of the central compartment (curved arrows).
- Small benign lymph nodes are seen in the neck on the STIR but without corresponding FDG uptake (arrowheads).
- Areas of increased FDG uptake have no abnormalities on the STIR or T2 images.

Discussion

One of the many pitfalls of PET FDG imaging is radiotracer accumulation in various organs secondary to physiological or non-neoplastic processes. FDG uptake in brown adipose tissue (BAT) is one such pitfall and its presence can lead to reporting of false-positive findings or obscuration of true neoplastic lesions in the inexperienced reader.

Adipose tissues in humans are of two types, brown adipose tissue and white adipose tissue. White adipose tissue serves as energy storage organ and for thermal insulation. On the other hand, BAT plays a role when there is need for extra body heat such as in neonates, during entry into a febrile state, and non-shivering thermogenesis. Similarly, when placed in cold waiting rooms or PET/MRI scanner rooms, BAT is activated in some patients. Since BAT utilizes glucose and fatty acids for thermogenesis, a patient with FDG in their circulation will demonstrate FDG uptake in BAT.

The most common locations for BAT are the neck, mediastinum, supraclavicular, axillary, and paravertebral regions. Less commonly FDG uptake in BAT is seen in the paraaortic, peridiaphragmatic, and perinephric regions. There are many factors that affect FDG accumulation in BAT. These include higher incidence and uptake in younger patients, more common in females, lower body mass index, and colder ambient temperature. Brown fat FDG uptake is observed more commonly in breast cancer and sarcoma patients and less commonly in patients with lymphoma and lung cancer. Comparison of the fused PET/MR images with non-fused MR images helps differentiate brown adipose tissue from

R. Gupta et al., *PET/MR Imaging*, https://doi.org/10.1007/978-3-319-65106-4_97

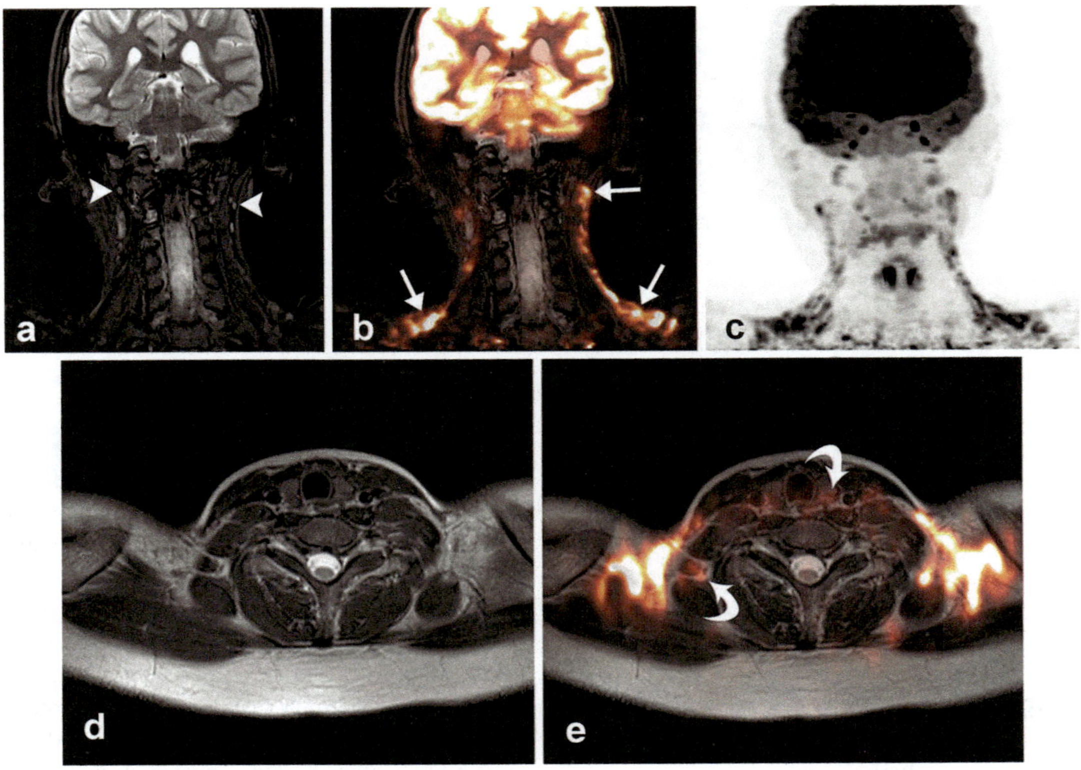

Fig. 97.1 STIR coronal (**a**), FDG PET/MR STIR coronal fusion (**b**), FDG PET MIP (**c**), T2 TSE axial (**d**), and FDG PET/MR T2 TSE axial fusion (**e**)

true lesions. In particular, this is important in the distinction of FDG abnormal uptake in the lymph nodes from surrounding BAT FDG activity. Appearance of BAT on MR is exactly the same as white adipose tissue elsewhere in the body. When the signal intensity on MR images is not clear, fat-suppressed images may be obtained to demonstrate absence or presence of a true lesion.

Suggested Reading

Cronin CG, Prakash P, Daniels GH, Boland GW, Kalra MK, Halpern EF, et al. Brown fat at PET/CT: correlation with patient characteristics. Radiology. 2012;263(3):836–42.

Townsend KL, Tseng YH. Brown fat fuel utilization and thermogenesis. Trends Endocrinol Metab. 2014;25(4):168–77.

Case 98
Squamous Cell Carcinoma of the Maxilla

James Bai and Lev Bangiyev

History

A 71-year-old man presents with painful sores in the upper oral cavity and difficulty eating (Fig. 98.1).

Diagnosis

Squamous cell carcinoma of the maxilla with lymph node metastasis

Findings

- T1 isointense, T2 mildly hypointense, and STIR mildly hypointense signal relative to normal mucosa corresponding to a mass the anterior superior aspect of the oral cavity centered along the hard palate and maxilla (thin arrow). The mass involves the upper lip and extends into anterior inferior nasal cavity.
- PET images show intense hypermetabolic activity associated with the mass (wide arrow) compatible with malignancy.
- Enlarged hypermetabolic left level II cervical lymph node (curved arrows) compatible with lymph node metastasis.

Discussion

Malignant lesions of the maxilla are rare. Squamous cell carcinoma is the predominant malignancy accounting for greater than 90% of the cases. These often result from direct tumor extension from adjacent structures such as gingiva, mucosa of the upper lip, maxillary sinuses, or nasal cavity. Tobacco, alcohol, and a poor diet account for the majority of risk factors. Squamous cell carcinoma spreads in three major ways: by direct extension, dissemination through the lymphatic drainage, and extension along the neurovascular bundle. Therefore, evaluation of all three pathways is necessary for accurate staging. MRI is more reliable in detecting bone marrow invasion, intracranial invasion, invasion of deep tongue muscle, and perineural spread. CT has been shown to be superior to MRI in evaluating cortical bone involvement and bone erosion.

R. Gupta et al., *PET/MR Imaging*, https://doi.org/10.1007/978-3-319-65106-4_98

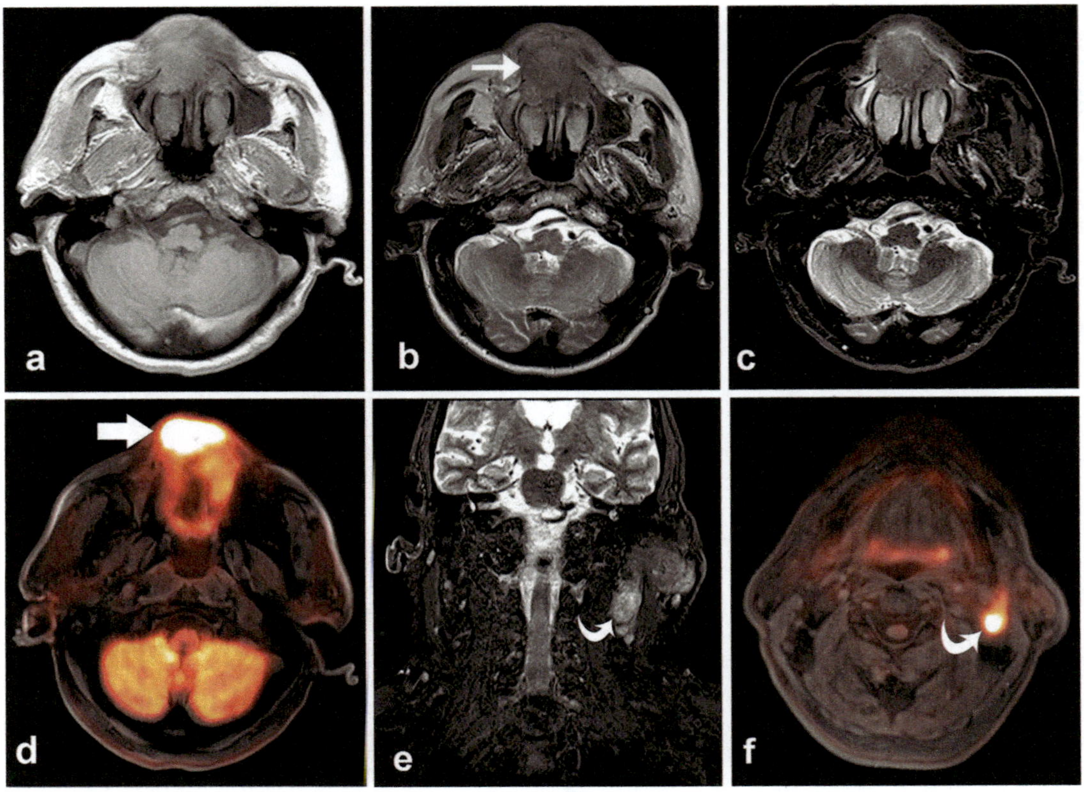

Fig. 98.1 T1 axial (**a**), T2 axial (**b**), STIR axial (**c**), FDG PET/MR T1 with fat suppression axial fusion (**d**), STIR coronal (**e**), and FDG PET/MR T1 VIBE with fat suppression axial fusion, at more inferior level (**f**)

FDG PET imaging has advantages over MRI and CT in detecting metastatic lymph nodes and distant metastases. Initial experience with PET/MR imaging has shown superior sensitivity in determination of N-stage with reported sensitivity and specificity of 85% and 92% respectively. In a separate clinical trial, PET/CT was reported to have sensitivity of 78% and a specificity of 58% for detecting spread to regional lymph nodes. Small metastases or micrometastases in morphologically normal lymph nodes however can be occult on PET and anatomic imaging and can only be diagnosed by histological evaluation. There is reasonable potential that the combined functional MR and PET can be better able to diagnose these micrometastases as well.

Suggested Reading

Lee JL, Seo HJ, Cheon GJ, Kim JH, Kim EE, Kang KW, et al. Usefulness of integrated PET/MRI in head and neck cancer: a preliminary study. Nucl Med Mol Imaging. 2014;48:98–105.

Queiroz MA, Huellner MW. PET/MR in cancers of the head and neck. Semin Nucl Med. 2015;45:248–65.

Trotta BM, Pease CS, Rasamny JJ, Raghavan P, Mukherjee S. Oral cavity and oropharyngeal squamous cell cancer: key imaging findings for staging and treatment planning. Radiographics. 2011;31(2):339–54.

Case 99
Physiological FDG Uptake in Tonsils

Jerrin Varghese and Amit Gupta

History

A 20-year-old male presents for lymphoma restaging (Fig. 99.1).

Diagnosis

Physiological FDG uptake in tonsils

Findings

- Prominent bilateral palatine tonsils that are homogenously isointense on T1 and mildly hyperintense on T2 without evidence of a mass (thin white arrow).
- Intense hypermetabolic activity in the palatine tonsils.
- Intense hypermetabolic activity in the pharyngeal tonsil (wide white arrow) with mild activity in the lingual tonsil (curved white arrow).
- Small reactive lymph nodes are seen in the neck (white arrowheads).
- PET MIP demonstrates hypermetabolic activity in the pharyngeal, palatine, and lingual tonsils forming a ring of lymphoid tissue (arrowheads).
- Loss of MRI signal in the anterior mouth due to metal-induced susceptibility artifact.

Discussion

The tonsils are a group of lymphoid structures involved in the first line of immune response to pathogens introduced to the oropharynx. They include the palatine, pharyngeal (or adenoid), and lingual tonsils and together are known as Waldeyer's ring. The tonsils are known to demonstrate avid FDG uptake, especially in pediatric and adolescent patients, with mean SUVs ranging from 3 to 5. As age increases, the tonsils are known to show progressive decrease in FDG uptake. In adenoidal hypertrophy, uptake increases, but usually in a symmetric pattern. Diffusely increased FDG activity in the tonsils is considered a normal variant, but may be seen with inflammation. In head and neck cancers such as lymphoma involving the tonsils, there may be unilateral or bilateral enlargement of the tonsils with prominent increased FDG uptake of the affected side.

On MRI, the tonsils demonstrate isointense signal on T1 sequences and hyperintense signal on T2 sequences when compared to muscle. They also demonstrate avid enhancement on post-contrast imaging. Tumors of the tonsils can be difficult to identify on MRI unless the mass is large and demonstrates mass effect. MRI can be most helpful in determining local invasion when tumor size is advanced. Adenoidal hypertrophy can be differentiated from malignancy

R. Gupta et al., *PET/MR Imaging*, https://doi.org/10.1007/978-3-319-65106-4_99

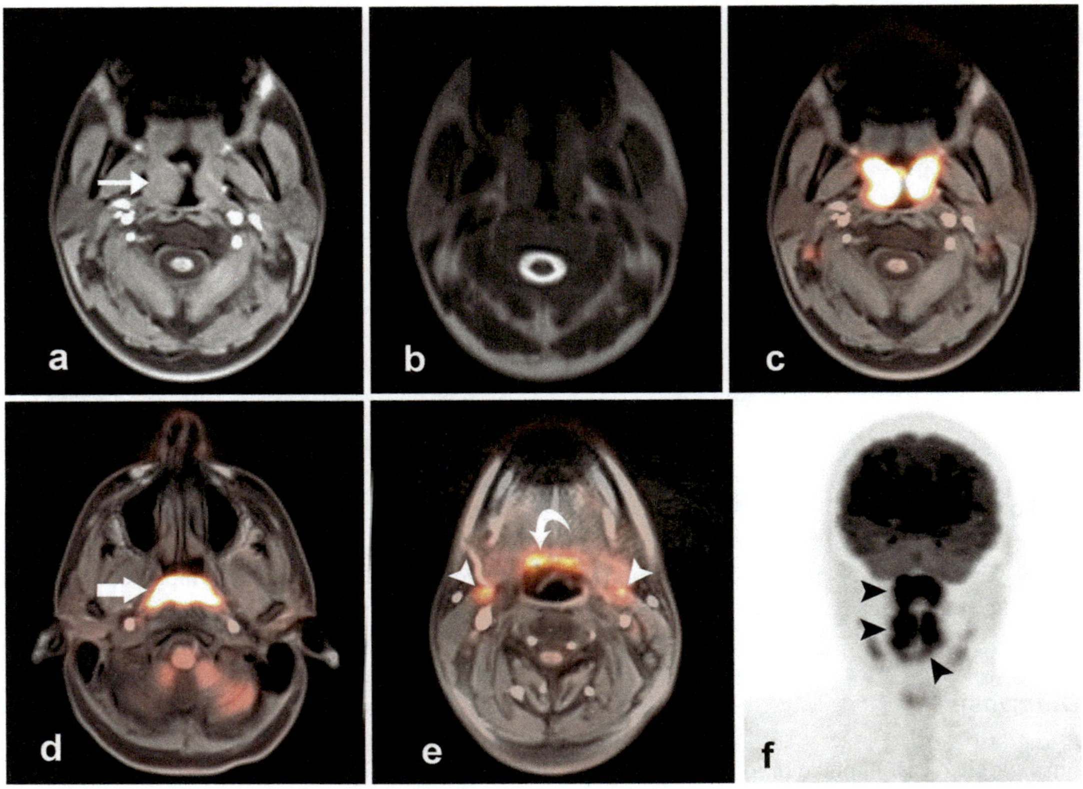

Fig. 99.1 T1 radial VIBE with fat suppression axial (**a**), T2 HASTE axial (**b**), FDG PET/MR T1 radial VIBE with fat suppression axial fusion (**c**), FDG PET/MR T1 radial VIBE with fat suppression axial fusion (**d**), FDG PET/MR T1 radial VIBE with fat suppression axial fusion (**e**), and FDG PET MIP coronal (**f**)

due to symmetric enlargement as well as the presence of hypointense stripes on T1-post contrast images, representing normal organization of adenoid tissue.

When used together, PET and MRI can complement each other. Indeterminate foci of increased FDG uptake may become more worrisome if associated with mass-like appearance or focal asymmetry on MRI. Otherwise, normal MRI appearance may become concerning if PET imaging reveals avid asymmetric or focal uptake. When tonsils appear suspicious on PET/MR imaging, visual assessment and biopsy are essential.

Suggested Reading

Bhatia KS, King AD, Vlantis AC, Ahuja AT, Tse GM. Nasopharyngeal mucosa and adenoids: appearance at MR imaging. Radiology. 2012;263(2):437–43.

Nakamoto Y, Tatsumi M, Hammoud D, Cohade C, Osman MM, Wahl RL. Normal FDG distribution patterns in the head and neck: PET/CT evaluation. Radiology. 2005;234(3):879–85.

Purohit BS, Ailianou A, Dulguerov N, Becker CD, Ratib O, Becker M. FDG-PET/CT pitfalls in oncological head and neck imaging. Insights Imaging. 2014;5(5):585–602.

Case 100
Recurrent Laryngeal Cancer

Rajesh Gupta

History

A 55-year-old male with resection of true vocal cord squamous cell carcinoma 15 months ago, and laser excision of recurrent lesion 4 months ago. Referred for restaging PET/MRI scan (Fig. 100.1).

Diagnosis

Recurrent laryngeal cancer

Findings

- Mass lesion in the left true vocal cord that bulges toward the midline. The lesion is hyperintense on T2 and STIR images (wide arrow) and isointense on T1 (black arrowhead).
- Mass lesion in the left true vocal cord shows avid homogeneous enhancement (white arrowhead).
- PET/MR fusion images show intense focal FDG uptake in the mass (curved arrow) compatible with malignancy.

Discussion

Laryngeal cancer accounts for up to 25% of all head and neck malignancies. The majority of laryngeal cancers, approximately 67%, are glottic; while supraglottic cancers are less common, with subglottic tumors being the least frequent. The glottis is lined with nonkeratinized squamous epithelium, and therefore over 90% of malignant laryngeal tumors are composed of squamous cell carcinomas. They are typically low-grade and frequently involve the anterior third of the true vocal cord. Cancers of the larynx often present in adults between 50 and 70 years of age. Notably, these tumors are identified on endoscopy, however integration with cross-sectional imaging is important as it improves the T staging accuracy by assessing local submucosal extent.

MRI has been shown to have a higher sensitivity and negative predictive value compared to CT in assessing malignant extension to laryngeal subsites, which include the anterior commissure, paraglottic space, thyroid, cricoid, as well as arytenoid cartilages. However, MR has a lower specificity than CT for laryngeal cartilage involvement as the cartilage can undergo osteoblastic transfor-

R. Gupta et al., *PET/MR Imaging*, https://doi.org/10.1007/978-3-319-65106-4_100

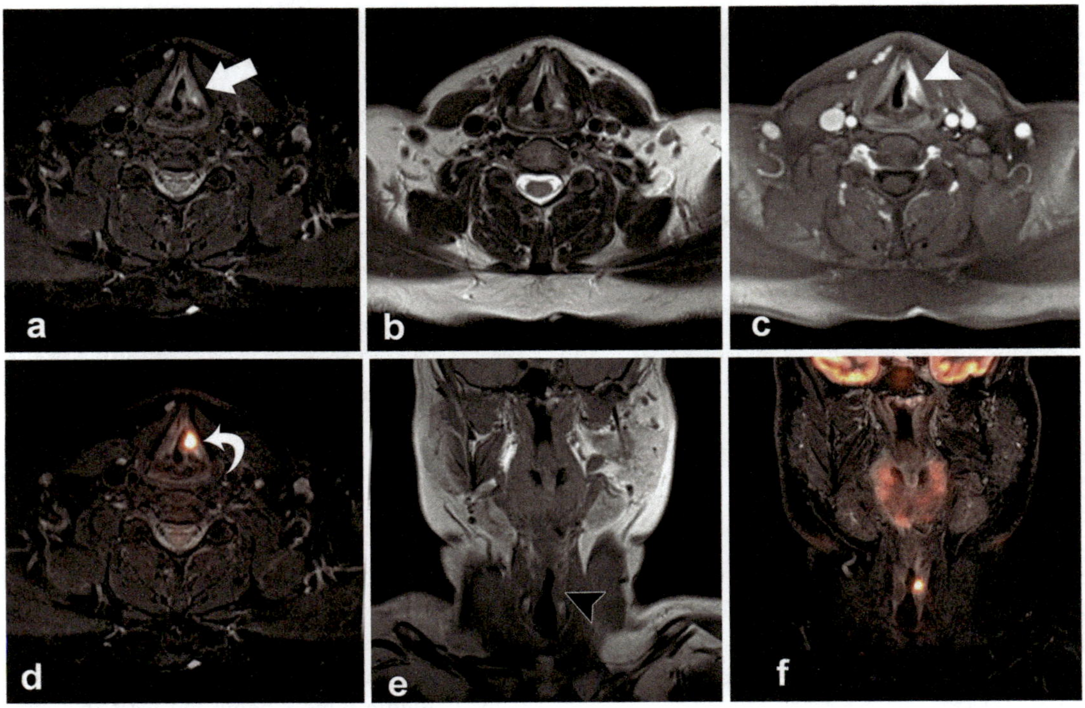

Fig. 100.1 STIR axial (**a**), T2 TSE axial (**b**), T1 radial VIBE post-gadolinium contrast axial (**c**), PET/MR STIR fusion axial (**d**), T1 TSE coronal (**e**), and PET/MR STIR fusion coronal (**f**)

mation with neoplastic invasion. Tumor tissue typically exhibits low-to-intermediate signal on T1 and high signal on T2-weighted images with enhancement after contrast administration.

Laryngeal tumors, as with other head and neck cancers, are FDG avid. The role of FDG PET is well established in the detection of regional nodal as well as distant metastases. FDG PET is also useful in evaluation of tumor volume for radiation therapy planning. The degree of metabolic activity can predict tumor behavior. It has been shown that patients with higher FDG uptake in neck lymph nodes should be considered at increased risk for poor outcome and therefore, may benefit from more aggressive treatment approaches. In the evaluation of treatment response and recurrence of laryngeal tumor, the high negative predictive value of FDG PET precludes unnecessary diagnostic invasive procedures and neck dissection in many patients. Combining superior MR soft tissue contrast and PET metabolic activity, FDG PET/MR imaging provides complimentary information in the evaluation of head and neck cancers that cannot be obtained by either modality alone.

Suggested Reading

Allegra E, Ferrise P, Trapasso S, Trapuzzano O, Barca A, Tamburrini S, et al. Early glottic cancer: role of MRI in the preoperative staging. Biomed Res Int. 2014;2014:890385.

Joshi VM, Wadhwa V, Mukherji SK. Imaging in laryngeal cancers. Indian J Radiol Imaging. 2012;22(3):209–26.

Kitajima K, Suenaga Y, Kanda T, Miyawaki D, Yoshida K, Ejima Y, et al. Prognostic value of FDG PET imaging in patients with laryngeal cancer. PLoS One. 2014;9(5):e96999.

Oe A, Kawabe J, Torii K, Kawamura E, Kotani J, Hayashi T, et al. Detection of local residual tumor after laryngeal cancer treatment using FDG-PET. Ann Nucl Med. 2007;21(1):9–13.

Case 101
Benign Sinus Disease

Frank Papik and Robert Matthews

History

A 45-year-old female with unexplained weight loss and mild cognitive changes (Fig. 101.1)

Diagnosis

Benign sinus disease

Findings

- Circumferential mucosal thickening (black arrowheads) of the maxillary sinuses bilaterally that is isointense on T1 and hyperintense on T2. More pronounced on the left side.
- STIR coronal image shows hyperintense mucosal thickening of the left maxillary sinus (curved arrow) with frothy mucous secretions, which represents active inflammation. Right maxillary sinus shows mild sinus disease (thin arrow).
- Mild FDG uptake in the sinus mucosa reflecting active inflammation or infection.

Discussion

Benign sinus disease is a term that includes infectious or inflammatory types of sinusitis, as well as non-malignant polyps or tumors. Infectious sinusitis is usually an acute process that is treated with antibiotics and anti-inflammatory medications. Chronic sinusitis is frequently related to structural abnormalities of the sinuses that affect drainage of the sinuses and make them more susceptible to infections and chronic inflammation. Chronic sinusitis may require surgical intervention in addition to antibiotics and anti-inflammatory treatment. In immunocompromised patients, the sinuses are also susceptible to fungal infections, which are more difficult to treat. Invasive fungal sinusitis is the most aggressive and frequently lethal infection that affects immunocompromised hosts with mortality ranging from 50% to 80%. Patients with asthma and aspirin allergies often develop benign polyps that block the sinuses causing secondary sinusitis that can be treated with oral steroids and sometimes surgery.

Non-malignant sinus tumors can present like sinusitis; however, they do not respond to the usual sinusitis treatment. These tumors are often diagnosed on endoscopy or imaging. An example of this are inverted papillomas, which are usually classified as benign tumors, but have an aggressive nature when they are found in the paranasal sinuses. Although rare, inverted papillomas have potential to transform into squamous carcinoma at a rate of 5–15%. Furthermore, they have a high rate of recurrence after surgical resection.

MRI can be helpful in the evaluation of paranasal sinuses differentiating mucosal disease from tumors. Typically mucosal thickening and polyps demonstrate homogeneous T2 hyperintense signal. Inverted papilloma shows a striated "cerebriform" appear-

R. Gupta et al., *PET/MR Imaging*, https://doi.org/10.1007/978-3-319-65106-4_101

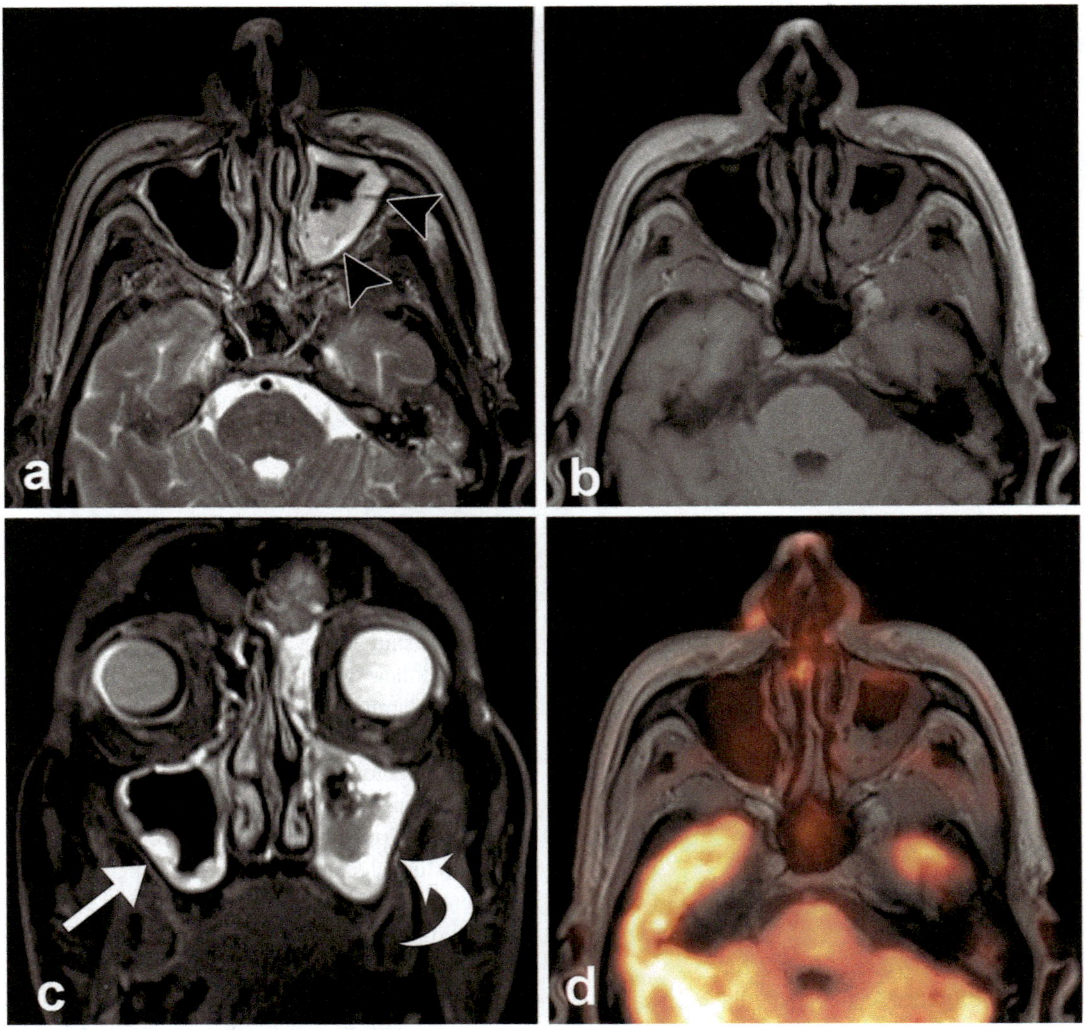

Fig. 101.1 T2 axial (**a**), T1 axial (**b**), STIR coronal (**c**), and PET/MR T1 axial fusion (**d**)

ance on the T2-weighted sequence. Frequently acute sinusitis will present on imaging with a fluid level within the affected sinus and frothy or bubbly secretions. After contrast administration, inflamed mucosa will demonstrate enhancement while fluid and secretions do not. Sinonasal tumors also enhance after contrast administration, however will demonstrate nodular or mass-like appearance.

On PET/MR imaging, benign sinusitis appears as thickened mucosa with mild diffuse FDG uptake reflecting inflammation and infection. This is often detected incidentally on PET whole-body imaging. In the acute phase, the FDG uptake may be prominent, and as it heals it will resolve before the mucosal thickening regresses. If there is focal uptake in the sinus on PET/MR, then other pathology such as tumor or fungal infection might be considered. Inverted papillomas have intense FDG uptake and PET/MR may be used in the diagnosis and detection of recurrence of this tumor, as well as, aid in the surgical planning.

Suggested Reading

Cohen EG, Baredes S, Zuckier LS, Mirani NM, Liu Y, Ghesani NV. 18F-FDG PET evaluation of sinonasal papilloma. AJR Am J Roentgenol. 2009;193(1):214–7.

Shojaku H, Fujisaka M, Yasumura S, Ishida M, Tsubota M, Nishida H, et al. Positron emission tomography for predicting malignancy of sinonasal inverted papilloma. Clin Nucl Med. 2007;32(4):275–8.

Yousem DM. Imaging of sinonasal inflammatory disease. Radiology. 1993;188(2):303–14.

Case 102
Recurrent Soft Palate Cancer

Dharmesh Tank

History

A 75-year-old male with squamous cell carcinoma of the soft palate treated with radiation and chemotherapy presents for restaging (Fig. 102.1).

Diagnosis

Recurrent soft palate cancer

Findings

- MRI shows mass-like soft tissue in the right soft palate that is isointense to tongue muscle on STIR and mildly hypointense on T1 (arrowheads).
- PET/MR fusion demonstrates intense FDG uptake within mass-like signal abnormality consistent with malignancy (thin arrows).

Discussion

Soft palate cancers are oropharyngeal malignancies that can be easily detected by visual inspection and thus are potentially diagnosed in its early stages. The preponderance of new oropharyngeal cancer cases are squamous cell carcinomas. Other oropharyngeal tumors such as minor salivary gland tumors, lymphoid tumors, sarcomas, and mixed cellularity tumors are rarer. The incidence of newly diagnosed oropharyngeal malignancy is closely associated with tobacco use, excessive alcohol use, as well as human papillomavirus infection. In the evaluation of initially diagnosed oropharyngeal cancer, PET is valuable in delineating the extent of the tumor and for the detection of nodal and distant metastatic disease. The addition of MRI provides superior soft tissue contrast resolution. The initial treatment depends on the local extent of disease and presence of metastases which determines staging of the disease, treatment options, and ultimately patient prognosis. Patients with early disease and those with persistent disease post treatment can receive surgical resection and neck dissection.

In the follow-up of patients post treatment for oropharyngeal cancer, there are no clear guidelines; however, it is important to include a multidisciplinary evaluation with clinical and imaging follow-up. The primary concern for patients with oropharyngeal cancer is regional recurrence. Detection of recurrence earlier through clinical and imaging surveillance potentially allows for increased likelihood of salvage therapy and potentially improved

R. Gupta et al., *PET/MR Imaging*, https://doi.org/10.1007/978-3-319-65106-4_102

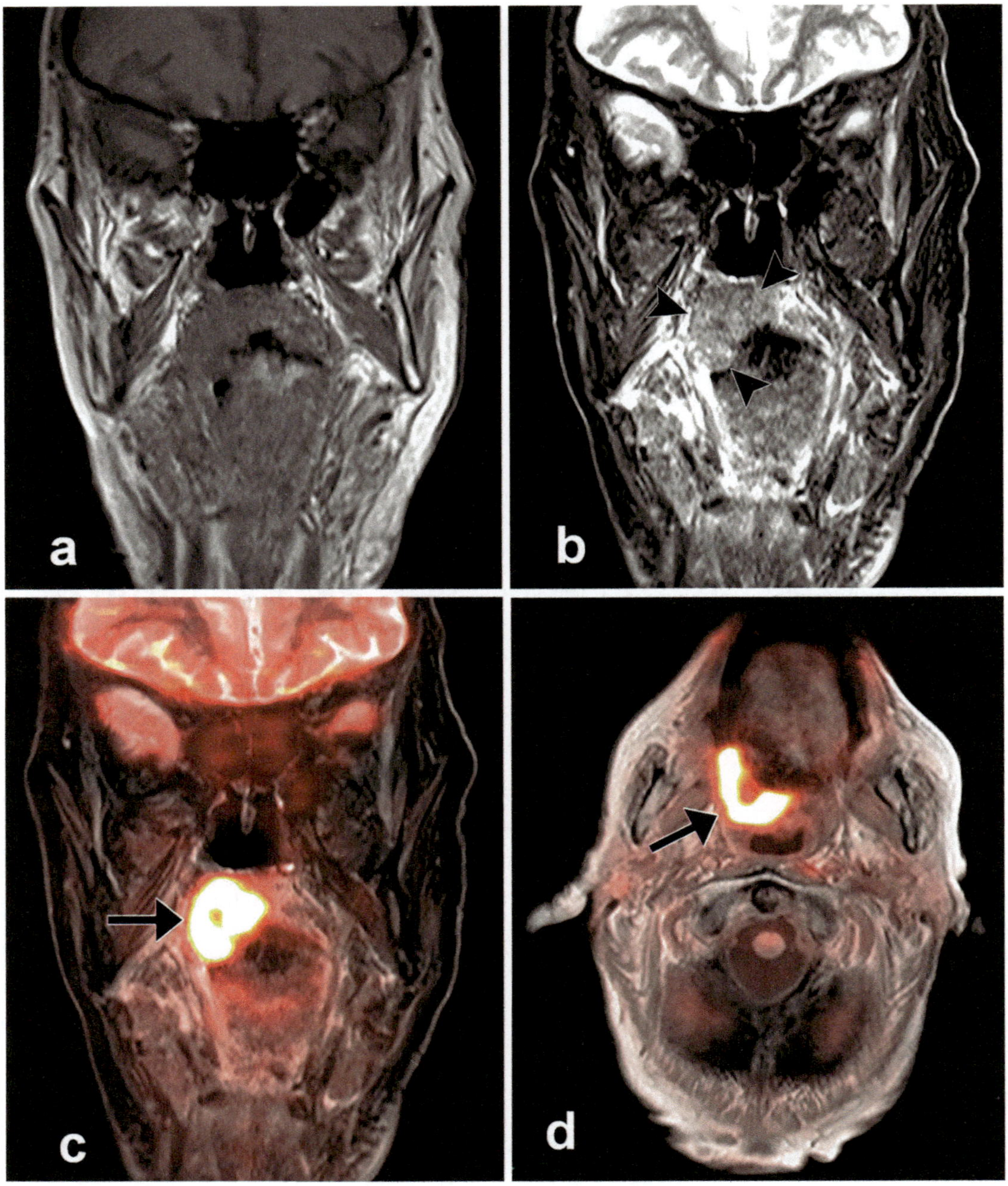

Fig. 102.1 T1 TSE coronal (**a**), STIR coronal (**b**), PET/MRI STIR coronal fusion (**c**), and PET/MRI T1 axial fusion (**d**)

survival. Especially in head and neck malignancies, the lack of any tumor marker increases the importance of imaging for surveillance for recurrence, and is supplemental to clinical exam. Although there is no clear recommendation for the type of imaging follow-up, the National Comprehensive Cancer Network recommends baseline cross-sectional imaging at 4–6 months following treatment of oropharyngeal cancer. In addition, if any any point there is clinical suspicion for recurrence, imaging should be obtained.

The reappearance of malignancy after 6 months of complete regression is the definition of recurrent disease. Imaging evaluation with CT, MRI, and FDG PET is essential for the investigation of treatment response, post-treatment changes, and disease recurrence. On MRI, recurrent disease may present as new or increasing in size, contrast enhancing mass-like soft tissue, which is iso- or hyperintense on T2-weighted sequences. Treatment-related change is often seen as T2 hypointense soft tissue. FDG PET/MR imaging adds accuracy to findings from CT and MRI alone because of the cancer FDG avidity. PET/MRI is limited in the immediate post-treatment period secondary to treatment-related inflammatory changes and granulation tissue that can be FDG positive and demonstrate enhancement, hence MR false positive as well. There should usually be a delay of approximately 3 months prior to imaging with PET/MRI to reduce false-positive findings, yet this still allows time for further surgical management if necessary. If there is a clinical concern for recurrence, or there is a palpable lesion on clinical examination, PET/MR imaging can be performed earlier.

Suggested Reading

Cohan DM, Popat S, Kaplan SE, Rigual N, Loree T, Hicks WL Jr. Oropharyngeal cancer: Current understanding and management. Curr Opin Otolaryngol Head Neck Surg. 2009;17:88–94.

De Felice F, Musio D, Tombolini V. Follow-up in head and neck cancer: a management dilemma. Adv Otolaryngol. 2015;2015:4.

Mukherji SK, Wolf GT. Evaluation of head and neck squamous cell carcinoma after treatment. AJNR Am J Neuroradiol. 2003;24(9):1743–6.

Case 103
Recurrent Salivary Gland Cancer

Ana M. Franceschi and Lev Bangiyev

History

An 86-year-old male treated for locally advanced salivary gland cancer by radiation and chemotherapy complains of a new lump under his jaw (Fig. 103.1).

Diagnosis

Recurrent salivary gland cancer

Findings

- Isointense T1 and isointense T2 thick-walled mass (thin arrow) in the left submandibular region with central heterogeneous T2 hyperintensity and T1 hypointensity consistent with necrosis.
- Extensive soft tissue infiltration with the lack of delineation of fat and muscle planes in the left mandibular region due to radiation therapy (arrowheads).
- PET/MR fusion shows markedly increased FDG uptake in the anterior periphery of the lesion consistent with tumor recurrence (curved arrows).

Discussion

Neoplasms of the salivary glands classically present as a painless, enlarging masses. The smaller the anatomic salivary gland, the higher chance of a tumor being malignant with a rate of malignancy being 50–80% in the sublingual and minor salivary glands, 40–50% in the submandibular gland, and 20–25% in the parotid gland. Due to its proportionally larger size, up to 70% of all salivary gland neoplasms occur in the parotid gland. The most common primary malignant neoplasm of the parotid gland is mucoepidermoid carcinoma, while adenoid cystic carcinoma typically involves the minor salivary glands and has a high propensity for perineural spread. In patients with malignant salivary gland tumors, surgical excision, lymph node dissection, and adjuvant chemoradiation therapy are typically employed due to their infiltrative nature and high affinity for perineural spread.

Characteristic imaging features of salivary gland tumors on FDG PET/MR imaging depends on tumor grade and histologic subtype. In general, benign and malignant salivary gland tumors demonstrate increased FDG uptake. However, malignant tumors typically show higher metabolic activity in comparison to benign lesions

R. Gupta et al., *PET/MR Imaging*, https://doi.org/10.1007/978-3-319-65106-4_103

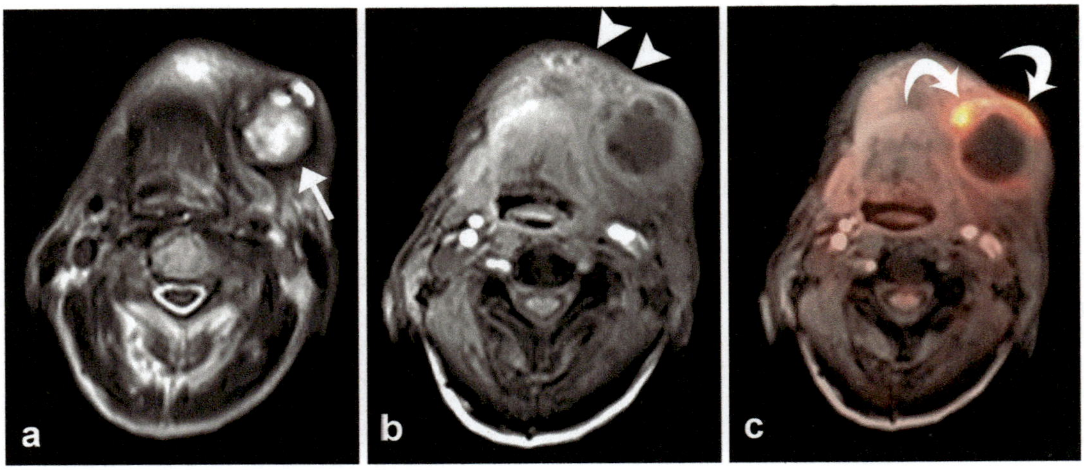

Fig. 103.1 T2 HASTE axial (**a**), T1 VIBE with fat suppression axial (**b**), and PET/MR T1 VIBE with fat suppression axial fusion (**c**)

with the exception of Warthin's tumors which have some overlap with malignant lesions. In patients with malignant salivary gland neoplasms, it is crucial to interrogate the cranial nerves with post-contrast, fat-saturated T1-weighted sequences due to their high propensity for perineural spread, particularly involving the CN VII facial nerve. While it may be difficult to differentiate low-grade mucoepidermoid carcinoma from the benign pleomorphic adenoma in the parotid glands, high-grade mucoepidermoid carcinomas present as poorly marginated, locally infiltrative lesions with low to intermediate signal on both T1 and T2-weighted sequences. Adenoid cystic carcinoma, which typically involves the minor salivary glands, demonstrates intermediate signal intensity on T1-weighted images, but is hyperintense on T2-weighted sequences with marked, homogeneous contrast enhancement and increased uptake on FDG PET imaging.

Suggested Reading

Freling N, Crippa F, Maroldi R. Staging and follow-up of high-grade malignant salivary gland tumours: the role of traditional versus functional imaging approaches—a review. Oral Oncol. 2016;60:157–66.

Sharma P, Jain TK, Singh H, Suman SK, Faizi NA, Kumar R, Bal C, Malhotra A, Kumar R. Utility of (18)F-FDG PET-CT in staging and restaging of patients with malignant salivary gland tumours: a single-institutional experience. Nucl Med Commun. 2013;34(3):211–9.

Yousem DM, Kraut MA, Chalian AA. Major salivary gland imaging. Radiology. 2000;216(1):19–29.

Case 104
Tonsillar Squamous Cell Carcinoma

James Bai and Lev Bangiyev

History

An 82-year-old female with right tonsil mass (Fig. 104.1). Human papillomavirus test was positive.

Diagnosis

Tonsillar squamous cell carcinoma

Findings

- Axial images at the palatine tonsils show right palatine mass that is T1 isointense and T2 mildly hyperintense (thin arrow). The mass effaces right glossopharyngeal sulcus with mild effacement of the adjacent airway.
- The mass demonstrates abnormal metabolic activity on the PET/MR fusion image, which is consistent with malignancy (curved arrow).
- Axial images at the base of tongue show pathologically enlarged right level IIa lymph node which is posterior to submandibular gland and demonstrates T1 isointense and T2 mildly hyperintense signal (wide arrow).
- PET/MR fusion image shows hypermetabolic activity associated with the abnormal lymph node consistent with metastasis.
- Metal induced susceptibility artifact with loss of signal in the anterior mouth due to dental hardware.

Discussion

Tonsillar cancer is a form of oropharyngeal cancer that involves the pharyngeal, palatine, or lingual tonsils. The two most common types of tonsillar cancer include squamous cell carcinoma (SCC) and lymphoma. Common symptoms include sore mouth or throat, mouth pain, swollen tonsils, earache, and difficulty or pain swallowing. In cases of SCC, it is important to distinguish human papillomavirus (HPV) positive cancer from cancer related to tobacco and alcohol use in order to develop specific treatment approaches, and more accurately predict prognosis. HPV-positive head and neck squamous cell carcinoma better responds to radiotherapy and chemotherapy.

Surgery and radiotherapy with complimentary chemotherapy remain the primary treatment options for early and regional advanced head and neck squamous cell carcinoma. Trans-oral endoscopic head and neck surgery allows surgeons to gain access through a minimally invasive technique with improved visualization of the tumor and avoiding disfiguring incisions and minimizing the risk of speech and swallow dysfunction. The effi-

R. Gupta et al., *PET/MR Imaging*, https://doi.org/10.1007/978-3-319-65106-4_104

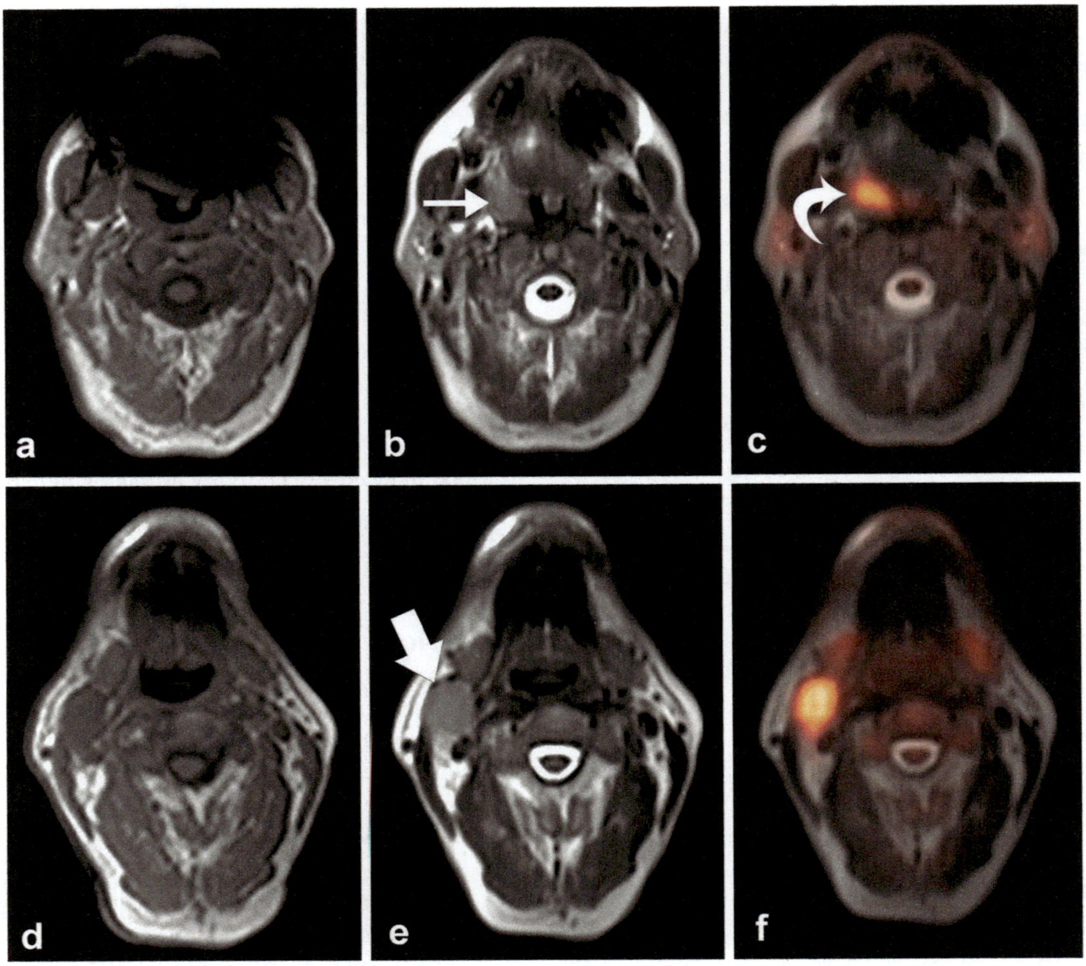

Fig. 104.1 T1 axial, at the palatine tonsils (**a**), T2 HASTE, at the palatine tonsils (**b**), FDG PET/MR T2 HASTE axial fusion, at the palatine tonsils (**c**), T1 axial, at the base of tongue (**d**), T2 HASTE axial, at the base of tongue (**e**), and FDG PET/MR T2 HASTE axial fusion, at the base of tongue (**f**)

cacy of radiotherapy of head and neck cancer has improved tremendously with introduction of intensity-modulated radiotherapy and the use of advanced imaging for target volume and organ at risk delineation, which renders an overall increase in head and neck cancer survival probability and improvement in quality of life.

Anatomic MRI imaging of the head and neck typically shows a soft tissue mass in the region of the oropharynx involving either of the tonsils, which is often isointense on T1-weighted images and isointense to mildly hyperintense on T2-weighted images, with intense homogeneous enhancement. Advanced tonsillar tumors may show areas of necrosis that are T1 hypointense and T2 hyperintense with heterogeneous enhancement. Furthermore, these tumors metastasize initially to ipsilateral lymph nodes and in the later stages to contralateral lymph nodes especially when tumors cross the midline. HPV positive tumors more frequently present at higher stages with larger metastatic lymph nodes, which often show a cystic or necrotic appearance on imaging.

Many FDG PET studies of head and neck cancers have shown that high SUV is associated with advanced stage, large tumor size, and poor differentiation. A meta-analysis study concluded that high primary tumor SUV max can serve as a prognostic marker in patients with head and neck SCC with high SUV max correlating with poorer outcomes. Patients with elevated SUV might be candidates for more aggressive therapy, whereas patients with a low SUV might be candidates for less aggressive treatment, although no exact SUV cutoff value could be defined. SUV cutoff values for malignant lymph nodes can vary depending on the size of the lymph nodes. Combined PET/MR imaging offers a better choice for these patients utilizing both anatomic and functional analysis to detect metastases and provide prognostic information.

Suggested Reading

Cantrell SC, Peck BW, Li G, Wei Q, Sturgis EM, Ginsberg LE. Differences in imaging characteristics of HPV-positive and HPV-negative oropharyngeal cancers: a blinded matched-pair analysis. AJNR Am J Neuroradiol. 2013;34(10):2005–9.

Loeffelbein DJ, Souvatzoglou M, Wankerl V, Dinges J, Ritschl LM, Mücke T, et al. Diagnostic value of retrospective PET-MRI fusion in head-and-neck cancer. BMC Cancer. 2014;14:846.

Rischin D, Ferris RL, Le QT. Overview of advances in head and neck cancer. J Clin Oncol. 2015;33(29):3225–6.

Xie P, Li M, Zhao H, Sun X, Fu Z, Yu J. 18F-FDG PET or PET-CT to evaluate prognosis for head and neck cancer: a meta-analysis. J Cancer Res Clin Oncol. 2011;137(7):1085–93.

Case 105
Benign Thyroid Adenoma

Laura L. Rosenkrantz and Robert Matthews

History

A 55-year-old female being evaluated for paraneoplastic sensory neuropathy (Fig. 105.1).

Diagnosis

Benign thyroid adenoma

Findings

- Right thyroid mass that is isointense on T1-weighted image with areas of hyperintensity and mildly heterogeneous, isointense on T2-weighted image (thin arrow).
- PET/MR fusion shows indeterminate focal FDG activity in the thyroid mass (curved arrow).
- Coronal images show the T2 mildly heterogeneous, isointense right thyroid mass (wide arrow) with focal hypermetabolic activity that is deviating the trachea (asterisk) toward the left side.
- Subsequent biopsy revealed a benign thyroid adenoma.

Discussion

Thyroid nodules are very common and appear in about half of the population at autopsy. Thyroid nodules vary in shape, texture, and mobility and are caused by many conditions including iodine deficiency, overgrowth of normal thyroid tissue, cysts, thyroiditis, multinodular goiter, or tumor. Most nodules do not cause any signs or symptoms and are instead incidentally found on physical exam or by imaging. However, if the nodule grows to a large size, then it can be seen and felt, and exert a mass effect on surrounding structures including the trachea and esophagus causing shortness of breath and difficulty in swallowing. Some nodules secrete thyroid hormone causing symptoms of hyperthyroidism such as tachycardia, tremor, weight loss, and intolerance to heat. About 95% of all thyroid nodules are benign. Thyroid malignancy is most prevalent among children, adults less than 30 years old or over 60 years old, and those with a family history of thyroid cancer or personal history of radiation to the head and neck.

Ultrasound is the gold standard in evaluating thyroid nodules and the most sensitive method for diagnosing intrathyroid lesions. MRI has a

R. Gupta et al., *PET/MR Imaging*, https://doi.org/10.1007/978-3-319-65106-4_105

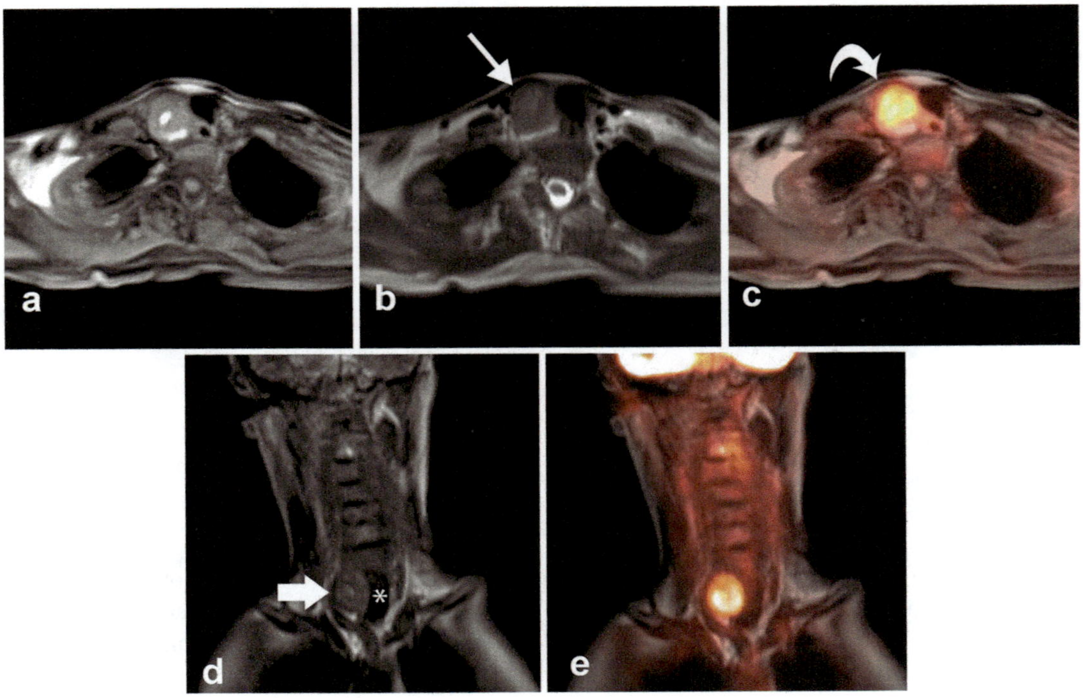

Fig. 105.1 T1 radial VIBE with fat suppression axial (**a**), T2 HASTE axial (**b**), PET/MR T1 radial VIBE with fat suppression axial fusion (**c**), T2 TSE coronal (**d**), and PET/MR T2 TSE coronal fusion (**e**)

limited role in the initial characterization of thyroid nodules but has been shown to be very effective in the assessment of thyroid cancer extension into adjacent structures including the trachea and esophagus as well as evaluating for regional metastatic lymphadenopathy. Relative to the neck muscles, the thyroid gland is slightly hyperintense on T1-weighted images and isointense to slightly hyperintense on T2-weighted images. Nodules are typically hyperintense masses and can either be homogeneous or heterogeneous.

Incidental focal FDG PET uptake within the thyroid gland has been reported in 1–4% of patients undergoing PET imaging. Diffusely increased uptake is typically consistent with benign disease and usually reflects chronic thyroiditis. Focal FDG uptake can frequently represent malignancy and warrants further investigation with ultrasound-guided FNA biopsy. The higher the SUV values, the more likely the thyroid nodule is malignant. FDG PET scanning is particularly useful for patients with undifferentiated thyroid cancer that no longer accumulates radioactive iodine. PET/MR imaging with a dedicated neck MRI is an excellent technique to assess for local thyroid cancer recurrence and distant metastases.

Suggested Reading

Chen L, Xu J, Bao J, Huang X, Hu X, Xia Y, et al. Diffusion-weighted MRI in differentiating malignant from benign thyroid nodules: a meta-analysis. BMJ Open. 2016;6(1):e008413.

Dong MJ, Liu ZF, Zhao K, Ruan LX, Wang GL, Yang SY, et al. Value of 18F-FDG-PET/PET-CT in differentiated thyroid carcinoma with radioiodine-negative whole-body scan: a meta-analysis. Nucl Med Commun. 2009;30:639–50.

Marcus C, Whitworth PW, Surasi DS, Pai SI. PET/CT in the Management of Thyroid Cancers. Nucl Med Mol Imaging. 2014;202:1316–29.

Tanpitukpongse TP, Grady AT, Sosa JA, Eastwood JD, Choudhury KR, Hoang JK. Incidental thyroid nodules on CT or MRI: discordance between what we report and what receives workup. AJR Am J Roentgenol. 2015;205(6):1281–7.

Case 106
Retropharyngeal Cancer

Matthew Comito and James Bai

History

An 80-year-old male presents for staging of head and neck cancer involving the retropharynx (Fig. 106.1).

Diagnosis

Retropharyngeal cancer

Findings

- MRI shows predominantly exophytic soft tissue mass in the inferior oropharynx arising from retropharyngeal wall that demonstrates T1 hypointense, T2 mildly hyperintense, and STIR hyperintense signal (wide arrow).
- Although there are edematous changes in the retropharyngeal space appearing as hyperintense signal on T2-weighted image (arrowheads), there is preservation of prevertebral space consistent with resectability.
- Post-gadolinium contrast MRI shows homogeneous enhancement of the mass.
- PET/MRI shows intense FDG uptake within the mass consistent with malignancy (curved arrow).

Discussion

Primary tumors of the retropharyngeal space (RPS) are fairly uncommon. Lipomas are the most common of these primary tumors and tend to conform to the shape of the RPS. Much more frequently, tumors of the oropharynx or nasopharynx will directly invade the RPS. The most common of these invading tumors is squamous cell carcinoma. Tumor extension beyond the RPS and into the prevertebral space is limited by the pharyngobasilar fascia. Within the RPS, there are no boundaries in the craniocaudal direction until the tumor contacts the buccopharyngeal fascia superiorly, as it attaches to the skull base. Squamous cell carcinoma is also the most prevalent primary malignancy involving the RPS. Other much less common malignancies include minor salivary gland tumors and lymphoma.

The TNM classification system is used in head and neck cancers to describe the extent of the cancer (T describes the size of the tumor, N indicates the spread to regional lymph nodes, and M describes spread of tumor to other organs of the body or distant metastases). The TNM staging system is ultimately used in treatment planning and to determine resectability of the tumor. The three major criteria that are considered to

R. Gupta et al., *PET/MR Imaging*, https://doi.org/10.1007/978-3-319-65106-4_106

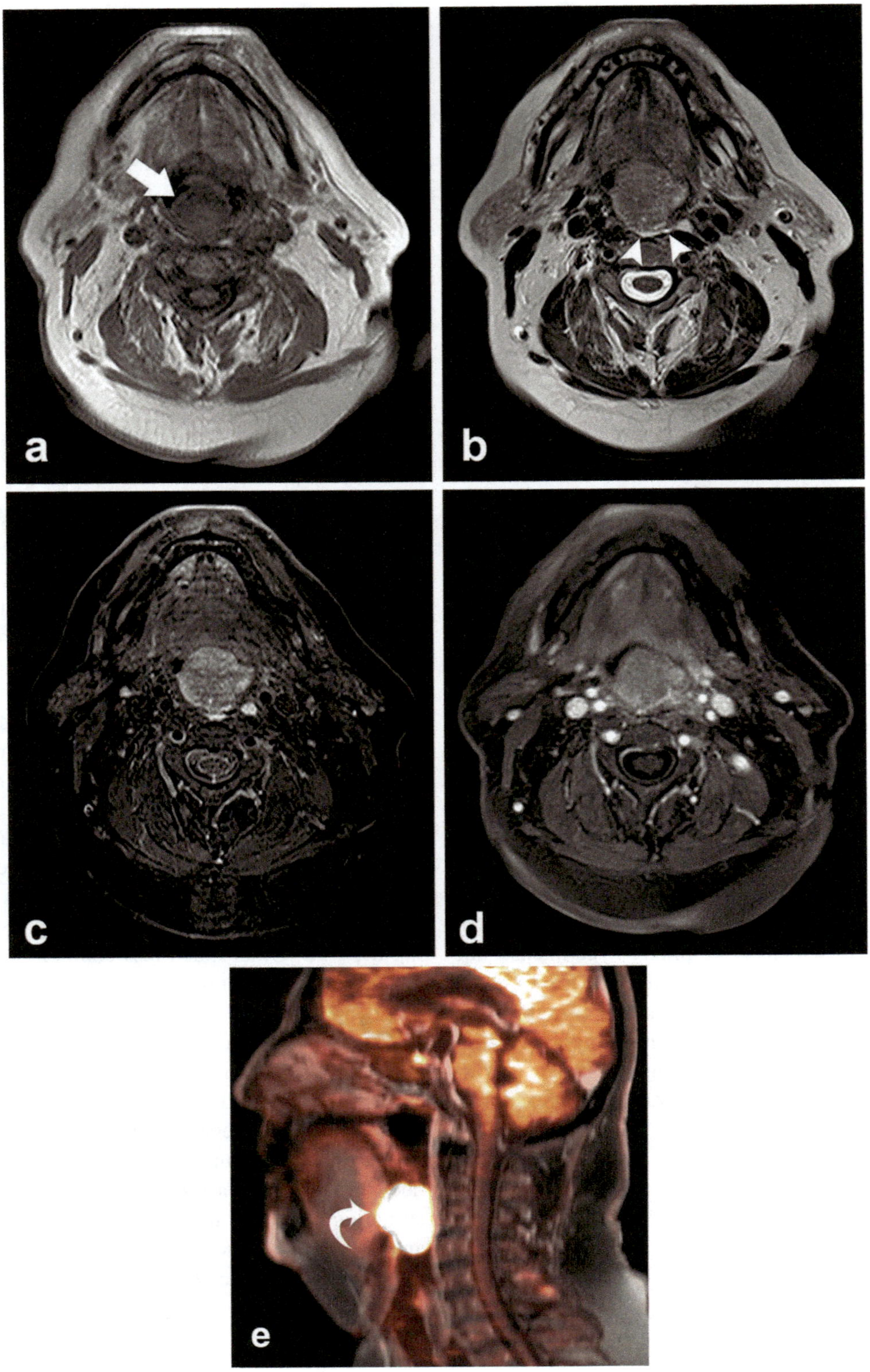

Fig. 106.1 T1 axial (**a**), T2 TSE axial (**b**), STIR axial (**c**), T1 radial VIBE with fat suppression post-gadolinium contrast axial (**d**), and PET/MR T1 radial VIBE with fat suppression post-gadolinium contrast sagittal fusion (**e**)

determine resectability of tumors in the aerodigestive tract include vascular invasion, prevertebral space invasion, and mediastinal invasion. However, it is crucial to recognize that tumors deemed unresectable are not necessarily incurable and these patients should be offered chemotherapy and radiation.

Invasion of the prevertebral space is defined clinically by fixation to the prevertebral musculature. Tumors extending to the prevertebral musculature and therefore beyond the prevertebral fascia are considered unresectable as resection along the longus colli musculature is exceedingly difficult with no survival benefit. In staging of head and neck cancers, the traditional imaging modalities, MRI, CT, and PET, have overlapping advantages. MRI has inherent superior tissue contrast resolution and more reliable detection of bone marrow invasion, intracranial invasion, invasion of deep tongue muscle, and perineural spread. Preservation of the T1 hyperintense retropharyngeal fat, on MRI, is considered as no invasion to the prevertebral space. Findings suggesting prevertebral musculature invasion include abnormal T2 signal intensity within the musculature and abnormal nodularity of the prevertebral musculature. CT has shown to be superior to MRI in detecting invasion of bony cortex.

FDG PET has advantage over MRI and CT in detecting metastatic lymph nodes (N stage) and distant metastases (M stage). In comparison with the conventional imaging modalities, FDG PET/MR imaging combines morphological information of complex head and neck anatomy from the MRI component with high sensitivity of metabolic imaging. FDG PET and MRI in combination allow for more accurate assessment of the primary tumor and TNM staging. Oropharyngeal and nasopharyngeal malignancies are FDG avid, and delineation of the tumor by PET can aid in the assessment of retropharyngeal extension.

Suggested Reading

Chong VF, Fan YF. The retropharyngeal space: route of tumour spread. Clin Radiol. 1998;53(1):64–7.

Debnam JM, Guha-Thakurta N. Retropharyngeal and prevertebral spaces: anatomic imaging and diagnosis. Otolaryngol Clin N Am. 2012;45(6):1293–310.

Hsu WC, Loevner LA, Karpati R, Ahmed T, Mong A, Battineni ML, et al. Accuracy of magnetic resonance imaging in predicting absence of fixation of head and neck cancer to the prevertebral space. Head Neck. 2005;27(2):95–100.

Case 107
Supraglottic Laryngeal Cancer

Apar Gupta

History

A 73-year-old male with dysphagia for several months and epiglottic mass detected on CT. Referred for PET/MR imaging to evaluate tumor extent and staging (Fig. 107.1).

Diagnosis

Supraglottic laryngeal cancer with metastatic lymph nodes

Findings

- Contrast enhancing soft tissue mass with increased STIR signal within the body and left leaflet of the epiglottis. It extends across the midline to also involve the right leaflet (wide arrow). The mass extends into pre-epiglottic space and is inseparable from the strap muscle.
- Epiglottic mass has intense FDG uptake on PET/MR fusion images (arrowhead).
- Enlarged left level IIA lymph node with increased signal on STIR (thin arrow). It is hypermetabolic only in its anterior aspect consistent with a predominantly necrotic metastatic lymph node.
- Enlarged, hypermetabolic right level IIA lymph node (curved arrow) consistent with metastasis.

Discussion

Supraglottic squamous cell carcinoma is less common than glottic laryngeal cancer, accounting for approximately 30–40% of the laryngeal cancers in the United States. It is treated differently than cancer originating in the glottis or subglottis, and because of its location, treatment can affect speech, swallowing, and breathing. The supraglottic larynx can be divided into four parts: the epiglottis, false cords, arytenoids, and aryepiglottic folds. Lymphatic vascularity is denser in the supraglottis, which leads to a higher incidence of cervical lymph node metastases compared to other parts of the larynx.

Cross-sectional imaging evaluation is important to determine spread to the preepiglottic space, thyroid cartilage invasion, or extralaryngeal submucosal extension which characterizes different T stages of the supraglottic cancer. MRI provides superior soft tissue contrast, allows to readily demonstrate invasion of the preepiglottic and paraglottic space which mainly contains fat, and is therefore best evaluated on T1-weighted images. Cartilage invasion and metastatic spread to lymph nodes can also be thoroughly evaluated with MRI. The tumor and metastatic deposits demonstrate isointense signal on T1, hyperintense signal on T2, and avid enhancement post-contrast administration. MR imaging has been shown to predict local outcome in the supraglottic carcinoma before curative radiation therapy

R. Gupta et al., *PET/MR Imaging*, https://doi.org/10.1007/978-3-319-65106-4_107

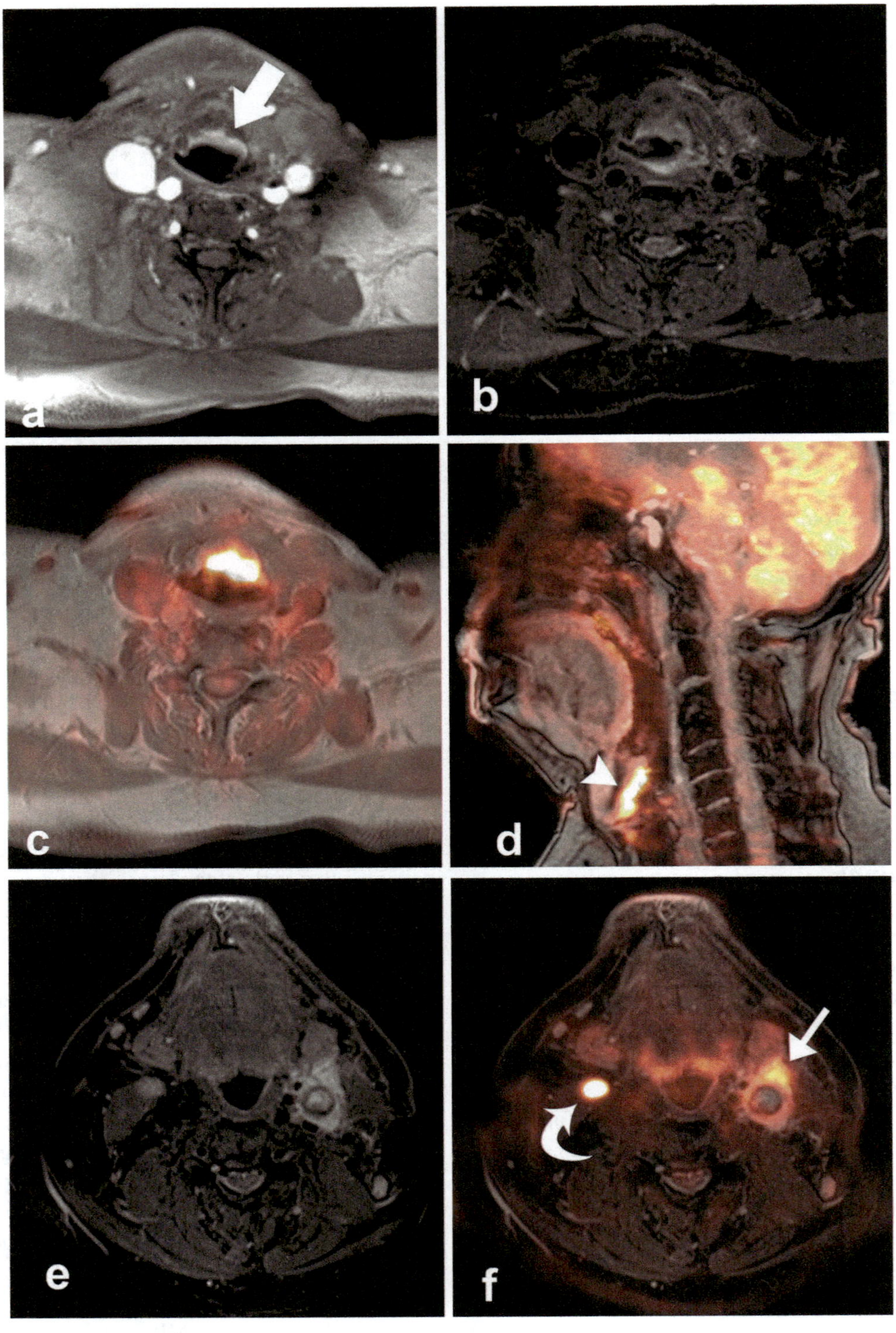

Fig. 107.1 T1 radial VIBE post-gadolinium contrast axial (**a**); STIR axial (**b**); PET/MR T1 axial fusion (**c**); PET/MR T1 GRE sagittal fusion (**d**); STIR axial, more superior level (**e**); and PET/MR STIR axial fusion, more superior level (**f**)

by demonstrating preepiglottic space extension or thyroid cartilage involvement.

Cervical lymph node involvement is one of the most important prognostic factors. High rates of false-negative results occur when based on size criteria and morphological assessment alone whether by CT or MRI. The primary role of FDG PET imaging in addition to determine the extent of the primary tumor is also to detect regional lymph node involvement and distant metastases. One limitation of PET/CT in evaluating supraglottic laryngeal carcinoma and other head and neck cancers is its inability to accurately assess the primary tumor site, extent of tumor spread, and relationship of the tumor and adjacent structures. This can be overcome by combining superb soft tissue contrast provided by MR imaging and metabolic information obtained by PET. In laryngeal cancer, functional identification of an occult primary tumor in patients with cervical lymph node metastasis can increase the radiotherapy target volume. It has been shown that the degree of hypermetabolic activity can predict tumor behavior and provide prognostic information in order to identify those patients who may need more aggressive therapy. Additionally, PET/MRI can be used to assess treatment response, as well as detect tumor recurrence, especially within the first year. FDG PET/MR imaging is an excellent tool in the staging, restaging, radiotherapy planning, and post-therapy follow-up assessment of laryngeal cancers.

Suggested Reading

Cacicedo J, Navarro A, Del Hoyo O, Gomez-Iturriaga A, Alongi F, Medina JA, et al. Role of fluorine-18 fluorodeoxyglucose PET/CT in head and neck oncology: the point of view of the radiation oncologist. Br J Radiol. 2016;89(1067):20160217.

Ljumanović R, Langendijk JA, Schenk B, Van Wattingen M, Knol DL, Leemans CR, et al. Supraglottic carcinoma treated with curative radiation therapy: identification of prognostic groups with MR imaging. Radiology. 2004;232(2):440–8.

Case 108 Recurrent Rhabdomyosarcoma of the Infratemporal Fossa

Matthew Comito

History

A 15-year-old male with rhabdomyosarcoma of the infratemporal fossa, status postsurgical resection, and radiation in 2010, presents for restaging (Fig. 108.1).

Diagnosis

Recurrent rhabdomyosarcoma of the infratemporal fossa

Findings

- Axial T1 image shows mildly hypointense mass (thin arrow) in the left infratemporal fossa which heterogeneously enhances on post-contrast image (white arrowheads).
- Increased diffusion restriction is demonstrated by high DWI and low ADC signals which is characteristic of rhabdomyosarcoma (wide white arrow).
- PET/MR fusion demonstrates abnormal hypermetabolic activity within the mass (white curved arrow).
- Three-month posttreatment PET/MR fusion image shows markedly decreased hypermetabolic activity of the mass consistent with treatment response.

Discussion

Lesions of the infratemporal fossa, also known as the masticator space, are predominantly primary tumors that may be benign or malignant. Rarely, infratemporal fossa lesions may be acquired as a sequela of prior intervention or trauma. The infratemporal fossa is bound anteriorly by the posterior wall of the maxilla, laterally by the zygoma and temporalis muscle, inferiorly by the medial pterygoid muscle, and superiorly by the greater wing of the sphenoid. The fossa is bound medially by the lateral pterygoid plate. As the space is somewhat concealed and not amenable to physical examination, tumors often present late. The most common primary malignant tumor of this space is adenoid cystic carcinoma. These tumors have an indolent course and are frequently unresectable due to perineural spread at the time of diagnosis. If they are amenable to resection, there is a high rate of recurrence. Other malignant tumors of the infratemporal fossa include Hodgkin's lymphoma, rhabdomyosarcoma, squamous cell carcinoma, and primary bone tumors. Benign tumors include schwannomas, meningiomas, nasopharyngeal fibromas, and hemangiomas.

MRI is an excellent imaging modality to evaluate this region due to its superior tissue contrast. It is important to scrutinize the trigeminal and facial nerves on MRI as tumor extension via perineural spread have a great impact on patient

R. Gupta et al., *PET/MR Imaging*, https://doi.org/10.1007/978-3-319-65106-4_108

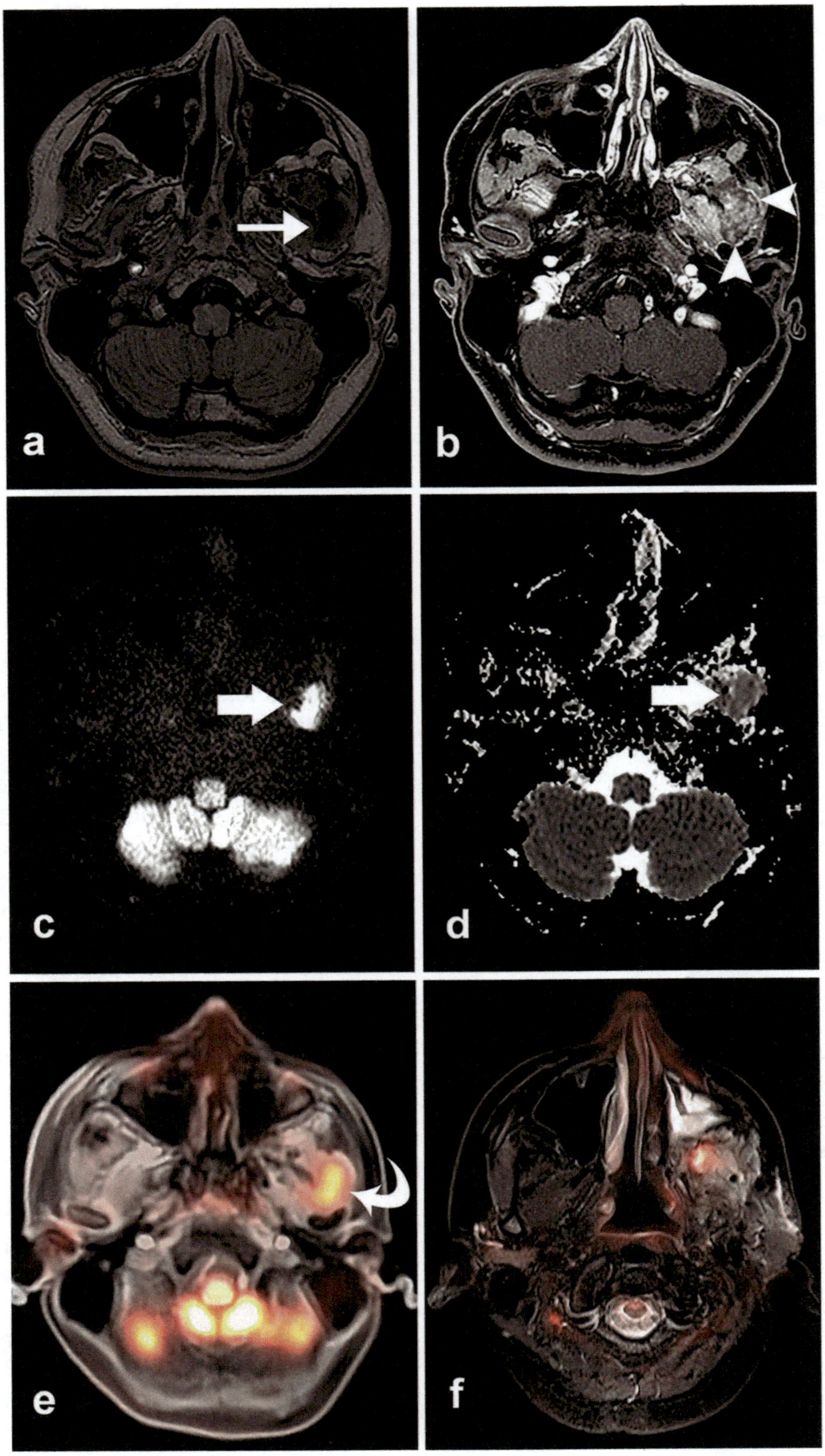

Fig. 108.1 T1 axial (**a**), T1-weighted with fat suppression post-gadolinium contrast axial (**b**), diffusion-weighted image axial (**c**), apparent diffusion coefficient axial (**d**), FDG PET/MR T1 radial VIBE with fat saturation axial fusion (**e**), and FDG PET/MR STIR axial fusion (3 months posttreatment) (**f**)

management. Perineural spread is said to occur when there is abnormal enhancement or thickening of a nerve. Rhabdomyosarcomas are the second most common primary tumor of the head and neck in pediatric patients and have a propensity to metastasize along nerve pathways. These are highly cellular tumors which commonly show low T2 signal with increased diffusion restriction and heterogeneous enhancement. In the infratemporal fossa, perineural spread occurs along the V2 and V3 (maxillary and mandibular, respectively) branches of the trigeminal nerve. Not infrequently, there will be expansion of the foramen rotundum if V2 is involved and expansion of the foramen ovale if V3 is involved. Furthermore, the trigeminal nerve has multiple connections with the facial nerve and therefore must also be carefully evaluated. It may be useful to compare the signal intensity and size of the nerve and foramina of the contralateral side to help ascertain a proper diagnosis.

Utilization of PET/MR imaging can provide additional information that was previously not available to the clinician while exposing younger patients to less radiation than PET/CT. MRI provides excellent soft tissue differentiation of masses from non-diseased tissue which ultimately has a direct impact on patient management. One of the shortcomings of MRI is relatively low sensitivity in determining metastatic involvement within normal, sub-centimeter lymph nodes as lymph node evaluation heavily relies on the size and morphology. PET is much more sensitive in the N-stage evaluation as it explores metabolic activity within the regional lymph nodes. Additionally, PET/MRI is also the modality of choice for serial evaluation of treatment response, detection of tumor recurrence, and differentiation of treatment-related changes from true disease progression or recurrence.

Suggested Reading

Freling NJ, Merks JH, Saeed P, Balm AJ, Bras J, Pieters BR, et al. Imaging findings in craniofacial childhood rhabdomyosarcoma. Pediatr Radiol. 2010;40(11):1723–38. quiz 1855

Majoie CB, Hulsmans FJ, Verbeeten B Jr, Castelyns JA, Oldenburger F, Schouwenburg PF, et al. Perineural tumor extension along the trigeminal nerve: magnetic resonance imaging findings. Eur J Radiol. 1997;24(3):191–205.

Platzek I, Beuthien-Baumann B, Schneider M, Gudziol V, Langner J, Schramm G, et al. PET/MRI in head and neck cancer: initial experience. Eur J Nucl Med Mol Imaging. 2013;40(1):6–11.

Tiwari R, Quak J, Egeler S, Smeele L, Waal IV, Valk PV, et al. Tumors of the infratemporal fossa. Skull Base Surg. 2000;10(1):1–9.

Case 109
Warthin Tumor

Ana M. Franceschi

History

An 82-year-old female presents with painless right parotid gland swelling concerning for neoplasm (Fig. 109.1).

Diagnosis

Warthin tumor

Findings

- Hyperintense T1-weighted and mildly hyperintense T2-weighted, well-circumscribed nodule that is protruding from the right parotid gland (white thin arrow).
- PET fusion image demonstrates intense hypermetabolic activity corresponding to the right parotid nodule (curved white arrow).
- PET fusion at a more inferior level demonstrates a second hypermetabolic nodule in the right parotid gland (white arrowhead).
- PET MIP shows the relationship of the two nodules in the right parotid gland (black arrowheads) representing Warthin tumor.

Discussion

The majority of salivary gland tumors occur in the parotid gland, likely related to its proportionally larger size. The most common benign salivary gland tumors are pleomorphic adenoma, also known as benign mixed tumor and Warthin tumor. In patients with benign salivary gland tumors, surgical excision is usually curative. Pleomorphic adenomas may recur at the surgical site due to it being poorly encapsulated and its propensity for seeding. Furthermore, pleomorphic adenomas have the potential for malignant transformation. Benign pleomorphic adenoma is typically hypointense on T1-weighted images; markedly hyperintense on T2-weighted images, especially the myxoid subtype; and heterogeneously enhancing on post-contrast T1-weighted imaging sequences. These tumors have increased FDG uptake in up to 25% of the cases. Carcinoma ex pleomorphic adenoma is the malignancy arising from pleomorphic adenomas. Its risk of development increases with time from 1.5% in the first 5 years reaching 9.5% after 15 years.

Warthin tumor is the second most common benign salivary gland tumor with a male predilection. As opposed to pleomorphic adenomas,

R. Gupta et al., *PET/MR Imaging*, https://doi.org/10.1007/978-3-319-65106-4_109

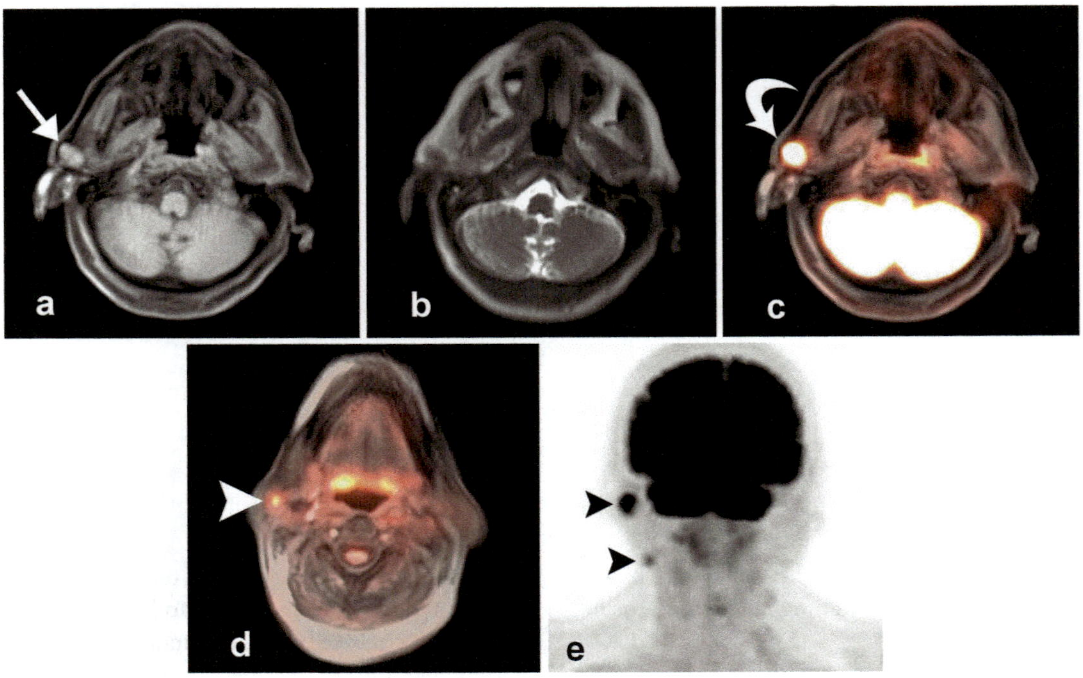

Fig. 109.1 T1 radial VIBE with fat suppression axial (**a**), T2 HASTE axial (**b**), FDG PET/MR T1 radial VIBE with fat suppression axial fusion (**c**), FDG PET/MR T1 radial VIBE axial fusion, at a more inferior level (**d**), and FDG PET MIP coronal (**e**)

Warthin tumors have an extremely low potential for malignant transformation. They are often multifocal or bilateral, with cholesterol-containing foci of cystic change in 30% of patients. These neoplasms typically demonstrate intermediate signal on T1-weighted images, especially their cystic areas, and intermediate signal on T2-weighted images without significant contrast enhancement. Warthin tumors are hypermetabolic on FDG PET imaging. Typically, pleomorphic adenomas show lower FDG uptake in comparison to malignant salivary gland neoplasms. However, Warthin tumors demonstrate overlap with malignant tumors in its degree of FDG uptake. These tumors can be identified incidentally on whole-body PET/MRI. Therefore, a hypermetabolic lesion in any of the salivary glands should be further investigated with fine needle aspiration biopsy to determine the type of the tumor, which in turn will determine further management. The advantage of whole-body FDG PET imaging is early detection of distant metastasis and, therefore, significant effect on management of patients with high-grade malignant salivary glands tumors. However, it is not recommended for the routine evaluation of low-grade malignant salivary gland tumors due to low avidity for FDG.

Suggested Reading

Freling N, Crippa F, Maroldi R. Staging and follow-up of high-grade malignant salivary gland tumours: the role of traditional versus functional imaging approaches - a review. Oral Oncol. 2016;60:157–66.

Sharma P, Jain TK, Singh H, Suman SK, Faizi NA, Kumar R, et al. Utility of (18)F-FDG PET-CT in staging and restaging of patients with malignant salivary gland tumours: a single-institutional experience. Nucl Med Commun. 2013;34(3):211–9.

Yousem DM, Kraut MA, Chalian AA. Major salivary gland imaging. Radiology. 2000;216(1):19–29.

Case 110
Squamous Cell Carcinoma of the Scalp

Laura L. Rosenkrantz and Robert Matthews

History

An 81-year-old male with skin cancer presents with scalp lesions for over a year (Fig. 110.1).

Diagnosis

Squamous cell carcinoma of the scalp

Findings

- MRI shows T1 isointense (wide arrow) and T2 hyperintense (curved arrows) bilateral head lesions that involve full thickness of the scalp.
- PET/MRI fusion images demonstrate intense FDG uptake within scalp lesions consistent with malignancy.
- No clear osseous invasion is seen.

Discussion

Squamous cell carcinoma (SCC) is the result of uncontrolled growth of abnormal cells in the upper layers of the skin. It is the second most common form of skin cancer, with more than 1 million cases diagnosed each year in the United States. It is mainly caused by cumulative ultraviolet (UV) exposure and therefore is most commonly found on areas frequently exposed to the sun such as the scalp, ear, lip, face, neck, hands, arms, and legs. Risk factors include fair skin, light hair, light eyes, male gender, age over 50 years old, history of excessive sun exposure, or those with an inherited UV-sensitive condition such as xeroderma pigmentosum. Clinically, SCC of the scalp can appear as scaly red patches, open sores, ulcerations, or warts which can crust or bleed. The diagnosis is mainly clinical, based on history and skin exam, and then confirmed with biopsy.

The initial diagnostic workup of squamous cell carcinoma of the head and neck is usually purely clinical. Occasionally, a CT scan is performed to evaluate for the extent of the depth of soft tissue involvement, potential bony invasion, and lymph node metastases. CT is superior at showing cortical disruption of the underlying bone. MR imaging is the preferred method to evaluate perineural invasion and orbital or intracranial extension. MR can help show the tumor extent in the skin since the tumor shows high signal intensity on T2-weighted images, isointense

R. Gupta et al., *PET/MR Imaging*, https://doi.org/10.1007/978-3-319-65106-4_110

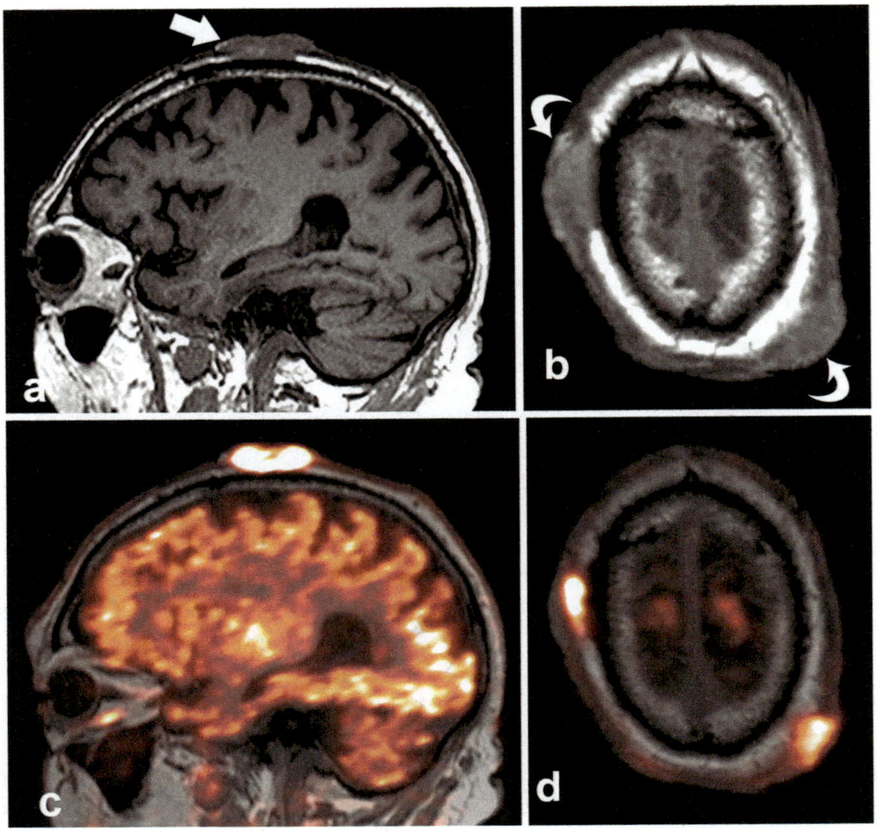

Fig. 110.1 MPRAGE sagittal (**a**), T2 axial (**b**), PET/MRI MPRAGE sagittal fusion (**c**), and PET/MRI MPRAGE axial fusion (**d**)

to muscle on T1-weighted images, and show contrast enhancement following administration of gadolinium.

On PET/MR imaging, these tumors show increased FDG uptake similar to other head and neck cancers. FDG PET is useful in baseline staging of squamous cell carcinoma, treatment planning, assessing response to therapy, and monitoring for recurrence. PET/MRI can delineate tumor extent but is most valuable in detecting metastatic lesions, especially regional lymph nodes and distant metastases outside the neck region.

Suggested Reading

Bhat V, Devere J, Ramakrishanan A, Kuriakose MA. Perineural spread in squamous cell carcinoma of the face: an overlooked facet of information on imaging. J Maxillofac Oral Surg. 2016;15(3):390–3.

Castaldi P, Leccisotti L, Bussu F, Miccichè F, Rufini V. Role of 18F-FDG PET-CT in head and neck squamous cell carcinoma. Acta Otorhinolaryngol Ital. 2013;33(1):1–8.

Lang PG Jr, Braun MA, Kwatra R. Aggressive squamous carcinomas of the scalp. Dermatol Surg. 2006;32(9):1163–70.

Case 111
Orbital Sarcoidosis

Dharmesh Tank and Anuj Rajput

History

A 53-year-old male with suspected orbital lymphoma (Fig. 111.1).

Diagnosis

Orbital sarcoidosis

Findings

- T1 isointense and T2 hypointense mass in the superolateral aspect of the right orbit in the region of the lacrimal gland (thin arrows).
- Orbital mass shows relatively homogenously enhancement following contrast administration.
- PET/MRI fusion demonstrates increased FDG uptake within the mass.
- Subsequent biopsy revealed multiple small noncaseating granulomas consistent with sarcoidosis.

Discussion

When considering solid orbital lesions, there is a wide differential diagnosis that includes various etiologies such as neoplastic (lymphoma, multiple myeloma, meningioma, metastasis, optic glioma), inflammatory (pseudotumor and thyroid ophthalmopathy), granulomatous (sarcoidosis and Wegener's granulomatosis), vascular (orbital varix, venolymphatic malformation), infectious, and congenital (infantile hemangioma). Lymphoma is the most prevalent orbital neoplasm in older adults, and choroidal melanoma is the most common primary adult ocular malignancy. Breast cancer is the most common malignancy to metastasize to the orbit.

Diplopia, proptosis, decreased visual acuity, and eye pain are all common presenting symptoms in patients with nontraumatic orbital pathology. In addition to clinical examination, imaging modalities requested include computed tomography and MRI. MRI provides valuable anatomic information in the evaluation of orbital lesions. Sarcoidosis is a multisystem granulomatous disease with orbital involvement seen in approximately 10–50% of patients. Uveitis is by far the most common presentation of orbital sarcoidosis and is typically bilateral. Orbital sarcoidosis may mimic metastatic disease and often involve the lacrimal gland, extraocular muscles, optic nerve, optic sheath, and optic chiasm.

Sarcoid involvement of the lacrimal glands on contrast-enhanced CT and MRI typically presents with enlargement and enhancement of the gland. The involved gland will usually demonstrate hypointensity on T1- and T2-weighted sequences; however, lesions may also be hyperintense on

R. Gupta et al., *PET/MR Imaging*, https://doi.org/10.1007/978-3-319-65106-4_111

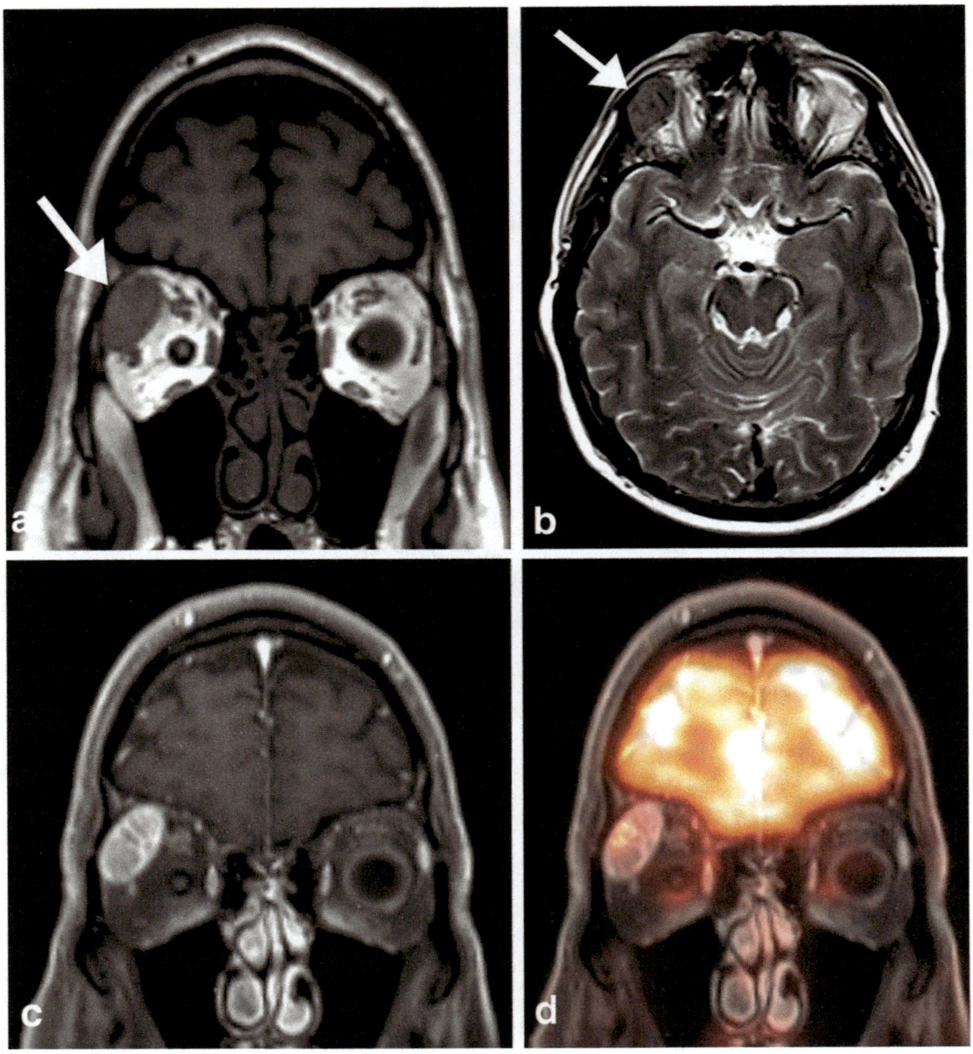

Fig. 111.1 T1-weighted coronal (**a**), T2-weighted axial (**b**), T1 VIBE with fat suppression post-gadolinium contrast coronal (**c**), and FDG PET/MRI T1 VIBE with fat suppression post-gadolinium contrast fusion (**d**)

T2-weighted sequences. On post-contrast sequences, there will be homogeneous enhancement. FDG PET/MR imaging shows increased FDG uptake in the structures involved with sarcoidosis. As increased SUV can also be seen in other processes such as lymphoma, metastasis, and other malignancies, biopsy is often necessary for diagnosis. It is also important to note that sarcoidosis can coexist in patients with malignancy. Regardless, FDG PET/MRI can help to identify sites and tissues of concern and be used as a guide for biopsy. In patient with orbital sarcoidosis being their initial presentation of the disease, whole-body PET imaging findings may reveal hilar lymphadenopathy and typical lung abnormalities in the thorax. The patients often show a good response to treatment with systemic steroids with resolution of FDG activity in the affected lesions.

Suggested Reading

Chowdhury FU, Sheerin F, Bradley KM, Gleeson FV. Sarcoid-like reaction to malignancy on whole-body integrated 18F-FDG PET/CT: prevalence and disease pattern. Clin Radiol. 2009;64:675–81.

Iannuzzi MC, Rybicki BA, Teirstein AS. Sarcoidosis. N Engl J Med. 2007;357:2153–65.

Tailor TD, Gupta D, Dalley RW, Keene CD, Anzai Y. Orbital neoplasms in adults: clinical, radiologic, and pathologic review. Radiographics. 2013;33(6): 1739–58.

Teirstein AS, Machac J, Almeida O, Lu P, Padilla ML, Iannuzzi MC. Results of 188 whole-body fluorodeoxyglucose positron emission tomography scans in 137 patients with sarcoidosis. Chest. 2007;132:1949–53.

Part VI

Neuroradiology

Case 112 High-Grade Glioma

Anuj Rajput, Michael Goodman, and Lev Bangiyev

History

A 59-year-old female presenting with seizures and found to have a left temporal lesion on recent brain MRI (Fig. 112.1).

Diagnosis

High-grade glioma

Findings

- T1 post-contrast image shows heterogeneously enhancing mass in the left temporal lobe (wide arrow).
- FLAIR shows hyperintense signal in the left mesial temporal lobe due to the mass and associated edema. There is some mass effect with mild medial displacement of the mesial temporal lobe (curved arrow) and effacement of the sulci and Sylvain fissure.
- PET/MR fusion shows intense hypermetabolic activity consistent with malignancy which is more extensive than the area of enhancement.
- The mass shows increased restricted diffusion with hyperintense DWI and low ADC signal (thin arrows).
- Spectroscopy demonstrates marked elevation of the choline peak and significant depression of the *N*-acetylaspartate peak.

Discussion

The conventional MRI sequences demonstrate a large left temporal lobe lesion that demonstrates a hyperintense signal on FLAIR, increased diffusion restriction, and ill-defined contrast enhancement. The lesion demonstrates prominent hypermetabolic activity on PET imaging consistent with malignancy. Given the location of the lesion and MR imaging characteristics, the differential diagnosis would include herpes encephalitis and primary high-grade glioma. MRS demonstrates marked elevation of choline peak with profound decrease in N-acetylaspartate (NAA) peak. NAA is a marker of neuronal tissue and typically decreased with destruction of normal brain parenchyma. Choline is the marker for cell turnover and therefore commonly elevated in neoplasms. Extension of choline elevation beyond the margin of enhancement is very characteristic of infiltrative tumors such as glioma.

The World Health Organization classifies central nervous tumors according to a histological grading system in which higher grades are more likely to be infiltrative and progressive in nature with a worse prognosis for patients. Although

R. Gupta et al., *PET/MR Imaging*, https://doi.org/10.1007/978-3-319-65106-4_112

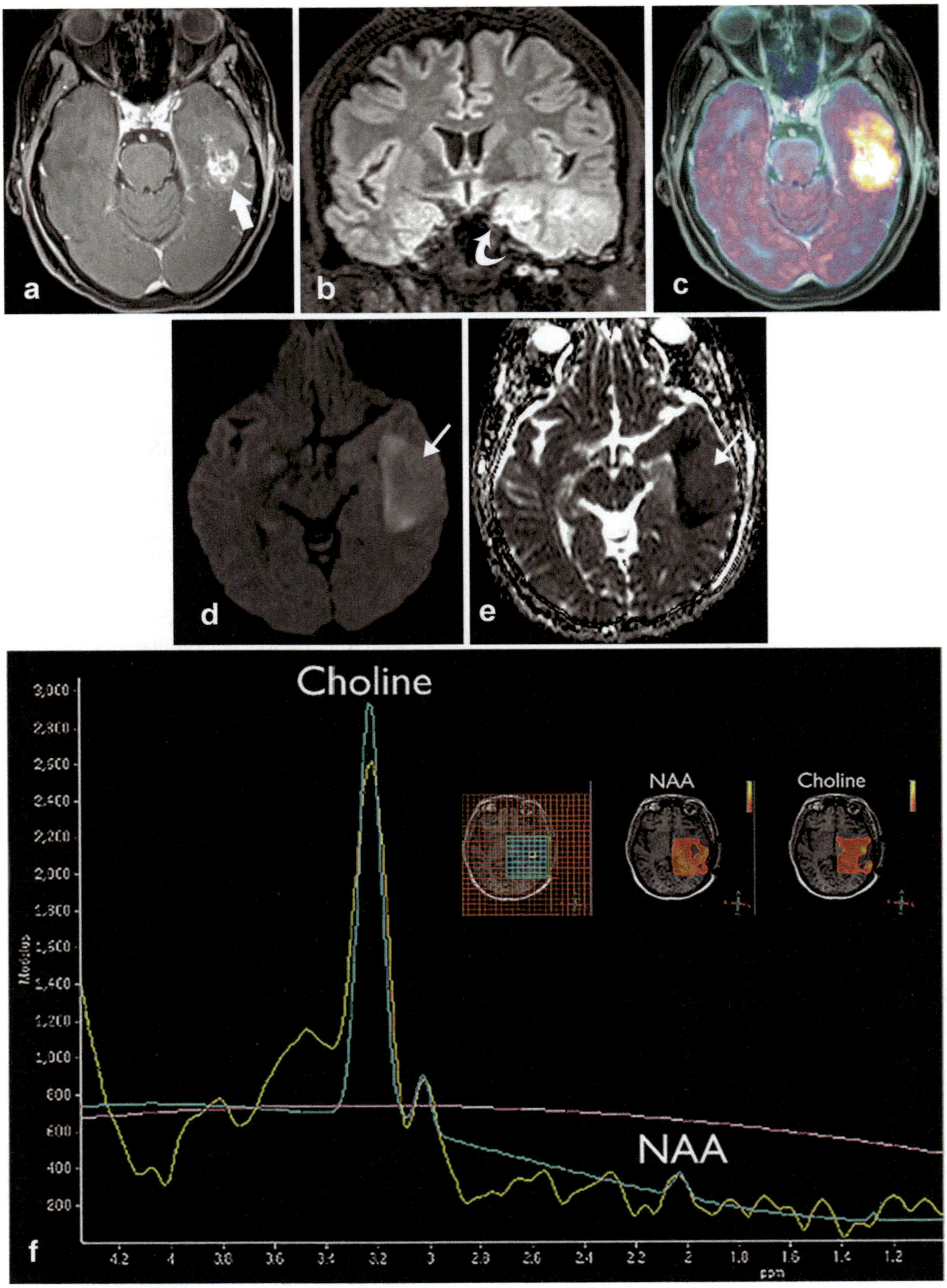

Fig. 112.1 T1 VIBE post-gadolinium contrast axial (**a**), FLAIR coronal (**b**), PET/MR T1 VIBE post-gadolinium contrast axial fusion (**c**), diffusion-weighted image axial (**d**), apparent diffusion coefficient axial (**e**), and MR spectroscopy (**f**)

definitive grading is done with biopsy, noninvasive imaging modalities can be used to evaluate the extent of these tumors with certain imaging characteristics to assign a grade Evaluation of these tumors is often performed utilizing advanced imaging techniques that are useful for tumor grading and distinguishing gliomas from metastases and are also utilized in the assessment of treatment response.

The use of PET in conjunction with MR often demonstrates the full extent of hypermetabolic tumor which is commonly beyond the area of enhancement and well coincides with infiltrative nature of primary brain neoplasms. Although FDG PET has been described as helpful in grading and prognosis of gliomas, it has certain limitations. The background activity of FDG in the brain is high. Therefore, for a tumor to be identifiable as malignant, FDG uptake should be higher than within surrounding normal brain. Low-grade gliomas have metabolic activity less or equal to normal brain and can be difficult to characterize on PET imaging. Hypermetabolic activity is also not specific just for tumor activity, as active infectious or inflammatory processes may show increased FDG uptake as well.

Suggested Reading

Bangiyev L, Rossi Espagnet MC, Young R, Shepherd T, Knopp E, Friedman K, et al. Adult brain tumor imaging: state of the art. Semin Roentgenol. 2014;49(1):39–52.

Padma MV, Said S, Jacobs M, Hwang DR, Dunigan K, Satter M, et al. Prediction of pathology and survival by FDG PET in gliomas. J Neuro-Oncol. 2003;64(3):227–37.

Puttick S, Bell C, Dowson N, Rose S, Fay M. FET, MRI, and simultaneous PET/MRI in the development of diagnostic and therapeutic strategies for glioma. Drug Discov Today. 2015;20(3):306–17.

Case 113
Alzheimer's Disease

Ana M. Franceschi, Michael J. Hoch,
and Timothy M. Shepherd

History

A 65-year-old female with progressive worsening short-term memory, comprehension, and judgment during the past 4 years (Fig. 113.1). No visual hallucinations, changes in behavior, or gait abnormality.

Diagnosis

Alzheimer's disease

Findings

- MPRAGE sagittal image shows atrophy of the precuneus (white wide arrow) with widening of the marginal ramus of the cingulate sulcus (white arrowhead).
- MPRAGE coronal image demonstrates temporoparietal atrophy (curved arrows).
- There is mesial temporal volume loss demonstrated on the MPRAGE coronal and axial FLAIR images (thin white arrows).
- PET and fusion images show global decreased FDG uptake which is worse in the right temporoparietal lobe (black arrowheads). There is preservation of the sensorimotor gyri (black thin arrows).

Discussion

Alzheimer's disease (AD) is the most common neurodegenerative disease, accounting for 60–80% of all dementia cases worldwide. There are multiple risk factors for the development of late-onset AD including advanced age, female sex, smoking, sleep apnea, apo-E4 allele status, positive family history particularly on the maternal side, and Down syndrome. Typically, patients will present with anterograde memory loss that slowly progresses over years to diminished ability to perform executive functions, decreased attention span, and neuropsychiatric symptoms.

Familial cases of AD demonstrate an autosomal dominant inheritance pattern, with typical mutations in one of at least three genes: presenilin 1, presenilin 2, and amyloid precursor protein. Histologically, AD is characterized by the accumulation of amyloid-B (AB) forming plaques, tau neurofibrillary tangles, and progressive neuronal loss. The only definitive test is brain biopsy, although typical clinical features and imaging findings are usually sufficient to make the diagnosis. In apo-E4 allele carriers, cerebral amyloid angiopathy is an important comorbidity, with increased risk of intracranial hemorrhage.

In the early stages of Alzheimer's disease, FDG PET/MR imaging demonstrates hypomet-

R. Gupta et al., *PET/MR Imaging*, https://doi.org/10.1007/978-3-319-65106-4_113

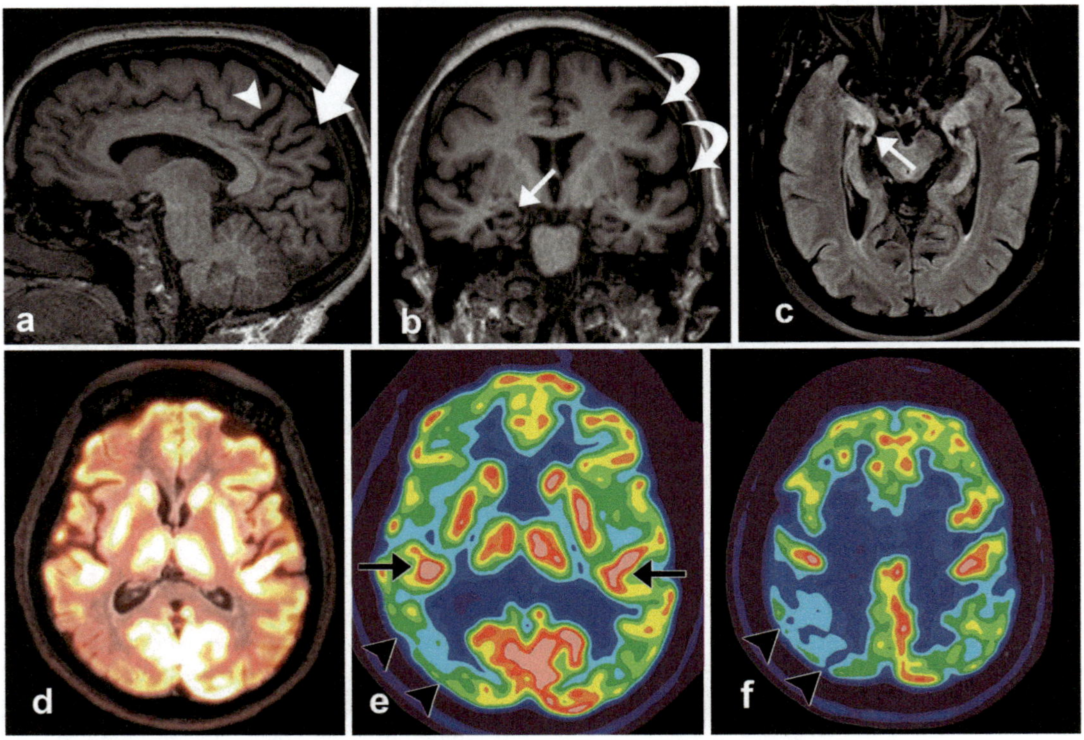

Fig. 113.1 MPRAGE sagittal (**a**), MPRAGE coronal (**b**), FLAIR axial (**c**), PET/MR FLAIR axial fusion (**d**), PET axial (**e**), and PET axial, at more superior level (**f**)

abolic activity in the parietotemporal cortices with associated decreased activity in the posterior cingulate and precuneus regions. In the normal elderly patient, the posterior cingulate will often have higher uptake than the other brain cortical regions. As the disease progresses, there is more global involvement including the frontal lobes. The hypometabolic regions of the cortex are commonly asymmetric. On PET imaging, there is preserved metabolic activity in the primary sensorimotor cortices, visual cortices, cerebellum, thalamus, and striatum. In the early stages, MRI findings are absent. As the disease progresses, there may be cortical atrophy in the associated region of hypometabolism. Combined FDG PET/MR imaging improves the diagnostic ability as the changes in FDG activity can be directly correlated to MRI findings.

Suggested Reading

Brown RK, Bohnen NI, Wong KK, Minoshima S, Frey KA. Brain PET in suspected dementia: patterns of altered FDG metabolism. Radiographics. 2014;34(3):684–701.

Jalbert JJ, Daiello LA, Lapane KL. Dementia of the Alzheimer type. Epidemiol Rev. 2008;30:15–34.

Case 114 Pituitary Adenoma

Jingyu Zhou

History

A 79-year-old male with squamous cell carcinoma of the head and neck presents with "nerve" pain (Fig. 114.1).

Diagnosis

Pituitary adenoma

Findings

- Heterogeneous signal on T1-weighted dominant MPRAGE image and mildly hyperintense on FLAIR image in the pituitary gland which is mildly enlarged (thin arrow)
- Intense FDG uptake within the pituitary gland on PET images (curved arrow)
- No suprasellar extension of pituitary tumor

Discussion

The pituitary gland is an endocrine organ at the base of the skull found within the sella turcica. The gland is divided into the anterior and posterior segments. The hormones secreted from the anterior pituitary have myriad of downstream effects that regulate growth, metabolism, and reproduction (adrenocorticotropic hormone, thyroid stimulating hormone, follicle stimulating hormone, luteinizing hormone, growth hormone, and prolactin). The two hormones produced in the posterior pituitary, oxytocin and vasopressin, induce uterine contraction and regulate blood pressure, respectively. The anterior pituitary gland appears isointense to gray matter on T1 and T2 sequences. The posterior pituitary appears hyperintense on T1 that is thought to be related to T1 shortening effect of vasopressin. The pituitary gland is the most vascular organ in the body, lays outside of the blood-brain barrier, and therefore demonstrates brisk and homogenous enhancement on post-contrast T1 sequence.

Pituitary adenoma is the most common pituitary tumor. This is a low-grade (WHO grade I), solid tumor that is often described as either microadenoma (less than 1 cm) or macroadenoma (larger than 1 cm). Pituitary adenomas can be endocrinologically active, secreting various hormones depending on the cell type from which they originate, thus leading to certain symptom manifestations and early discovery. However, most microadenomas are inactive, asymptomatic, and therefore incidentally discovered. These

R. Gupta et al., *PET/MR Imaging*, https://doi.org/10.1007/978-3-319-65106-4_114

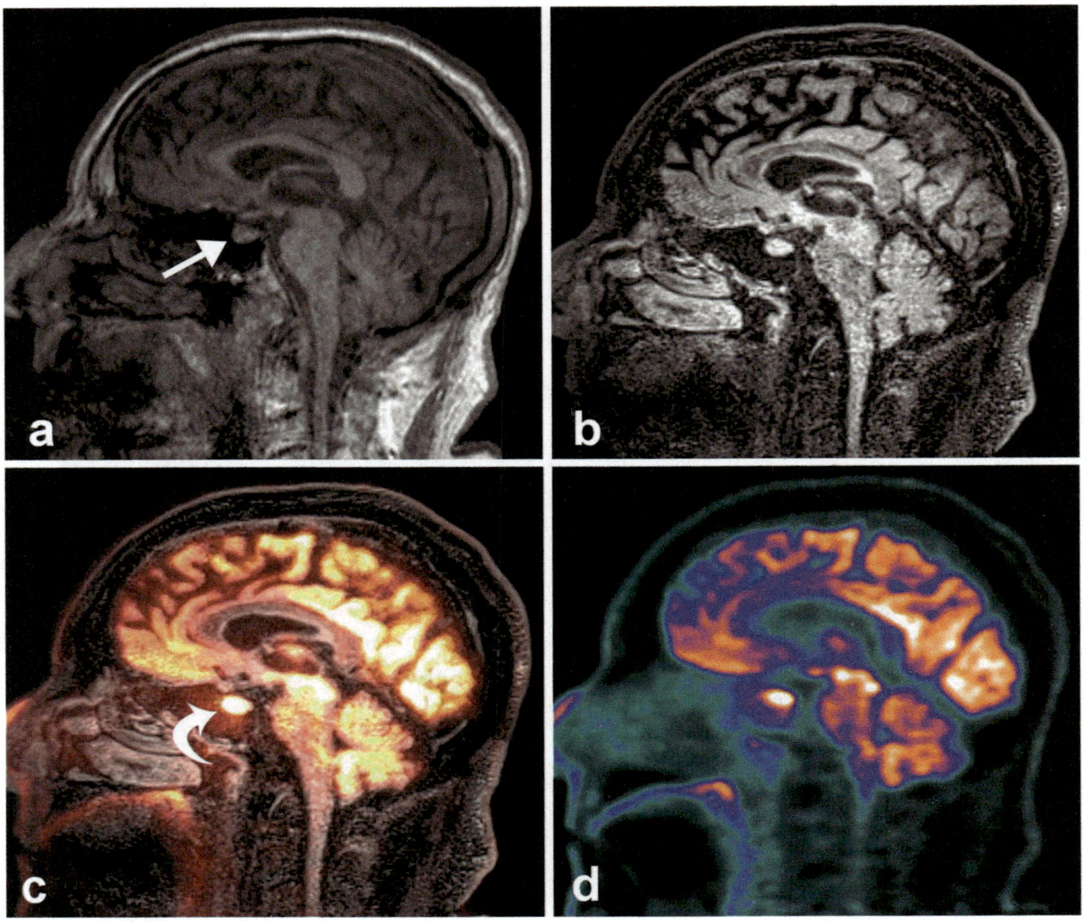

Fig. 114.1 MPRAGE sagittal (**a**), FLAIR with fat suppression sagittal (**b**), PET/MR FLAIR with fat suppression sagittal fusion (**c**), and PET sagittal (**d**)

small lesions are often T1 and T2 isointense to the surrounding pituitary gland. Some adenomas may hemorrhage leading to various signal intensity on T1 and T2 depending on the age of the blood products. Most frequently, 70–90% of adenomas enhance slower than normal pituitary tissue and thus will be hypointense to the pituitary gland on dynamic post-contrast T1-weighted images.

Macroadenomas, due to their size, often expand and extend out of the sella turcica and, when large, can be described as a "snowman" or "figure of 8" shape on coronal view. The T1 hyperintense posterior pituitary is often displaced. Like microadenomas, they are often isointense to the surrounding pituitary on T1 and T2 sequences. The tumor usually enhances heterogeneously with contrast. Large pituitary macroadenomas extend into the suprasellar cistern and exert mass effect on optic chiasm leading to temporal hemianopsia. Macroadenomas may also extend laterally and invade adjacent cavernous sinuses with encasement of the internal carotid arteries (ICAs). However, they do not narrow the ICAs like meningioma.

A large percentage of pituitary adenomas may demonstrate focal increased FDG uptake on PET. Increase in size (macroadenoma) and hormone secretion (functional adenomas) correlate with higher tendency for FDG avidity. Other differentials to consider in focal pituitary FDG uptake include metastatic lesions and lymphoma. On PET/MR imaging pituitary adenomas are uncommon but can be easily detected as an incidental finding in asymptomatic patients due to their high FDG uptake.

Suggested Reading

Chaudhry AA, Gupta R, Woroch L, Filatov A, Peyster R, Bangiyev L. Making sense of Sellar region pathology: image-based diagnostic algorithm. Contemp Diagn Radiol. 2015;38(22):1–7.

Hyun SH, Choi JY, Lee KH, Choe YS, Kim BT. Incidental focal 18F-FDG uptake in the pituitary gland: clinical significance and differential diagnostic criteria. J Nucl Med. 2011;52(4):547–50.

Seok H, Lee EY, Choe EY, Yang WI, Kim JY, Shin DY, et al. Analysis of 18F-fluorodeoxyglucose positron emission tomography findings in patients with pituitary lesions. Korean J Intern Med. 2013;28(1):81–8.

Case 115
Oligodendroglioma

Michael J. Hoch, Ana M. Franceschi,
and Timothy M. Shepherd

History

A 47-year-old patient with a right frontal intra-axial mass (Fig. 115.1). PET/MR imaging requested by neurosurgery for preoperative biopsy planning.

Diagnosis

Oligodendroglioma (biopsy target)

Findings

- MRI shows a right frontal lobe infiltrative tumor with a small focus of faint posterior enhancement.
- Perfusion rCBV map reveals a focus of hyperperfusion (white arrow) along the posterior margin of the tumor.
- PET/MRI fusion and PET show increased FDG uptake associated with the area of hyperperfusion (red circle) indicating the best place to biopsy for detecting the highest grade of tumor.

Discussion

Oligodendroglioma is a primary brain tumor that commonly presents as a partially calcified cortical or subcortical mass in middle-aged adults or children. Oligodendroglioma represents 5–10% of all primary intracranial neoplasms and is generally dichotomized into WHO grade II (low grade) and WHO grade III (high grade) tumors. Patients often present with seizures, headaches, and personality changes. They generally grow slowly, so they can be quite large before symptoms occur. On histologic examination, the tumor often demonstrates a 1p19q codeletion which predicts a favorable response to chemotherapy and radiation. However, the primary treatment of choice is surgical resection with or without adjuvant chemoradiation. Local recurrence is common with a median survival time of 10 years for WHO grade II tumors and 3.5 years for WHO grade III tumors. Treatment may differ depending on the pathologic grade of the tumor. Patients with lower grade tumor are often treated with surgical resection followed by watchful waiting. This option is chosen because of the indolent nature of the tumor and potential morbidity

R. Gupta et al., *PET/MR Imaging*, https://doi.org/10.1007/978-3-319-65106-4_115

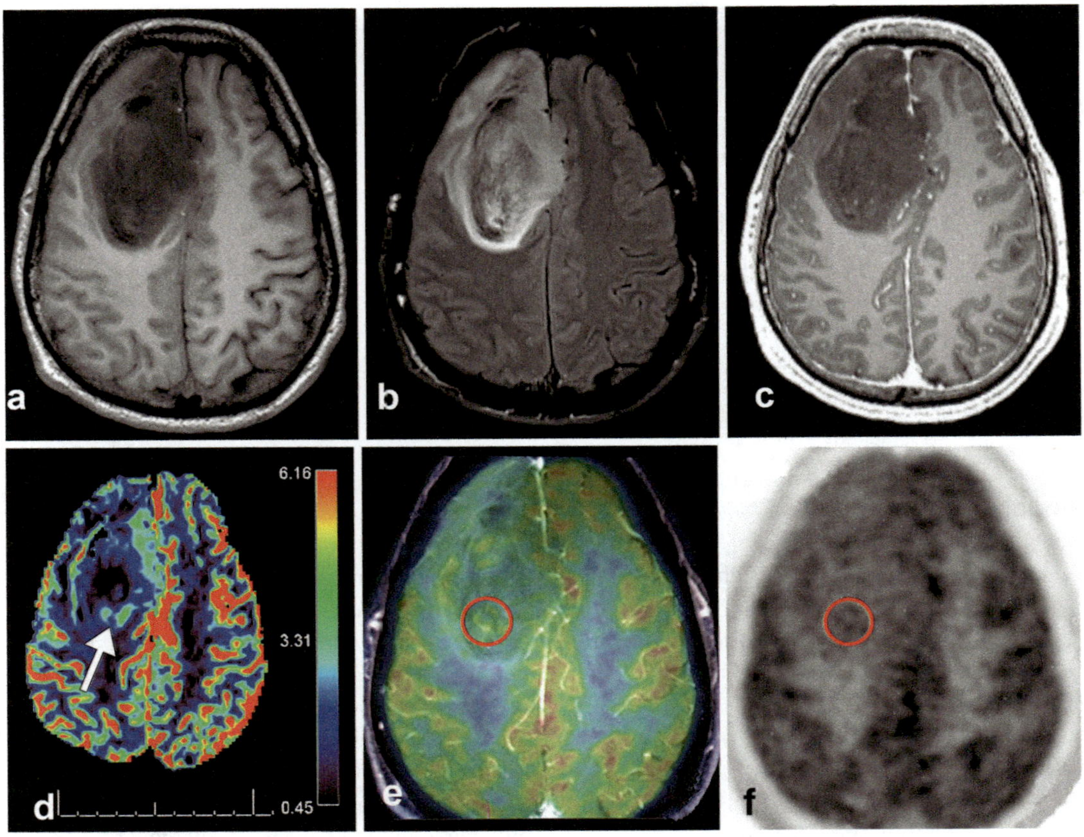

Fig. 115.1 MPRAGE axial (**a**), FLAIR axial (**b**), MPRAGE axial post-gadolinium contrast (**c**), Relative cerebral blood volume (rCBV) perfusion map (**d**), PET/MRI T1 post-gadolinium contrast fusion (**e**), and FDG PET axial (**f**)

related to chemotherapy and radiation. WHO grade III tumors are significantly more aggressive with greater rate of recurrence requiring adjuvant chemotherapy and radiation after surgical resection to improve patient survival. Therefore, identification of higher grade tumors on imaging is essential to guide biopsy and treatment planning.

At least 70–90% of oligodendrogliomas demonstrate calcifications on imaging. Associated remodeling of the calvarium suggests slower tumor growth. Conversely, patients with elevated relative cerebral blood volume on MR perfusion over 1.75 typically show more rapid progression, with a classic "chicken wire" pattern of tumor neovascularity. Classic findings of oligodendroglioma on neuroimaging with PET/MRI include areas of susceptibility or "blooming artifact" on T2*-weighted MRI sequences (such as GRE and SWI) in the areas of calcification. The tumor is typically T1 hypointense and T2 hyperintense and in 50% of patients may demonstrate heterogeneous enhancement following contrast. On FDG PET, the uptake is similar to background normal white matter in low-grade tumors. New or increased FDG uptake that is similar to normal gray matter suggests progression to anaplastic (WHO grade III) oligodendroglioma. Alternative PET agents such as C-11 methionine can be used to monitor disease progression.

Suggested Reading

Giammarile F, Cinotti LE, Jouvet A, Ramackers JM, Saint Pierre G, Thiesse P, et al. High and low grade oligodendroglioma (ODG): correlation of amino-acid and glucose uptakes using PET and histological classifications. J Neurooncol. 2004;68(3):263–74.

Law M, Yang S, Wang H, Babb JS, Johnson G, Cha S, et al. Glioma grading: sensitivity, specificity, and predictive values of perfusion MR imaging and proton MR spectroscopic imaging compared with conventional MR imaging. AJNR Am J Neuroradiol. 2003;24(10):1989–98.

Jenkinson MD, du Plessis DG, Smith TS, Joyce KA, Warnke PC, Walker C. Histological growth patterns and genotype in oligodendroglial tumours: correlation with MRI features. Brain. 2006;129(Pt):1884–91.

Case 116
Vascular Dementia

Priya Sharma and Rajesh Gupta

History

A 77-year-old female with a history of multiple strokes presents with confusion, short-term memory loss, depression, and visual hallucinations (Fig. 116.1).

Diagnosis

Vascular dementia

Findings

- DWI shows high signal intensity within the medial left occipital lobe indicating restricted diffusion (corresponding low ADC signal not shown), consistent with acute infarct 3 weeks earlier (curved arrow).
- FLAIR image demonstrates decreasing signal intensity in the left occipital lobe consistent with evolving chronic infarct (thin arrow).
- PET/MR shows decreased uptake in the left occipital lobe corresponding to the chronic infarct, as well as other focal areas of decreased activity in the bilateral cerebral cortices (arrowheads).

Discussion

Vascular dementia (VaD) is the second most common cause of dementia after Alzheimer's disease. The incidence of VaD is strongly correlated with age, presenting in only 1% of patients at 55 years of age but in over 4% of patients 71 years of age or older. VaD primarily occurs in patients with vascular risk factors who have had a single large stroke or multiple small strokes. Cerebral infarcts in certain locations or strategic infarcts are strongly associated with cognitive decline. These include infarcts in the dominant hemisphere involving temporoparietal region, posterior cerebral artery territory, and watershed infarctions. Also, bilateral anterior cerebral territory infarcts and bilateral lacunar infarcts in the thalami are at risk. Although symptoms overlap, VaD can be clinically distinguished from Alzheimer's by a sudden decline in cognitive function with temporal association to one or more cerebrovascular events. However, patients with chronic white matter small vessel disease may have a more gradual or stepwise deterioration. It is also important to note that VaD and Alzheimer's disease can coexist at the same time.

In addition to neuropsychological testing, imaging is essential for aiding in the diagnosis of

R. Gupta et al., *PET/MR Imaging*, https://doi.org/10.1007/978-3-319-65106-4_116

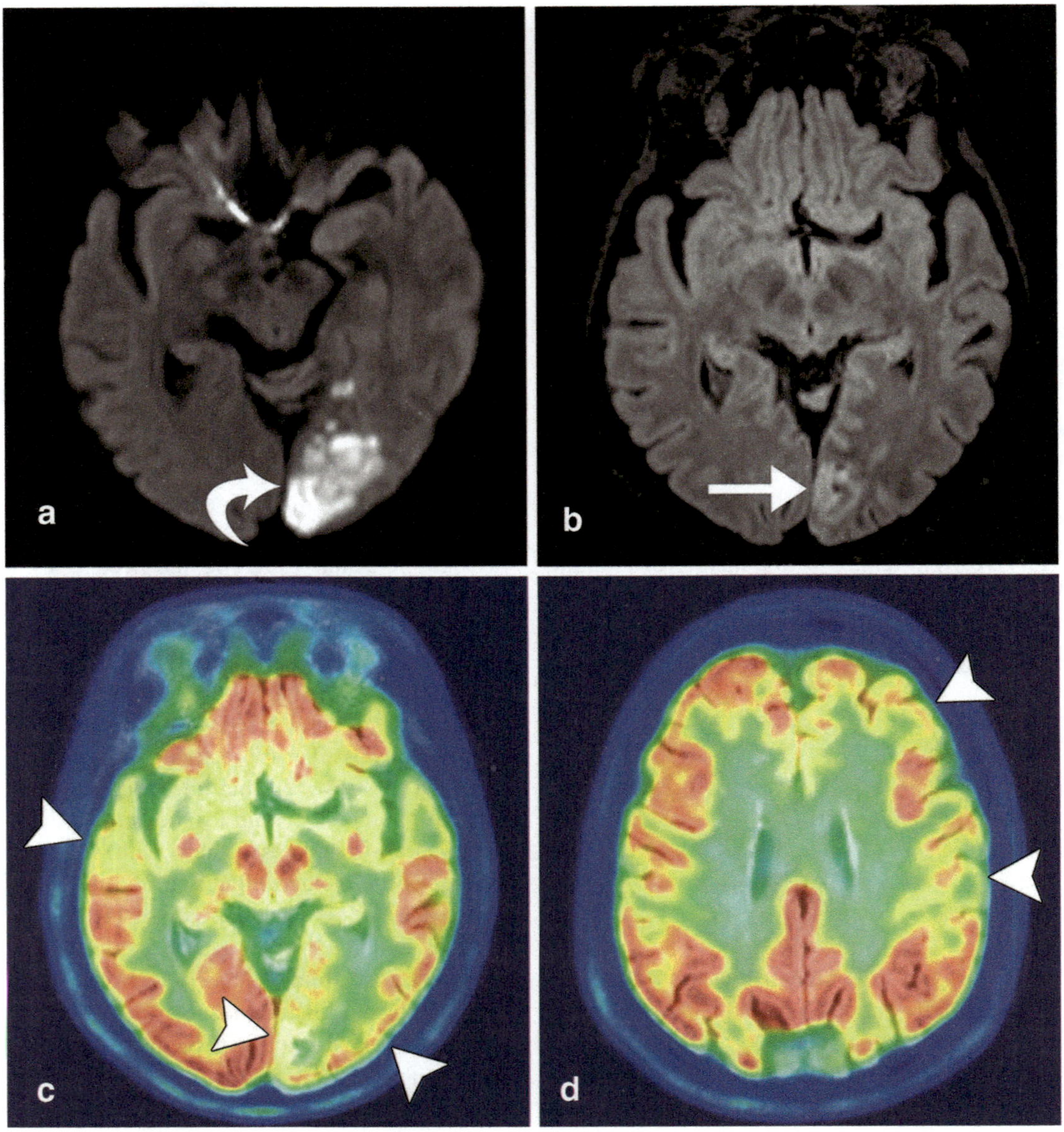

Fig. 116.1 Diffusion-weighted image axial from 3 weeks earlier (**a**), FLAIR axial (**b**), PET/MR FLAIR axial fusion (**c**), and PET/MR FLAIR axial fusion, at more superior level (**d**)

VaD. MRI is excellent at evaluating contributing vascular lesions, which include large vessel strokes, small vessel disease involving more than 25% of the white matter, and multiple lacunar infarcts. Utilizing specific MR sequences, the timing of ischemic strokes can be elucidated. Acute and subacute (1–3 weeks) lesions demonstrate restricted diffusion, with high b1000 diffusion-weighted and low ADC signal for up to 2 weeks which then eventually reverses as they become chronic. Infarcts demonstrate hyperintense T2 and FLAIR signal in the acute and subacute phase; however once tissue gliosis and encephalomalacia set in, the signal follows fluid characteristics being hypointense on T1, hyperintense on T2, and hypointense on FLAIR. Parenchymal enhancement may occur post-gadolinium administration starting approximately 1 week after a complete infarction and may last for a couple of months. Infrequently, an infarct could be mistaken for neoplastic process if found incidentally.

FDG PET/MR imaging can be useful in differentiating VaD from other forms of dementia, as it can more accurately localize contributing lesions and identify specific areas of cortical hypometabolism. PET imaging often identifies areas of infarct that are overlooked on conventional MRI imaging and shows more extensive vascular compromise than estimated by anatomical imaging. In VaD, altered brain metabolism can be more variable; however small subcortical infarcts in the basal ganglia or thalamus have been shown to be associated with large areas of frontal cortex hypometabolism. Larger subacute to chronic cortical infarcts demonstrate focal hypometabolism. Periventricular white matter small vessel disease may also demonstrate decreased frontal cortical metabolism. The overall severity of neurocognitive symptoms in VaD is associated with the extent of white matter injury.

Suggested Reading

Allen LM, Hasso AN, Handwerker J, Farid H. Sequence-specific MR imaging findings that are useful in dating ischemic stroke. Radiographics. 2012;32(5):1285–97.

Sultzer DL, Mahler ME, Cummings JL, Van Gorp WG, Hinkin CH, Brown C. Cortical abnormalities associated with subcortical lesions in vascular dementia. Clinical and position emission tomographic findings. Arch Neurol. 1995;52(8):773–80.

van Straaten EC, Scheltens P, Knol DL, van Buchem MA, van Dijk EJ, Hofman PA, et al. Operational definitions for the NINDS-AIREN criteria for vascular dementia: an interobserver study. Stroke. 2003;34(8):1907–12.

Case 117
Tumor Progression

Anuj Rajput, Michael Goodman, and Lev Bangiyev

History

An 80-year-old male with glioblastoma, treated with surgery, radiation, and chemotherapy completed 6 months ago (Fig. 117.1).

Diagnosis

Tumor progression

Findings

- FLAIR shows a mixed high signal intensity cavity, reflecting blood products, in the right parietal lobe due to surgical resection (wide arrow). There is diffuse increased signal around the surgical bed representing postradiation change.
- T1-weighted post-contrast image demonstrates three foci of nodular enhancement, one abutting the anterior surgical bed wall and two foci adjacent to the medial wall of the surgical cavity (thin arrows).
- PET fusion image shows prominent abnormal focal increased FDG uptake, greater than adjacent gray matter, in the anterior surgical bed wall nodule. Additional increased uptake is seen in the nodular foci adjacent to the medial wall. This is consistent with tumor progression.
- PET axial images demonstrate diffuse decreased FDG uptake in the right hemisphere due to postradiation changes (arrowheads).

Discussion

Gliomas are the most common primary malignant brain tumors with an incidence of 7 per 100,000. Over time there has been an increase in the 5-year survival for all malignant central nervous system tumors, due to better diagnostic imaging and improved treatment options. The World Health Organization classifies gliomas into four different grades from low grade to high grade. Glioblastoma is a WHO grade IV tumor that is the most common and most aggressive cancer originating within the brain. Its peak incidence is between 65 and 75 years of age. Symptoms often occur rapidly with headache, nausea, stroke-like symptoms, and personality changes. The prognosis is usually poor.

Histopathologic evaluation is the most accurate method for evaluating tumor type and extent; however, often tumor location prevents biopsies from being safely performed leading to greater reliance on noninvasive imaging methods, especially when evaluating lesion response to treatment. Contrast MRI plays an important role in the evaluation of glioblastomas and brain tumors. Glioblastomas are lesions located in the white matter that are hypo- to isointense on T1-weighted images with central heterogeneity due to necrosis

R. Gupta et al., *PET/MR Imaging*, https://doi.org/10.1007/978-3-319-65106-4_117

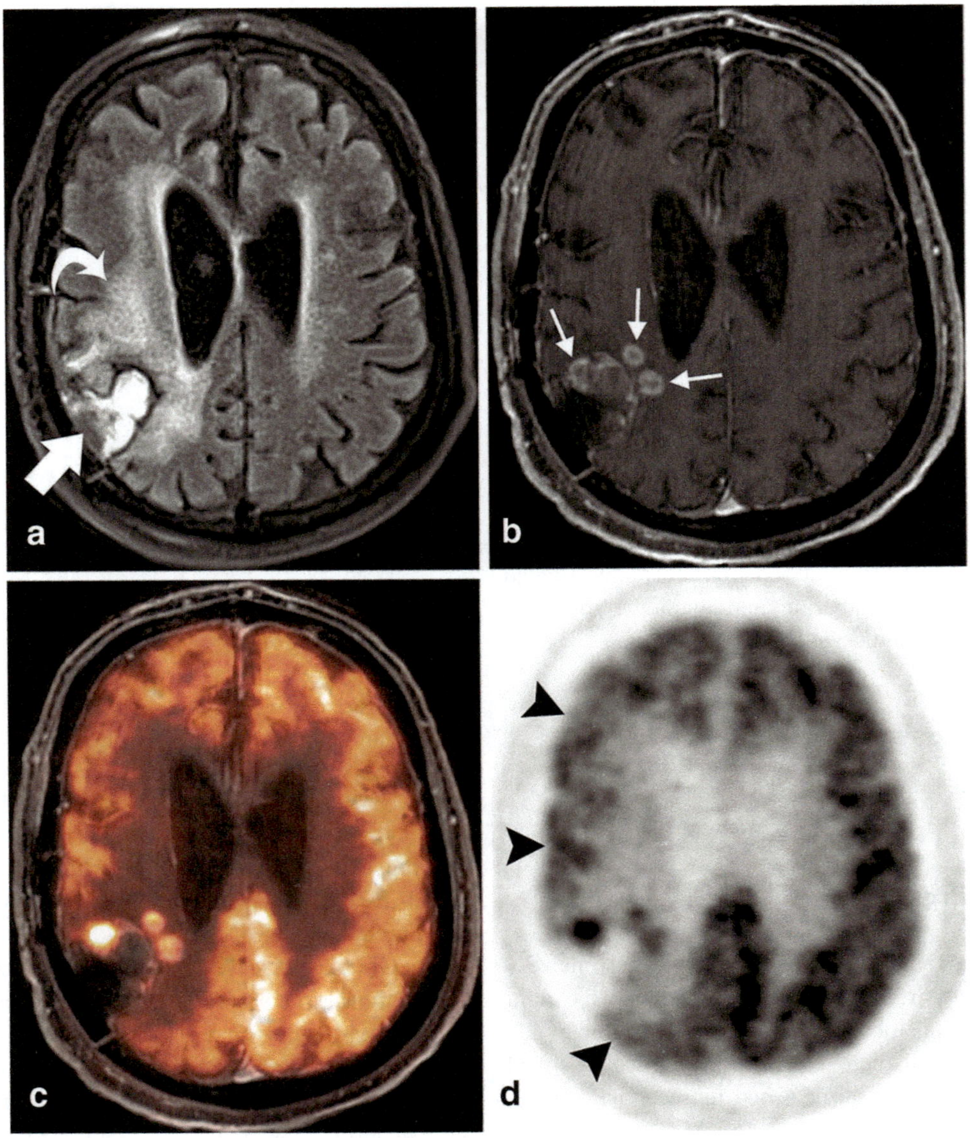

Fig. 117.1 FLAIR axial (**a**), T1 VIBE post-gadolinium contrast axial (**b**), PET/MR T1 VIBE post-gadolinium contrast axial fusion (**c**), and PET axial (**d**)

and hemorrhage. They demonstrate T2 hyperintensity and enhance with gadolinium contrast. However, brain tumor characterization based on MRI morphologic appearance, size, and enhancement patterns is often nonspecific.

PET/MRI combines anatomic imaging with physiologic imaging that has a great potential for advanced characterization of brain tumors and distinguishing treatment related changes from tumor progression. High-grade tumors like glioblastomas have higher FDG uptake compared to background gray matter on PET imaging. PET/MR imaging acquired simultaneously provides excellent anatomical and physiological details allowing for better delineation of the area of interest. MRI also allows for advanced imaging techniques such as diffusion-weighted imaging, diffusion tensor imaging, and perfusion imaging using dynamic susceptibility contrast technique. PET/MR findings characteristic of tumor recurrence include posttreatment enhancement, increased FDG uptake, increased cerebral blood volume, and increased diffusion restriction. Postradiation changes may demonstrate lesion enhancement; however, the FDG uptake is usually lower than the contralateral normal appearing cortex.

Suggested Reading

Kao HW, Chiang SW, Chung HW, Tsai FY, Chen CY. Advanced MR imaging of gliomas: an update. Biomed Res Int. 2013;2013:970586.

Singhal T, Narayanan TK, Jacobs MP, Bal C, Mantil JC. 11C-methionine PET for grading and prognostication in gliomas: a comparison study with 18F-FDG PET and contrast enhancement on MRI. J Nucl Med. 2012 Nov;53(11):1709–15.

Case 118
Meningioma

Priya Sharma and Rajesh Gupta

History

A 56-year-old female with follicular lymphoma presents with headache (Fig. 118.1).

Diagnosis

Meningioma

Findings

- Extra-axial mass in the left anterior temporal region is isointense on T1 and T2-weighted images (curved black arrow).
- Mass has a central T1 hypointensity that can be seen in both necrosis and calcification (black arrowhead).
- A T2-hyperintense CSF cleft (white arrowheads) is a classic finding of extra-axial tumor.
- Mass demonstrates very mild FDG uptake, markedly lower in comparison with the high uptake in the normal cerebral gray matter (asterisk).

Discussion

Meningiomas are the most common benign extra-axial tumors of the central nervous system, accounting for 16–20% of all intracranial tumors. They are non-glial neoplasms that arise from meningothelial cells of the arachnoid mater. Meningiomas are common after the 5th decade of life and have a female predominance. The majority are idiopathic; however risk factors include radiation exposure, neurofibromatosis type 2, a genetic disorder where the tumors may be multiple, and head injury. These tumors are often asymptomatic but can have a variety of symptoms depending on tumor location and adjacent mass effect.

There are several characteristic imaging features of meningiomas on MRI. They typically appear as well-circumscribed, lobular extra-axial masses. Meningiomas usually have a broad-based dural attachment and, if large, show inward displacement of the cortical gray matter. In relation to gray matter, meningiomas are isointense to slightly hypointense on T1-weighted images and isointense to slightly hyperintense on T2-weighted sequences. Meningiomas homogenously enhance post-gadolinium contrast administration. They may have central areas of necrosis or calcification which do not enhance. Two common MR features of extra-axial tumors are an enhancing dural tail, where the dura infiltrates away from the lesion, and a T2-hyperintense CSF cleft between the tumor and the underlying brain cortex. Hyperostosis is a common reactive bone change associated with meningiomas that arise in the skull base and anterior cranial fossa.

FDG PET can detect meningiomas; however it can be difficult to delineate tumor margins as its

R. Gupta et al., *PET/MR Imaging*, https://doi.org/10.1007/978-3-319-65106-4_118

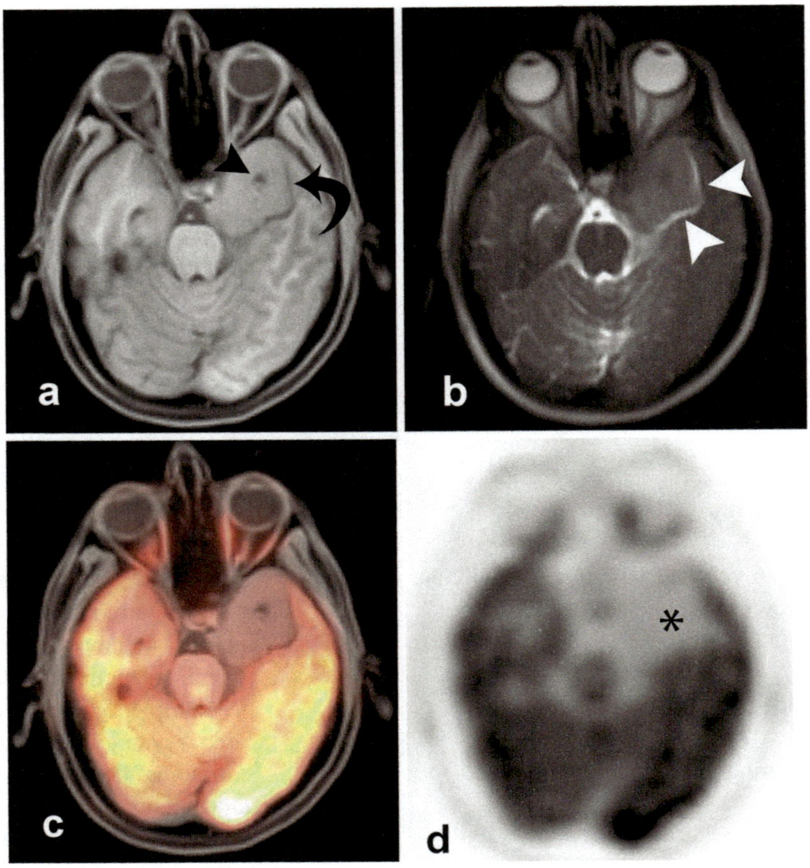

Fig. 118.1 T1 radial VIBE axial with fat suppression (**a**), T2 HASTE axial (**b**), PET/MR T1 radial VIBE with fat suppression axial fusion (**c**), and PET axial (**d**)

uptake is lower than that of normal brain gray matter. Additionally, FDG PET has a low sensitivity to differentiate between low- and high-grade tumors. This is because the high FDG uptake in normal brain gray matter leads to relatively small differences in the FDG uptake of the normal brain and low-grade tumors. The simultaneous acquisition of FDG PET and MR provides superior detection, localization, and characterization of meningiomas. Although benign, intracranial meningiomas can recur, and it has been shown that recurrent or regrowing tumors have higher glucose metabolic rates compared to nonrecurrent ones. Therefore, FDG PET/MR may provide prognostic information when the metabolic activity of a meningioma is quantified, helping with treatment considerations.

Suggested Reading

Lee JW, Kang KW, Park SH, Lee SM, Paeng JC, Chung JK, et al. 18F-FDG PET in the assessment of tumor grade and prediction of tumor recurrence in intracranial meningioma. Eur J Nucl Med Mol Imaging. 2009;36(10):1574–82.

Singh V, Bluestone A, Chen D, Shah A, Linden C, Bangiyev L. Meningiomas: variations and clinical presentations. Contemp Diagn Radiol. 2014;37(24):1–5.

Watts J, Box G, Galvin A, Brotchie P, Trost N, Sutherland T. Magnetic resonance imaging of meningiomas: a pictorial review. Insights Imaging. 2014;5(1):113–22.

Case 119
Mesial Temporal Lobe Sclerosis

Ana M. Franceschi, Michael J. Hoch, and Timothy M. Shepherd

History

A 28-year-old right-handed female with a remote history of encephalitis and subsequent medically refractory temporal lobe epilepsy by semiology and EEG (Fig. 119.1). Previous MRI demonstrated isolated right mesial temporal sclerosis.

Diagnosis

Mesial temporal lobe sclerosis with bilateral temporal seizure foci

Findings

- FLAIR and T2-weighted images show right hippocampus atrophy with mild increased signal (curved black arrow).
- PET coronal image shows decreased FDG uptake in the right mesial temporal lobe (black wide arrow). In addition, there is mesial and lateral temporal lobe hypometabolism on the left side without structural MRI changes.
- PET surface rendering images on lateral views show decreased radiotracer activity in the left lateral temporal lobe (wide white arrow) with more diffuse mild decrease of FDG uptake in the temporoparietal region. Right cerebral hemisphere has preserved FDG uptake with exception of the mesial temporal lobe.
- Overall PET findings show bilateral temporal lobe seizure foci that were confirmed by responsive neurostimulator placement in both hippocampi demonstrating bilateral epileptiform discharges and decreased seizure frequency.

Discussion

Mesial temporal sclerosis (MTS) is the most common cause of intractable complex partial seizures (temporal lobe epilepsy) in adults. Histologic specimens demonstrate neuronal loss, gliosis, and mossy fiber sprouting involving the hippocampal formation, particularly the dentate gyrus, CA1, CA3, and CA4 sections. Approximately 10% of cases are bilateral, and there is often dual pathology even when only unilateral MTS is present. Antiepileptic agents are the initial treatment of choice. Surgical lobectomy is reserved for medically refractory cases, with 70–95% success rates reported following temporal lobectomy if imaging findings consistent with MTS were present.

Clear MRI signs of MTS in the nondominant hemisphere with concordant clinical signs and electroencephalogram (EEG) localization might be resected without further workup in some patients but would not have led to seizure-free outcome in this patient. Responsive neurostimu-

R. Gupta et al., *PET/MR Imaging*, https://doi.org/10.1007/978-3-319-65106-4_119

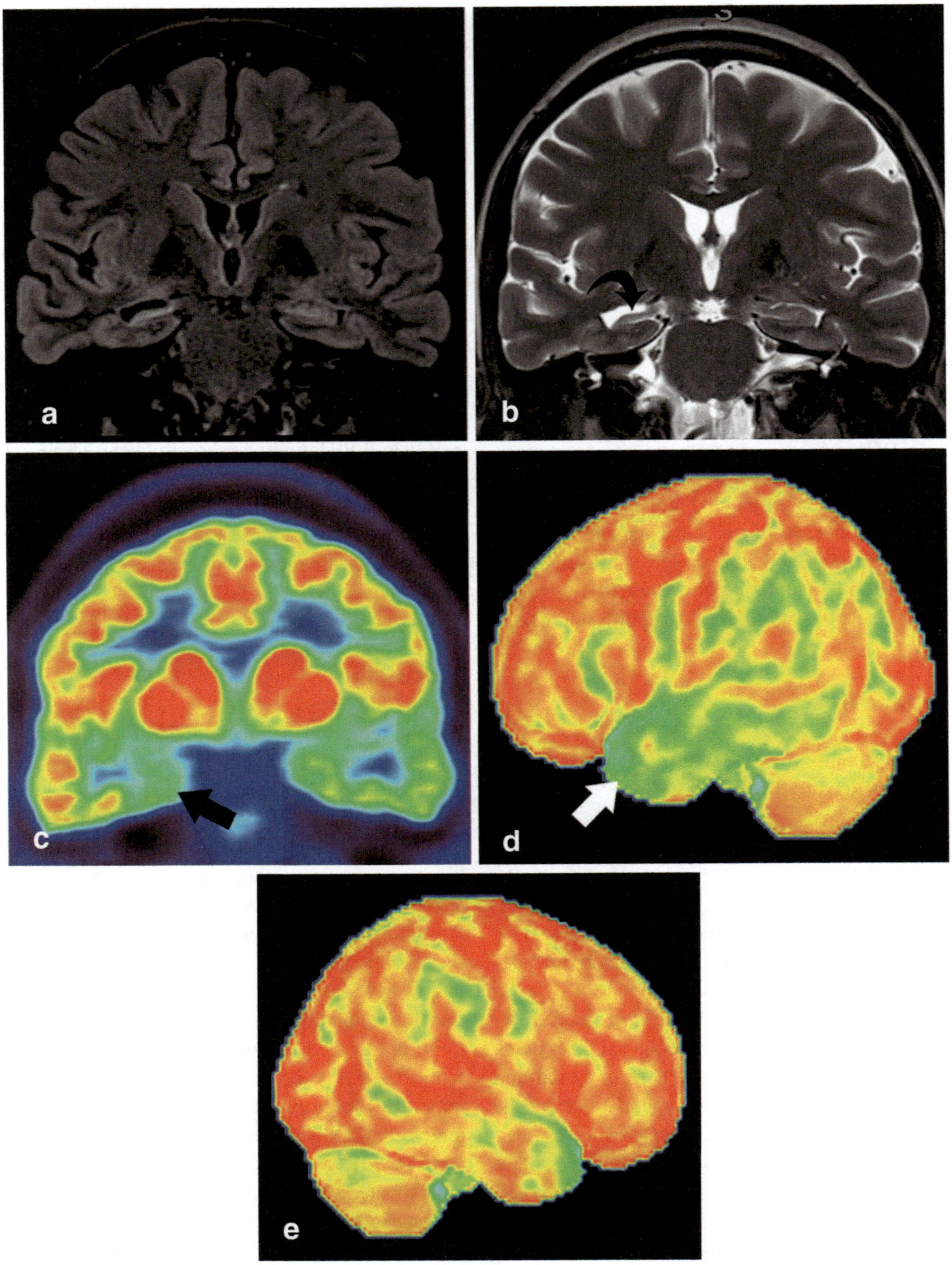

Fig. 119.1 FLAIR coronal (**a**), T2 coronal (**b**), PET coronal (**c**), PET surface rendering left lateral view (**d**), and PET surface rendering right lateral view (**e**)

lators are a new treatment option in patients with refractory epilepsy. The device continually monitors brain activity and delivers an electric stimulus when abnormal activity is detected. This treatment is well tolerated by patients and effectively decreases frequency of seizures.

Classic findings on neuroimaging with PET/MRI include a morphologic MRI triad of atrophy, loss of internal architecture, and increased T2 signal in the affected hippocampus. Additional clues on brain MRI include volume loss in the ipsilateral fornix, mammillary body, temporal stem, and collateral eminence white matter. The imaging findings may be subtle and are often limited to a subregion of the hippocampus such as the head or tail that is less obvious to cursory review.

Characteristic findings on FDG-PET obtained interictally include corresponding hypometabolism in the abnormal mesial temporal lobe as well as within the ipsilateral anterior thalamic nuclei. The degree of hypometabolism parallels the severity of hippocampal atrophy, although the extent of hypometabolism usually involves a much larger area of the mesial temporal lobe than the atrophy visualized on MRI. This illustrates a benefit of imaging with PET/MR that can allow more precise localization of the seizure focus. When FDG is injected during the initiation of an ictal state, the seizure focus would demonstrate increased metabolic activity.

Suggested Reading

Camacho DL, Castillo M. MR imaging of temporal lobe epilepsy. Semin Ultrasound CT MR. 2007;28(6):424–36.

Carne RP, O'Brien TJ, Kilpatrick CJ, Macgregor LR, Litewka L, Hicks RJ, et al. 'MRI-negative PET-positive' temporal lobe epilepsy (TLE) and mesial TLE differ with quantitative MRI and PET: a case control study. BMC Neurol. 2007;7:16.

Chan S, Erickson JK, Yoon SS. Limbic system abnormalities associated with mesial temporal sclerosis: a model of chronic cerebral changes due to seizures. Radiographics. 1997;17(5):1095–110.

Thomas GP, Jobst BC. Critical review of the responsive neurostimulator system for epilepsy. Med Devices (Auckl). 2015;8:405–11.

Case 120
Brain Abscess

James Bai and Lev Bangiyev

History

An 83-year-old man with right ocular basal cell carcinoma treated with resection, radiotherapy, and implantation of an ocular prosthesis. Recent imaging showed an indeterminate lesion in the brain (Fig. 120.1).

Diagnosis

Brain abscess

Findings

- MR images demonstrate diffuse T1 hypointense signal with extensive FLAIR hyperintense signal in the right frontal lobe characteristic of edema.
- Post-contrast image shows irregular heterogeneously enhancing lesion in the right anterior frontal lobe with small satellite enhancing lesion (thin arrows).
- PET/MR fusion image shows abnormal FDG activity associated with the lesion (wide arrow). There is decreased normal right frontal lobe gray matter activity due to radiation therapy (arrowhead).
- At a more inferior level, PET/MR fusion image demonstrates mild increased FDG uptake corresponding to an enhancing temporal lobe lesion (curved arrow).
- Extensive postsurgical changes are seen in the right orbit.

Discussion

The typical appearance of a brain abscess on MRI imaging is a ring-enhancing lesion that shows low or intermediate T1 signal intensity with central T2 hyperintense signal. A mature abscess has low signal intensity capsule on T2-weighted sequence. Commonly brain abscess demonstrates extensive edema with high T2 signal and associated mass effect. The mere presence of a classic ring-enhancing lesion in the brain, however, does not always represent an abscess. Other etiologies may produce a ring-enhancing cerebral lesion including primary and secondary necrotic tumors, subacute infarct, radiation necrosis, and postoperative changes.

Diffusion-weighted imaging can be helpful in differentiation between abscess and necrotic neoplasm. Pus in a brain abscesses demonstrates increased diffusion restriction with marked hyperintense signal on DWI and low ADC values in the center of the lesion. Necrotic tumors typically show the center of the lesion to be hypointense on DWI and hyperintense on ADC signal. The periphery of the necrotic tumor that is still viable and hypercellular may show some increased diffusion restriction. In patients with

R. Gupta et al., *PET/MR Imaging*, https://doi.org/10.1007/978-3-319-65106-4_120

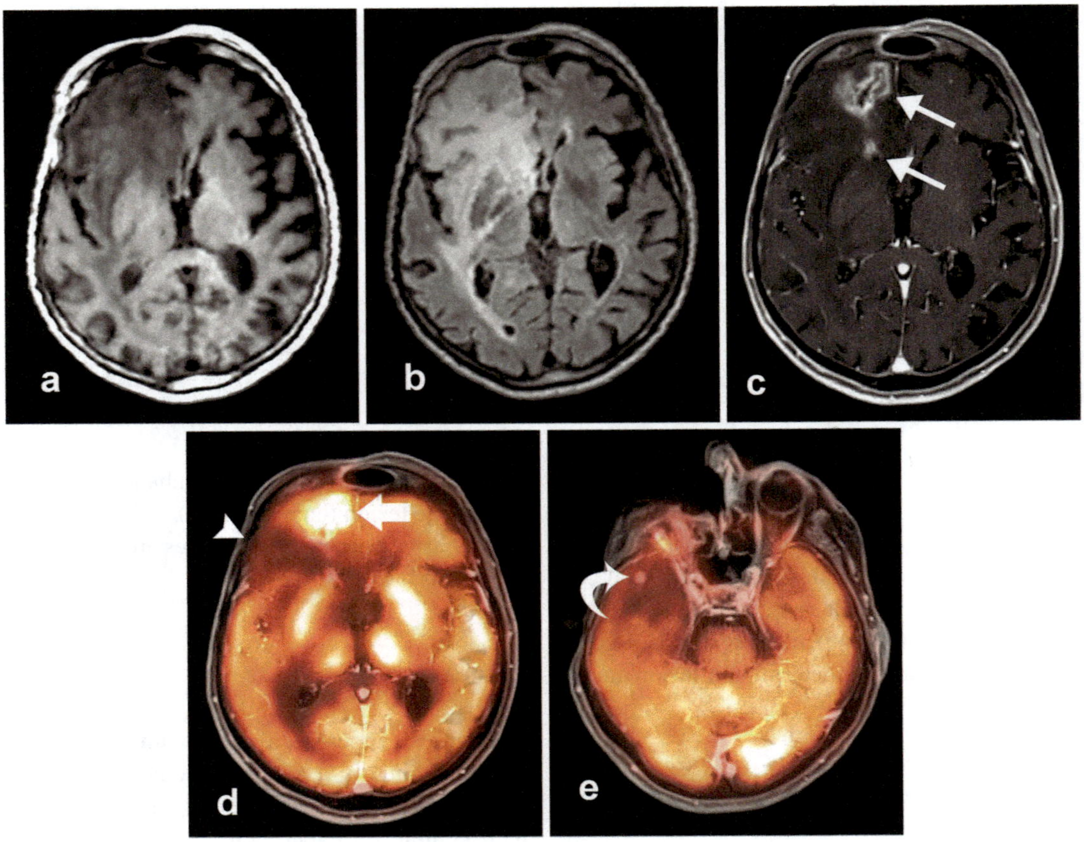

Fig. 120.1 T1-weighted axial (**a**), FLAIR axial (**b**), T1 radial VIBE post-gadolinium contrast axial (**c**), FDG PET/MR radial VIBE axial fusion (**d**), and FDG PET/MR radial VIBE axial fusion, at more inferior level (**e**)

prior radiation therapy, radiation necrosis is another differential consideration that may appear as a heterogeneous peripherally enhancing lesion that resembles a necrotic mass.

Hybrid PET/MR imaging can thoroughly evaluate brain abscesses by combining MR sequences with metabolic information. On FDG PET imaging, both abscesses and necrotic tumors show hypermetabolic activity; thus using PET imaging alone to differentiate between the two may not be useful. However, in cases of radiation necrosis, subacute infarct, or postoperative changes, PET imaging would not show increased FDG uptake. Furthermore, PET/MR imaging can be helpful in assessing the favorable effect of antibiotic therapy for an abscess by demonstrating resolution of FDG uptake.

Suggested Reading

Cartes-Zumelzu FW, Stavrou I, Castillo M, Eisenhuber E, Knosp E, Thurnher MM. Diffusion-weighted imaging in the assessment of brain abscesses therapy. AJNR Am J Neuroradiol. 2004;25(8):1310–7.

Chang SC, Lai PH, Chen WL, Weng HH, Ho JT, Wang JS, et al. Diffusion-weighted MRI features of brain abscess and cystic or necrotic brain tumors: comparison with conventional MRI. Clin Imaging. 2002;26(4):227–36.

Park SH, Lee SW, Kang DH, Hwang JH, Sung JK, Hwang SK. The role of f-fluorodeoxyglucose positron emission tomography in the treatment of brain abscess. J Korean Neurosurg Soc. 2011;49(5):278–83.

Case 121 Glioblastoma Recurrence with Negative FDG PET

Anuj Rajput, Michael Goodman, and Lev Bangiyev

History

A 71-year-old male with history of glioblastoma being evaluated for recurrence (Fig. 121.1).

Diagnosis

Glioblastoma recurrence with negative FDG PET

Findings

- Initial posttreatment follow-up pre- and post-contrast MR imaging demonstrates a new focal area of enhancement within the left frontal lobe (curved white arrow).
- PET/MR fusion image from the same exam demonstrates no discernible FDG uptake within the small enhancing lesion that is nonspecific (curved black arrow).
- 1-month follow-up MRI demonstrates increase in size of the enhancement (white thin arrow), highly suspicious for tumor progression.
- 3-month follow-up MRI demonstrates continuous increase in size of brain lesion with abnormal enhancement (white arrowheads). This is significantly worse at 5 months, consistent with tumor progression.

Discussion

Glioblastoma (GBM) is the most common primary CNS malignancy. GBM is histologically characterized by infiltrative growth commonly extending beyond visible enhancement on neuroimaging. The typical MR findings include an irregular T2 hyperintense, T1 hypointense to isointense lesion with heterogeneous enhancement related to destruction of the blood-brain barrier. There is usually surrounding increased T2 white matter signal that might represent either edema or tumor infiltration. Due to its infiltrative nature and rapid growth pattern, these tumors tend to outgrow its blood supply, with resultant central necrosis and hemorrhage. These findings can be seen on conventional MR with central heterogeneous low T1 and increased T2 signal with lack of central enhancement. Rapidly growing and more aggressive parts of the tumor commonly show increased diffusion restriction related to tumor cellularity.

FDG PET has been investigated in the initial evaluation and follow-up of glioblastoma with promising results. However, these studies have also discovered limitations in utility of FDG. In a patient undergoing treatment for high-grade gliomas, any new enhancing lesion can be considered as true disease progression or pseudoprogression, which is a treatment-related change. Enhancement

R. Gupta et al., *PET/MR Imaging*, https://doi.org/10.1007/978-3-319-65106-4_121

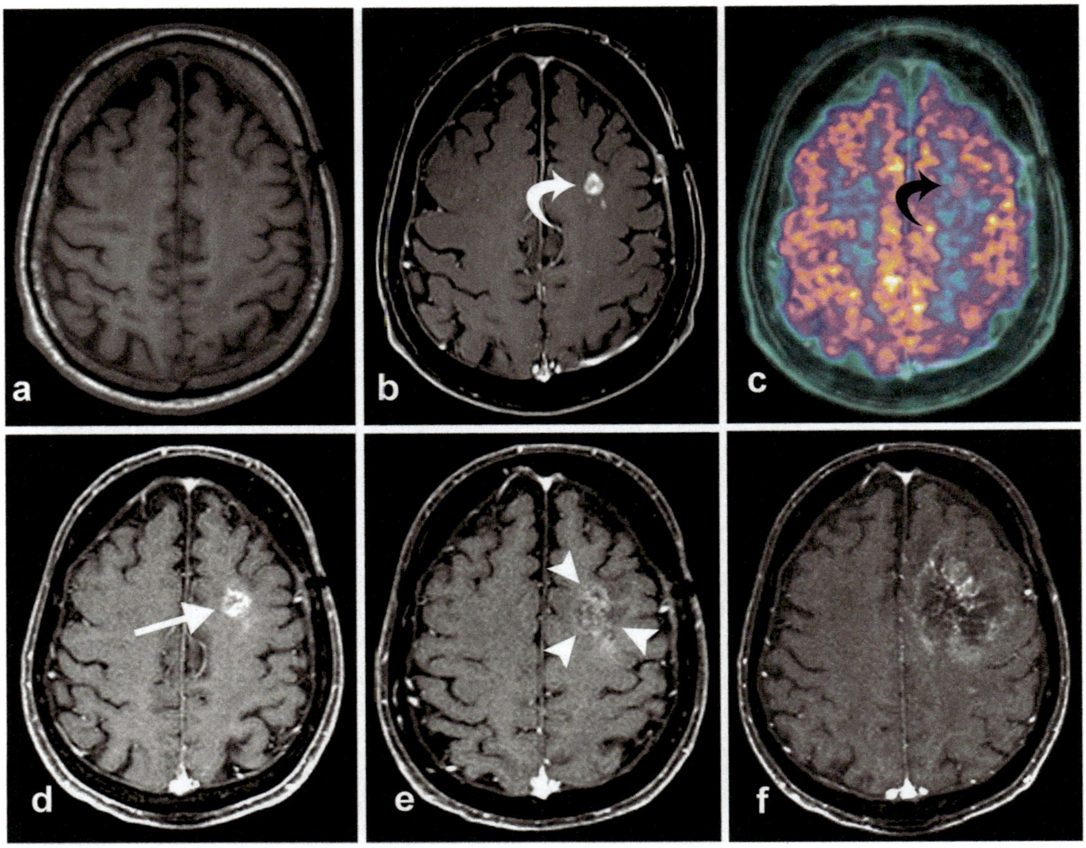

Fig. 121.1 T1 axial (**a**); T1 post-gadolinium contrast axial (**b**); PET/MR T1 post-gadolinium contrast axial fusion (**c**); T1 post-gadolinium contrast axial, 1-month follow-up (**d**); T1 post-gadolinium contrast axial, 3-month follow-up (**e**); and T1 post-gadolinium contrast axial, 5-month follow-up (**f**)

on post-contrast images simply reveals areas of blood-brain barrier breakdown, which is in itself a nonspecific finding. Although the use of FDG has been very helpful in evaluating tumor recurrence as it is sensitive in metabolic tissues due to its mechanism as a glucose analog, FDG lacks specificity thereby imposing limitations. In addition, there is high background FDG uptake by gray matter brain parenchyma decreasing visualization of neoplasms. Furthermore, glioblastoma is a pathologically and genetically heterogeneous tumor containing more aggressive and rapidly growing components along with less aggressive but still malignant areas. The regions of the tumor that are rapidly growing and show more aggressive behavior typically show much higher than normal brain FDG uptake and are readily recognizable on imaging. However, parts of the tumor that show less aggressive characteristics may demonstrate similar or only mildly increased metabolic activity in comparison to the background activity of the brain. Other limitations of FDG include the known difficulty in distinguishing malignancy from inflammatory or infectious changes. There are suggested threshold standardized uptake values that have been considered for certain processes, however these are not strict. Small sized recurrent lesions in GBM, as this case demonstrates, may only show no or mild uptake despite being an aggressive tumor.

These limitations of FDG have led to the development of more specific radiotracers that are based on amino acids which are essential in dividing proliferating cells. These amino acid labelled tracers can be more sensitive and specific to detect cerebral gliomas. The use of PET with C-11 methionine has demonstrated a sensitivity of 76–95% in the diagnosis and extent of gliomas. However the half-life of C-11 is very short and requires an on-site cyclotron, which makes it impractical for wide clinical use. The F-18 labelled radiotracers are more practical due to their longer half-life and therefore do not require an on-site cyclotron. One such radiotracer is F-18-dihydroxyphenylalanine (F-DOPA). The mechanism of F-DOPA is different than FDG as it uses an amino acid transporter to take up the radiotracer. Several studies have come to the conclusion that higher uptake values of amino acid tracers correlated with higher grade of gliomas and that F-DOPA demonstrated similar uptake to that of C-11 methionine. With this in mind, F-DOPA can be used instead of C-11 methionine. Thus, the use of more specific markers such as F-DOPA could also be considered instead of FDG when assessing gliomas in an initial evaluation to delineate tumor extent as well as in tumor follow-up.

Suggested Reading

Becherer A, Karanikas G, Szabó M, Zettinig G, Asenbaum S, Marosi C, et al. Brain tumour imaging with PET: a comparison between [18F]fluorodopa and [11C]methionine. Eur J Nucl Med Mol Imaging. 2003;30(11):1561–7.

Kracht LW, Miletic H, Busch S, Jacobs AH, Voges J, Hoevels M, et al. Delineation of brain tumor extent with [11C]L-methionine positron emission tomography: local comparison with stereotactic histopathology. Clin Cancer Res. 2004;10(21):7163–70.

Singhal T, Narayanan TK, Jain V, Mukherjee J, Mantil J. 11C-L-methionine positron emission tomography in the clinical management of cerebral gliomas. Mol Imaging Biol. 2008;10(1):1–18.

Villani V, Carapella CM, Chiaravalloti A, Terrenato I, Piludu F, Vidiri A, et al. The role of PET [18F]FDOPA in evaluating low-grade Glioma. Anticancer Res. 2015;35(9):5117–22.

Case 122
Logopenic Primary Progressive Aphasia

Michael J. Hoch, Lev Bangiyev,
and Timothy M. Shepherd

History

An 80-year-old male with progressive memory loss over 3 years dominated by word finding difficulties, slow speech, and alexia (Fig. 122.1). Patient unable to repeat complete sentences.

Diagnosis

Logopenic primary progressive aphasia

Findings

- MPRAGE and FLAIR images show mild global atrophy which is more severe in the left parietal lobe (wide arrows).
- PET surface rendering lateral view images show severe left parietal and left posterior temporal lobe hypometabolism (curved arrow), which is less severe on the right side.
- PET surface rendering view of the medial right hemisphere demonstrates decreased FDG activity in the right precuneus (thin arrow).

Discussion

Logopenic primary progressive aphasia (lvPPA) is often considered as an atypical variant of Alzheimer's disease (AD) characterized by decreased rate of spontaneous language production. The term logopenic is from Greek meaning "lack of words." The disease can be thought of as a more asymmetric or "language variant" AD at initial presentation. In primary progressive aphasias, like lvPPA, language impairment should be almost the exclusive symptom for the first 1–2 years of the dementia syndrome. Initially, there should be little or no memory impairment. Histology studies show most patients with lvPPA have underlying Alzheimer's pathology.

This dementia subtype shows similarity to AD that is demonstrated by increased PET amyloid radiotracer activity in the brain, and increased amyloid beta peptides (Aβ42) and tau in CSF. Early in disease development patients demonstrate length-dependent impaired sentence repetition, phonological errors, alexia, and anomia. As the dementia progresses, the disease overlaps with other primary progressive aphasia variants. In the late stages of the disease, patients

R. Gupta et al., *PET/MR Imaging*, https://doi.org/10.1007/978-3-319-65106-4_122

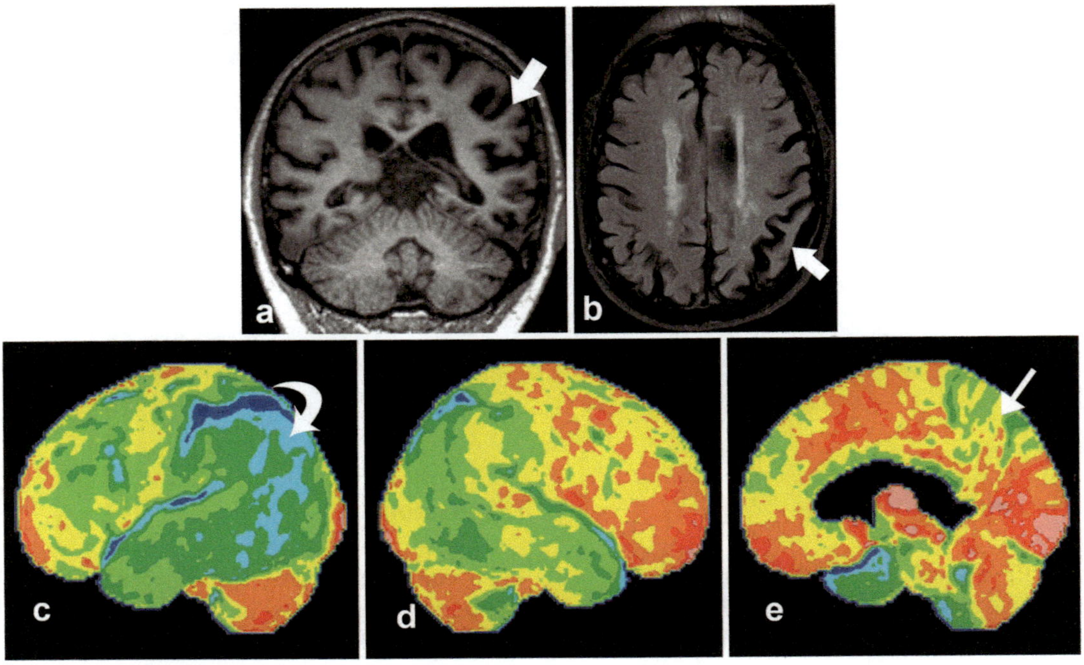

Fig. 122.1 MPRAGE coronal (**a**), FLAIR axial (**b**), PET surface rendering left lateral view (**c**), PET surface rendering right lateral view (**d**), and PET surface rendering medial right hemisphere view (**e**)

develop apraxia, semantic memory deficits, and jargon aphasia. Preservation of single word comprehension helps to distinguish logopenic aphasia from semantic variant of primary progressive aphasia.

Imaging findings for lvPPA on FDG PET/MRI show characteristic decreased metabolic activity in the temporal lobe, parietal lobe, and posterior cingulate gyrus with accompanied cortical volume loss on MRI similar to Alzheimer's disease. Areas of hypometabolism correspond well to areas of cortical atrophy. The area of the most severe decreased FDG uptake and cortical atrophy is in the left lateral temporoparietal region which is associated with repetition and phonological clinical defects. This is likely where the pathology initially appears before spreading to other areas of the brain.

Suggested Reading

Henry ML, Gorno-Tempini ML. The logopenic variant of primary progressive aphasia. Curr Opin Neurol. 2010;23(6):633–7.

Leyton CE, Villemagne VL, Savage S, Pike KE, Ballard KJ, Piguet O, et al. Subtypes of progressive aphasia: application of the international consensus criteria and validation using β-amyloid imaging. Brain. 2011;134:3030–43.

Madhavan A, Whitwell JL, Weigand SD, Duffy JR, Strand EA, Machulda MM, et al. FDG PET and MRI in logopenic primary progressive aphasia versus dementia of the Alzheimer's type. PLoS One. 2013;8(4):e62471.

Case 123 Crossed Cerebellar Diaschisis

Michael J. Hoch, Ana M. Franceschi, and Timothy M. Shepherd

History

A 71-year-old male with a history of multiple falls (Fig. 123.1). Now presenting with change in mental status after another fall.

Diagnosis

Crossed cerebellar diaschisis from subacute on chronic subdural hematoma

Findings

- SWI and MPRAGE images show a large mixed hyperintense subdural fluid collection consistent with a subacute hematoma (large arrow) with midline shift and effacement of the right lateral ventricle.
- Pseudoseptations from hemosiderin deposits indicating an older chronic bleed (arrowheads).
- Coronal MPRAGE and axial FLAIR images show no appreciable atrophy of the left cerebellum.
- PET image shows a severe focal defect in the right frontoparietal region from the hematoma (thin arrow). Much of the right cerebral hemisphere shows relatively decreased FDG uptake compared to the contralateral side as a result of the hematoma.
- Decreased radiotracer uptake in the left cerebellum with no MRI findings is compatible with cross cerebellar diaschisis (curved arrows).

Discussion

Crossed cerebellar diaschisis (CCD) is a well-recognized entity characterized by depressed blood flow, decreased metabolism, and resulting atrophy of a cerebellar hemisphere caused by injury or lesion involving the contralateral supratentorial cerebral hemisphere. This phenomenon has been described with various intracranial pathologies including supratentorial infarction, vascular malformation, trauma, epilepsy, and brain tumors. This case is a result of trauma causing a subdural hematoma with the MRI showing a blood collection between the dura and arachnoid mater of the meninges in a crescent shape and mixed signal seen with rebleeding in a chronic hematoma.

The postulated pathophysiologic mechanism behind CCD is disruption of the corticopontocerebellar pathway caused by the supratentorial injury or lesion. Of note, CCD is commonly clinically occult with no separate discernable movement disorder or cognitive dysfunction apart from the cerebral injury or lesion.

On neuroimaging with FDG PET/MRI, the functional PET findings are typically more pronounced than the corresponding structural abnor-

R. Gupta et al., *PET/MR Imaging*, https://doi.org/10.1007/978-3-319-65106-4_123

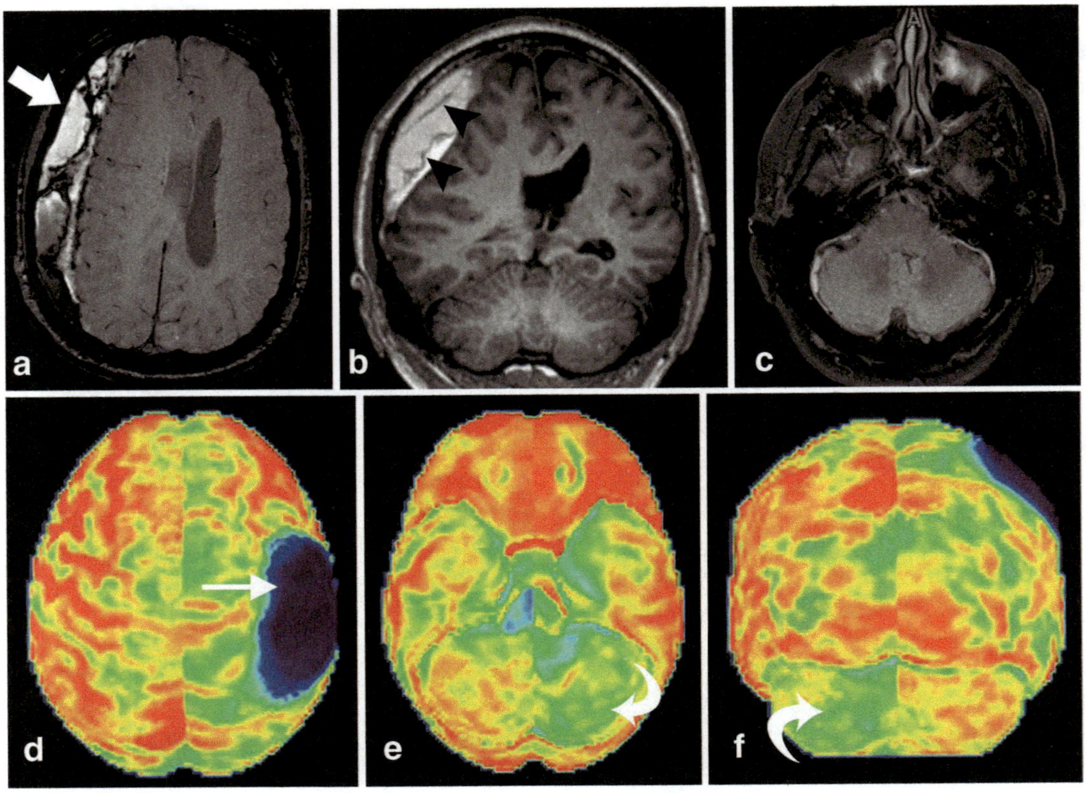

Fig. 123.1 Susceptibility-weighted imaging axial (**a**), MPRAGE coronal (**b**), FLAIR axial (**c**), PET surface rendering superior view (**d**), PET surface rendering inferior view (**e**), and PET surface rendering posterior view (**f**)

malities on MRI, with depressed metabolism in the affected cerebellar hemisphere. MRI sequences may demonstrate mild volume loss and atrophy in the affected cerebellum. Traditional MRI obtained for cognitive impairment is focused on the detection of treatable causes of CCD such as supratentorial tumor with mass effect, hydrocephalus, or intracranial hemorrhage, as in this case.

Suggested Reading

Alavi A, Mirot A, Newberg A, et al. Fluorine-18-FDG evaluation of crossed cerebellar diaschisis in head injury. J Nucl Med. 1997;38:1717–20.

Tien RD, Ashdown BC. Crossed cerebellar diaschisis and crossed cerebellar atrophy: correlation of MR findings, clinical symptoms, and supratentorial diseases in 26 patients. AJR Am J Roentgenol. 1992;158(5):1155–9.

Case 124
Amyloid Plaques in Alzheimer's Disease

Ana M. Franceschi and Robert Matthews

History

An 80-year-old female with short-term memory loss and cognitive changes to evaluate for the presence of amyloid plaques (Fig. 124.1).

Diagnosis

Amyloid plaques in Alzheimer's disease

Findings

- Cerebral cortical atrophy in the temporal and parietal lobes (arrowheads) with sparing of the frontal and occipital lobes
- Normal florbetapir binding to the cerebral white matter on PET with abnormal uptake in the cortical gray matter leading to loss of gray-white matter contrast
- Elevated amyloid plaque burden throughout the cortical gray matter (arrows)

Discussion

Florbetapir is a radiotracer used to evaluate the amyloid plaque burden in the brain of patients with memory decline and a clinical suspicion for Alzheimer's disease (AD). Amyloid-β peptide (Aβ) which is known to accumulate in excess in patients with Alzheimer's disease is released from the cells and form oligomers that are neurotoxic to the brain. These oligomers form larger insoluble β-sheet fibrils that in turn are the main component of dense amyloid plaques. These dense amyloid plaques are the ones associated with AD inducing neuronal inflammation.

Amyloid deposition is not always pathologic and occurs in up to 25% of patients age 70 years or older. Amyloid plaques can also be found in cerebral amyloid angiography, dementia with Lewy body, as well as Parkinson's disease. Currently there are three commercially available F-18 amyloid radiotracers including florbetapir that demonstrate general nonspecific cerebral white matter binding that was not seen with the historic C-11 Pittsburgh compound B (PIB). Patients with AD undergoing F-18 amyloid imaging show accumulation of the radiotracer in the gray matter of the brain indicating an elevated Aβ load. Florbetapir combined with other F-18 amyloid radiotracer demonstrates a 92% sensitivity for the detection of significant cortical amyloid burden and a 95% specificity. PIB historically showed a 73% sensitivity and 100% specificity.

A positive florbetapir PET/MRI indicates moderate to severe amyloid plaque accumulation in the cerebral cortex. While a positive scan does not necessarily indicate Alzheimer's disease, all patients with AD have above-normal amyloid plaque burden in their brain. A negative florbetapir scan means that few or no amyloid plaques

R. Gupta et al., *PET/MR Imaging*, https://doi.org/10.1007/978-3-319-65106-4_124

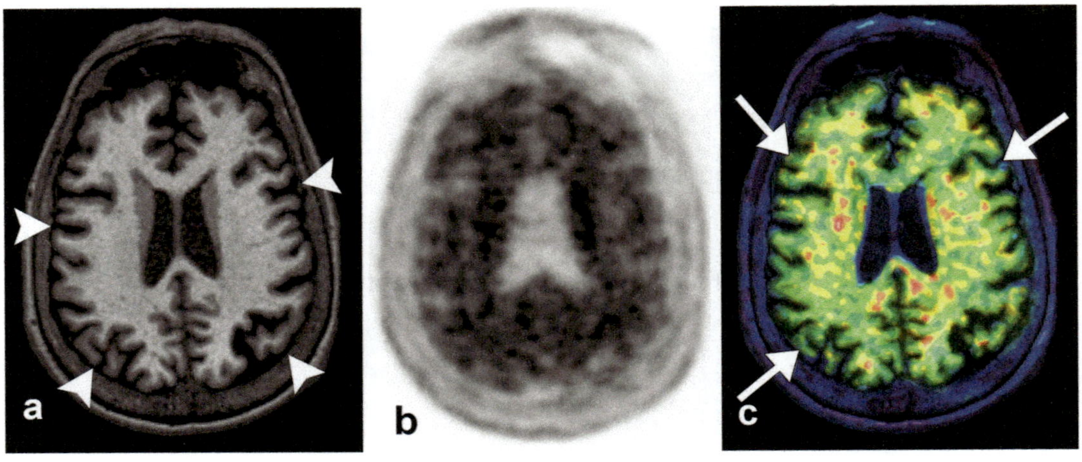

Fig. 124.1 MPRAGE axial (**a**), Florbetapir PET axial (**b**), and PET/MR Florbetapir axial fusion (**c**)

are detected in the cerebral cortex, and it is significantly less likely that the patient's cognitive impairment is related to underlying Alzheimer's pathology. Most patients with Lewy body dementia have a normal amyloid plaque scan, but a small percentage will have a positive scan with overall lower plaque burden compared to AD. Frontal lobe dementia patients have a normal florbetapir scan, while patients with posterior cortical atrophy, considered a variant of AD, have an abnormal amyloid plaque scan. Using PET/MR for amyloid plaque imaging provides underlying structural assessment to the radiotracer distribution allowing for a more accurate interpretation. The MR component shows clear depiction of the cerebral cortex while accurately discerning the white and gray matter border which on CT is difficult to distinguish when cerebral atrophy is present. In addition, MR correctly identifies cortical atrophy which complements the interpretation of AD. As AD progresses, cortical atrophy will begin in the temporoparietal region of the brain, as well as, the posterior cingulate and precuneus regions. In severe cases, the frontal lobes will be involved.

Suggested Reading

Del Sole A, Malaspina S, Magenta BA. Magnetic resonance imaging and positron emission tomography in the diagnosis of neurodegenerative dementias. Funct Neurol. 2016;31(4):205–15.

Mallik A, Drzezga A, Minoshima S. Clinical amyloid imaging. Semin Nucl Med. 2017;47(1):31–43.

Weiner MW, Veitch DP, Aisen PS, Beckett LA, Cairns NJ, Cedarbaum J, Alzheimer's Disease Neuroimaging Initiative, et al. 2014 update of the Alzheimer's disease neuroimaging initiative: a review of papers published since its inception. Alzheimers Dement. 2015;11(6):e1–120.

Wojtylak P, Faulhaber P, O'Donnell J. Initial experiences in PET/MRI for imaging dementia. J Nucl Med. 2014;55(Suppl 1):2514.

Case 125
Posterior Cortical Atrophy

Michael J. Hoch, Ana M. Franceschi,
and Timothy M. Shepherd

History

A 70-year-old male presents with progressive memory deficit and ataxia. He has difficulty recognizing objects and familiar faces (Fig. 125.1). He could not remember taking in the neighbor's cat, which his wife found hiding in their apartment.

Diagnosis

Posterior cortical atrophy

Findings

- FLAIR axial and MPRAGE coronal images show bilateral moderate to severe parietal atrophy with widening of the sulci (wide arrows).
- MPRAGE sagittal image demonstrates atrophy of the posterior hemispheres with widening of the marginal ramus of the cingulate sulcus (curved arrow) and parieto-occipital sulcus (thin arrow).
- PET surface rendering lateral view shows mild to moderate hypometabolic activity in the bilateral parietal, occipital, and temporal lobes. Normal FDG uptake is seen in the bilateral frontal lobes (asterisks).

Discussion

Posterior cortical atrophy (PCA) is a progressive neurodegenerative disorder that predominantly affects the occipital, temporal, and parietal cortex. It is referred to as a "visual variant of Alzheimer's disease (AD). The syndrome is characterized by visuospatial and visuoperceptual impairment. Approximately 60–80% PCA cases have identical histology to AD. Onset is earlier than typical AD, usually between 50–65 years. Early clinical features include visual agnosia, apraxia, and optic ataxia. PCA patients are often initially seen by an ophthalmologist who cannot find any visual abnormality on their exam. Common presenting symptoms are difficulty with reading and writing, running into objects, or getting into motor vehicle accidents.

Neuroimaging with PET/MRI in patients with PCA demonstrates areas of hypometabolism predominately in the parieto-occipital areas with relative posterior cingulate sparing compared to the precuneus and cuneus regions. In addition, there are specific areas of hypometabolism involving the bilateral frontal eye fields, Brodmann area 8, which is related to loss of input from occipitoparietal regions. There is considerable regional overlap on PET imaging when

R. Gupta et al., *PET/MR Imaging*, https://doi.org/10.1007/978-3-319-65106-4_125

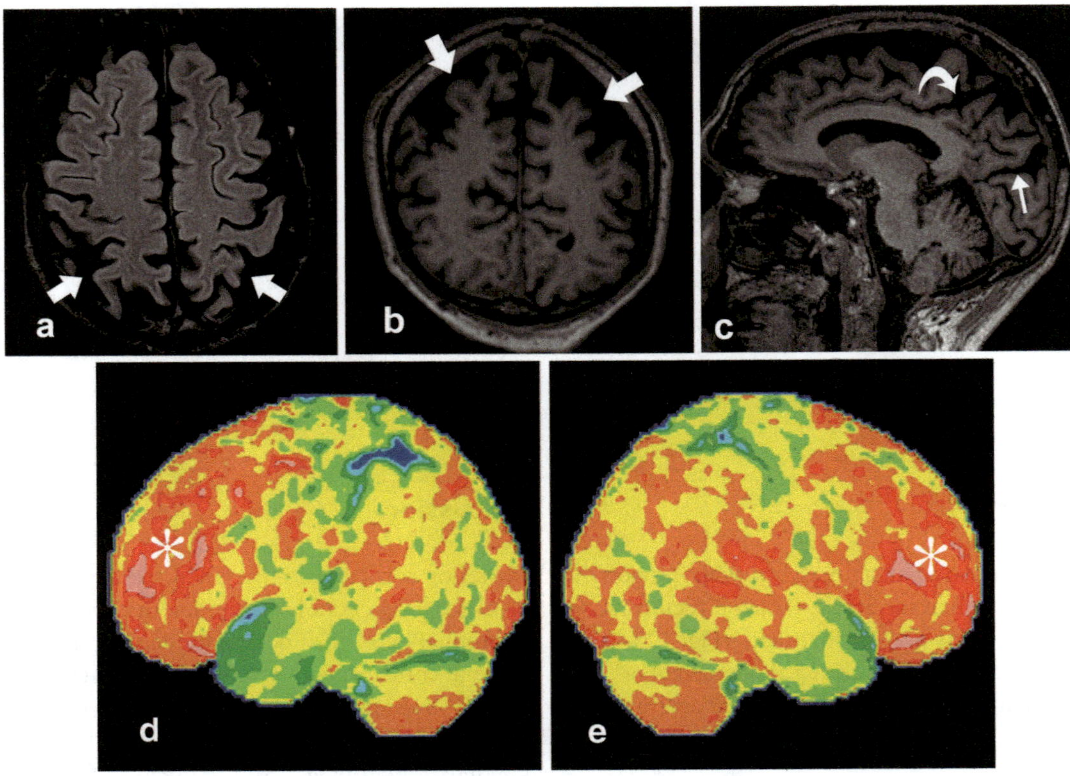

Fig. 125.1 FLAIR axial (**a**), MPRAGE coronal (**b**), MPRAGE sagittal (**c**), PET surface rendering left lateral view (**d**), and PET surface rendering right lateral view (**e**)

compared to patients with Lewy body dementia. Patients with PCA are amyloid positive.

Although early MRI findings may be normal, more severe cases may demonstrate asymmetric, cortical volume loss in the parietal and to a lesser degree medial temporal lobes that commonly affects the right side more than the left. Like with FDG PET imaging, there is considerable overlap of findings with AD.

Suggested Reading

Aharon-Peretz J, Israel O, Goldsher D, Peretz A. Posterior cortical atrophy variants of Alzheimer's disease. Dement Geriatr Cogn Disord. 1999;10(6):483–7.

Benson DF, Davis RJ, Snyder BD. Posterior cortical atrophy. Arch Neurol. 1988;45(7):789–93.

Singh TD, Josephs KA, Machulda MM, Drubach DA, Apostolova LG, Lowe VJ, et al. Clinical, FDG and amyloid PET imaging in posterior cortical atrophy. J Neurol. 2015;262(6):1483–92.

Case 126
Primary CNS Lymphoma

Anuj Rajput, Michael Goodman, and Lev Bangiyev

History

A 53-year-old male presents with a right cerebellar mass (Fig. 126.1).

Diagnosis

Primary CNS lymphoma

Findings

- MRI images show right cerebellar masses at the level of the right middle cerebellar peduncle that is T1 hypointense and heterogeneously T2 hyperintense with mild mass effect effacing right lateral recess of the fourth ventricle.
- Hyperintense T2 signal adjacent to the tumor is consisent with edema (arrowheads).
- The tumors demonstrate avid homogeneous enhancement on the post contrast image (curved arrows).
- The larger tumor shows increased DWI signal with corresponding low ADC signal consistent with increased diffusion restriction (wide arrows).
- PET/MRI fusion demonstrates multiple abnormal foci of increased FDG uptake consistent with malignancy (thin arrows).

Discussion

CNS lymphoma represents 6.6% of primary brain tumors and can occur at all ages, however the elderly population is affected the most. Patients commonly present with focal neurological deficits or altered mental status. These lesions are most commonly supratentorial, clustered around the ventricles, and may extend along the ependymal surfaces to involve the corpus callosum. Primary CNS lymphoma may also involve the leptomeninges and present as multifocal lesions.

On conventional MRI, CNS lymphomas typically demonstrate low signal on T2-weighted imaging due to its high cellularity. On T1-weighted images, lesions are commonly hypointense with avid homogeneous contrast enhancement. In lymphoma the cells are tightly packed with high nuclei to cytoplasm ratios and hence demonstrate increased diffusion restriction with low apparent diffusion coefficient values. MR spectroscopy will demonstrate increased choline and lipid peaks with very low NAA peak. Like all tumors, lymphoma of the brain is associated with edema and peritumoral high T2 signal. Although these findings are typical of CNS lymphoma, they are not pathognomonic. High-grade gliomas and metastatic lesions may demonstrate similar

R. Gupta et al., *PET/MR Imaging*, https://doi.org/10.1007/978-3-319-65106-4_126

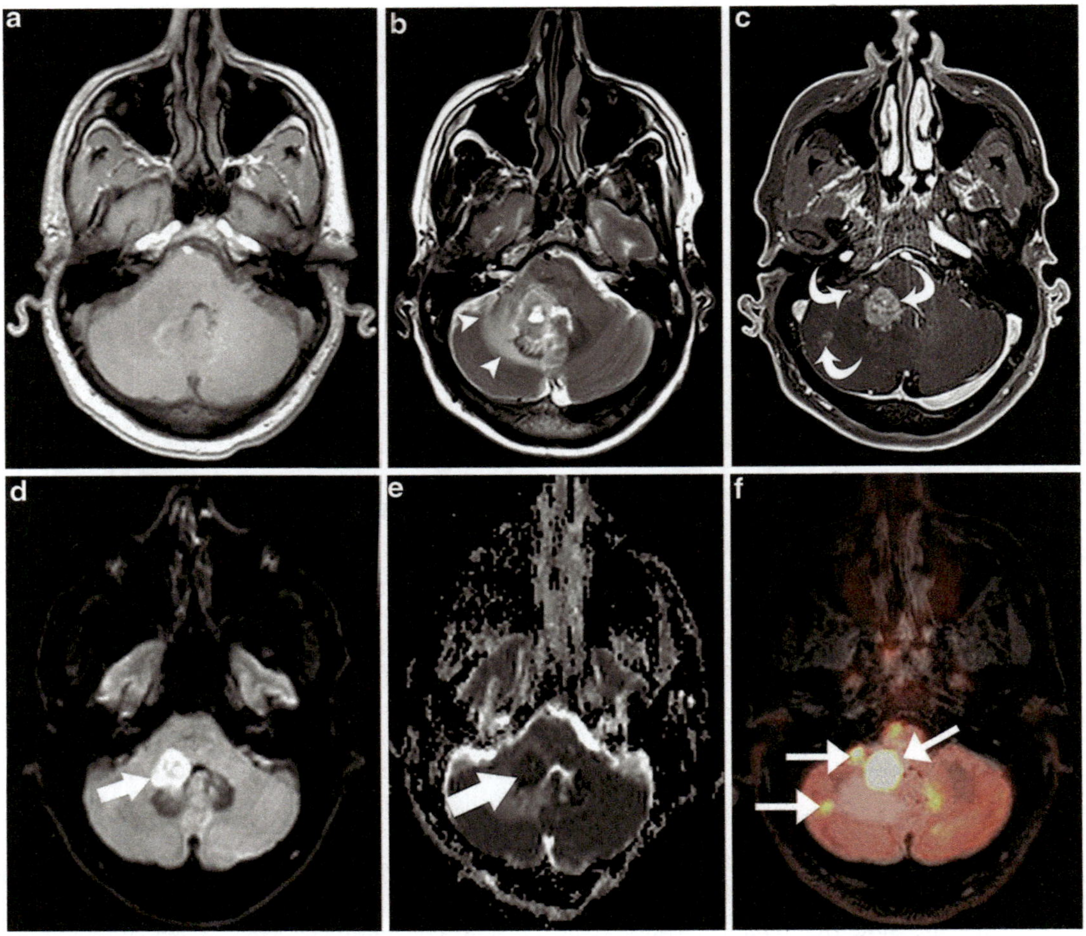

Fig. 126.1 T1 axial (**a**), T2 axial (**b**), T1 post-gadolinium contrast axial (**c**), diffusion-weighted imaging axial (**d**), apparent diffusion coefficient axial (**e**), and PET/MRI FLAIR axial fusion (**f**)

findings creating a diagnostic dilemma. Differentiating between lymphoma and other neoplasms is critical since lymphoma does not require surgical resection. It should also be noted that even though lymphoma is a high-grade neoplasm, it does not demonstrate hyperperfusion which can be used as a clue to differentiate from high-grade glioma.

The use of FDG PET/MR imaging exploits the hypermetabolic properties of primary CNS lymphoma and is helpful in providing both the initial characterization of the tumor, and a tool to monitor treatment response and surveillance for tumor recurrence. PET can be useful in identifying multifocal or multicentric disease. Furthermore, FDG PET imaging of lymphoma generally demonstrates significantly higher SUV values with primary brain lymphoma compared to gliomas or metastatic brain lesions.

Suggested Reading

Koeller KK, Smirniotopoulos JG, Jones RV. Primary central nervous system lymphoma: radiologic-pathologic correlation. Radiographics. 1997;17(6):1497–526.

Kosaka N, Tsuchida T, Uematsu H, Kimura H, Okazawa H, Itoh H. 18F-FDG PET of common enhancing malignant brain tumors. AJR Am J Roentgenol. 2008;190(6):W365–9.

Mansour A, Qandeel M, Abdel-Razeq H, Abu Ali HA. MR imaging features of intracranial primary CNS lymphoma in immune competent patients. Cancer Imaging. 2014;14:22.

Case 127
Creutzfeldt-Jakob Disease

Ana M. Franceschi, Michael J. Hoch,
and Timothy M. Shepherd

History

A 72-year-old female with progressive dementia over 4 months (Fig. 127.1). Her husband states she has increasing difficulty remembering names and speaks in incomplete sentences with poor articulation. Co-workers have noticed severe confusion.

Diagnosis

Creutzfeldt-Jakob disease

Findings

- Axial DWI and ADC show left cerebral cortex (white curved arrows) and basal ganglia (thin white arrow) diffusion restriction.
- Axial FLAIR demonstrates corresponding subtle hyperintensity.
- PET/MR fusion with decreased FDG uptake in the left parietal and temporal lobe (wide white arrows).
- FDG-PET shows corresponding hypometabolism in the affected left cerebral cortex (white arrowheads) and left thalamus (black arrowhead).

Discussion

Creutzfeldt-Jakob disease (CJD) is a type of spongiform encephalopathy caused by an infectious protein agent termed a prion. The disease progresses as the misfolded prion protein causes adjacent normally folded proteins to convert to the malformed one resulting in abnormal accumulation around neurons leading to cell death. CJD is characterized clinically by rapidly progressive dementia, myoclonus, and death usually within a year of presentation, with a mean survival time of 7 months. Currently, there is no known treatment for this disease.

There are four subtypes of CJD: sporadic (sCJD: most common, 85% of cases), variant (vCJD: "mad cow disease," Kuru), familial (fCJD: inherited with a PRPc mutation, 10% of cases), and iatrogenic (corneal and meningeal transplants). The CSF marker typically elevated in patients with CJD is the 14-3-3 protein, although brain biopsy is required for a definitive diagnosis. The patients with sporadic CJD also demonstrate a typical generalized periodic sharp wave pattern on electroencephalography.

The most common finding of CJD on imaging with FDG PET/MR imaging is T2 and FLAIR hyperintensity in the basal ganglia most commonly affecting the putamen and caudate

R. Gupta et al., *PET/MR Imaging*, https://doi.org/10.1007/978-3-319-65106-4_127

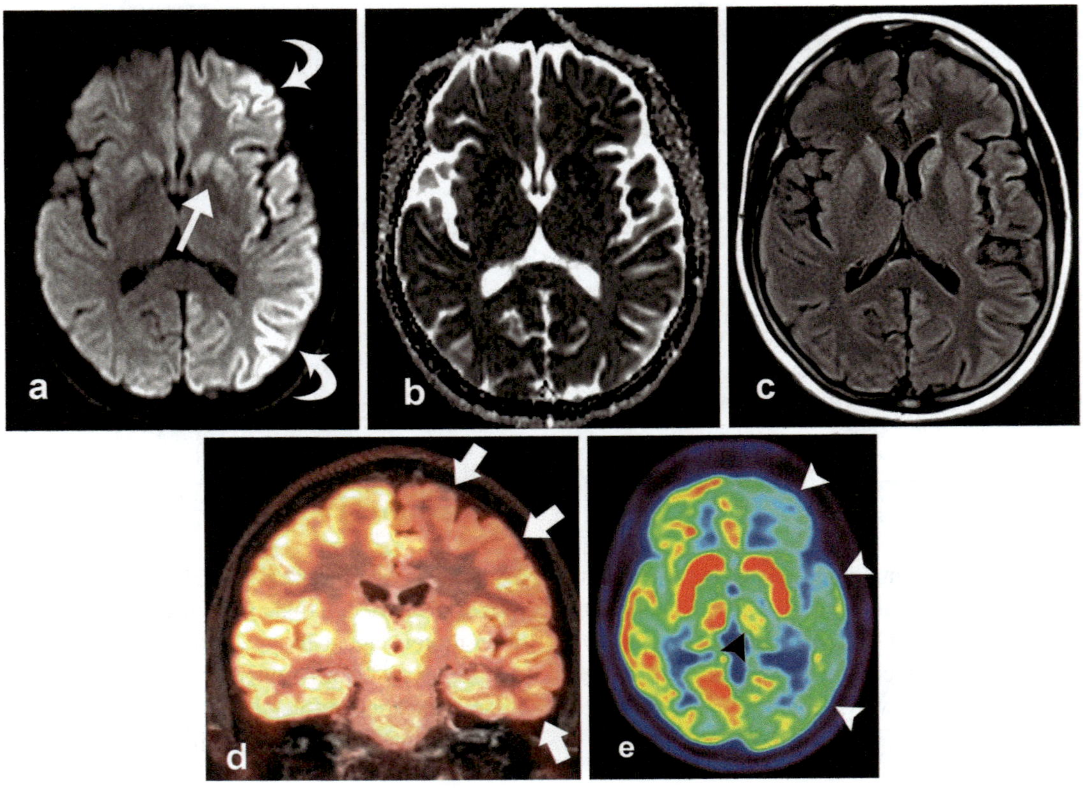

Fig. 127.1 Diffusion-weighted image axial (**a**), apparent diffusion coefficient axial (**b**), FLAIR axial (**c**), PET/MR FLAIR coronal fusion (**d**), and PET axial (**e**)

nucleus. Cerebral cortical findings are also common with hyperintense signal on T2 and FLAIR sequences that may be asymmetric. On PET these areas demonstrate decreased FDG uptake. Additional abnormalities may be seen within the thalamus with T2 and FLAIR hyperintensities and corresponding hypometabolism. Rapid progression of cerebral atrophy on subsequent exams is expected. Persistent restricted diffusion on DWI has been shown to be more sensitive than FLAIR in patients with CJD. Early in the disease, brain MRI may be without significant abnormalities and some cases of CJD have no definable MR changes. Therefore, isolated cortical hypometabolism or isolated cortical T2 hyperintensity on FDG PET/MR imaging can be a suspicious finding for CJD in a patient with rapid cognitive decline.

Suggested Reading

Henkel K, Zerr I, Hertel A, Gratz KF, Schroter A, Tschampa HJ, et al. Positron emission tomography with [(18)F] FDG in the diagnosis of Creutzfeldt-Jakob disease (CJD). J Neurol. 2002;249(6):699–705.

Kallenberg K, Schulz-Schaeffer WJ, Jastrow U, Poser S, Meissner B, Tschampa HJ, et al. Creutzfeldt-Jakob disease: comparative analysis of MR imaging sequences. AJNR Am J Neuroradiol. 2006;27:1459–62.

Shiga Y, Miyazawa K, Sato S, Fukushima R, Shibuya S, Sato Y, et al. Diffusion-weighted MRI abnormalities as an early diagnostic marker for Creutzfeldt-Jakob disease. Neurology. 2004;63:443–9.

Case 128
Calvarial Hemangioma

Rajesh Gupta and Priya Sharma

History

A 48-year-old male with headache presents for evaluation of a lesion in the occipital calvarium identified on prior imaging (Fig. 128.1).

Diagnosis

Calvarial hemangioma

Findings

- Midline lesion within the occipital calvarium that is hyperintense on T1-weighted image, heterogeneously hyperintense on FLAIR, and demonstrates heterogeneous enhancement post-contrast administration (curved arrows).
- No FDG uptake within the lesion on PET/MR fusion image.

Discussion

Hemangiomas of the calvaria are benign slow-growing vascular neoplasms that account for 0.2% of all bone neoplasms. They are more common in women and can affect any age group. The more common sessile type extends through the diploe of the skull. Rarely, calvarial hemangiomas can be of the globular type, which can be expansile. The frontal and parietal bones are most frequently affected. Calvarial hemangiomas are usually solitary, however, multifocal lesions have been reported. Hemangiomas are usually found incidentally but can present as a painless, palpable scalp mass if they expand the outer table of the skull.

MR imaging is useful in evaluating for intra-diploic or intracranial extension as well as involvement of adjacent neurovascular structures. Calvarial hemangiomas are typically hyperintense on T1-weighted images due to internal fat. They exhibit heterogeneous T2-weighted and FLAIR hyperintensity with hypointense borders. The tumor matrix has a stippled appearance. The mass will enhance heterogeneously after administration of gadolinium contrast material.

Benign intraosseous lesions demonstrate minimal to no FDG uptake on PET imaging. Hemangiomas fall into this category and have a narrow range of SUV measurements related to blood retention. Blood vessels within calvarial hemangioma are also the reason for post-contrast enhancement and can sometimes provide a diagnostic dilemma when excluding malignancy. The evaluation of hemangiomas with PET/MR imaging is not typically performed, however, it can provide superior anatomical and functional lesion characterization to differentiate them from malignant bone lesions.

R. Gupta et al., *PET/MR Imaging*, https://doi.org/10.1007/978-3-319-65106-4_128

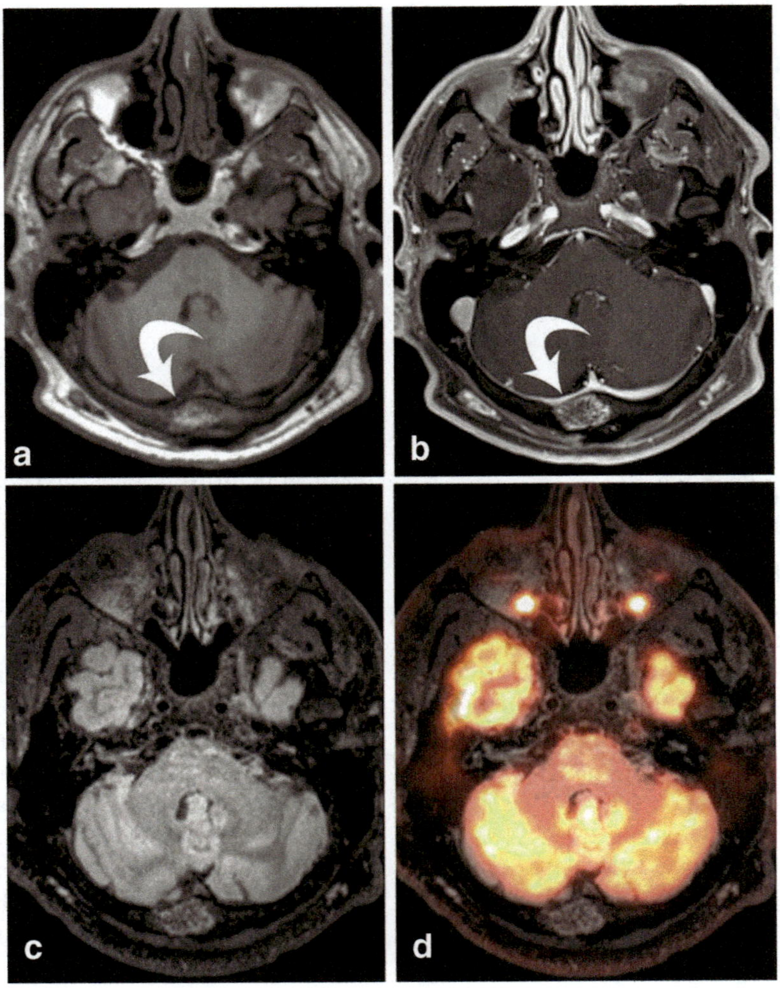

Fig. 128.1 T1 axial (**a**), T1 post-gadolinium contrast axial (**b**), FLAIR axial (**c**), and PET/MR FLAIR axial fusion (**d**)

Suggested Reading

Bastug D, Ortiz O, Schochet SS. Hemangiomas in the calvaria: imaging findings. AJR Am J Roentgenol. 1995;164(3):683–7.

Hatayama K, Watanabe H, Ahmed AR, Yanagawa T, Shinozaki T, Oriuchi N, et al. Evaluation of hemangioma by positron emission tomography: role in a multimodality approach. J Comput Assist Tomogr. 2003;27(1):70–7.

Case 129
Dementia with Lewy Body

Ana M. Franceschi, Michael J. Hoch,
and Timothy M. Shepherd

History

An 84-year-old female with macular degeneration, presents with fluctuating alertness, memory loss, and visual hallucinations for 6 months (Fig. 129.1). Patient reports seeing a stuffed rabbit growing to the size of an adult person in her living room.

Diagnosis

Dementia with Lewy body

Findings

- T1 and T2 images show prominent sulci and fissures consistent with cerebral volume loss.
- PET fusion and axial images show severe decreased FDG uptake in bilateral parietal and occipital lobes. Mild decreased uptake is seen in the frontal and posterior temporal lobes.
- Preservation of the metabolic activity in the sensorimotor cortex (thin arrows).
- PET surface rendering with threshold images show areas with the most intense decreased activity (blue-purple) located in the parietal (large black arrow) and occipital lobes (large white arrow).

Discussion

Dementia with Lewy body (DLB) is the second most common neurodegenerative disease following Alzheimer's disease and accounts for 20–30% of all dementias. The onset of the disease is approximately 50–60 years old. The disease is characterized by cognitive impairment, visual hallucinations, and motor Parkinsonism. Distinguishing dementia with Lewy body from Alzheimer's disease is difficult since many clinical and imaging features are similar. The underlying cause of DLB is the accumulation of Lewy bodies within the brain which are clumps of alpha-synuclein protein in neurons. Dementia usually precedes or accompanies Parkinson features in DLB. In Parkinson's disease, the dementia usually occurs many years after the onset of the movement disorders. Compared to Parkinson's disease, DLB is less responsive to levodopa and the drug may worsen psychiatric features.

MR has a limited role in diagnosing DLB since its imaging findings are often vague and nonspecific. In severe cases, there is less pronounced global atrophy in DLB as compared to Alzheimer's disease. This is most evident with less medial temporal lobe volume loss with Lewy body dementia. Hybrid FDG PET/MR allows better correlation of hypometabolism with

R. Gupta et al., *PET/MR Imaging*, https://doi.org/10.1007/978-3-319-65106-4_129

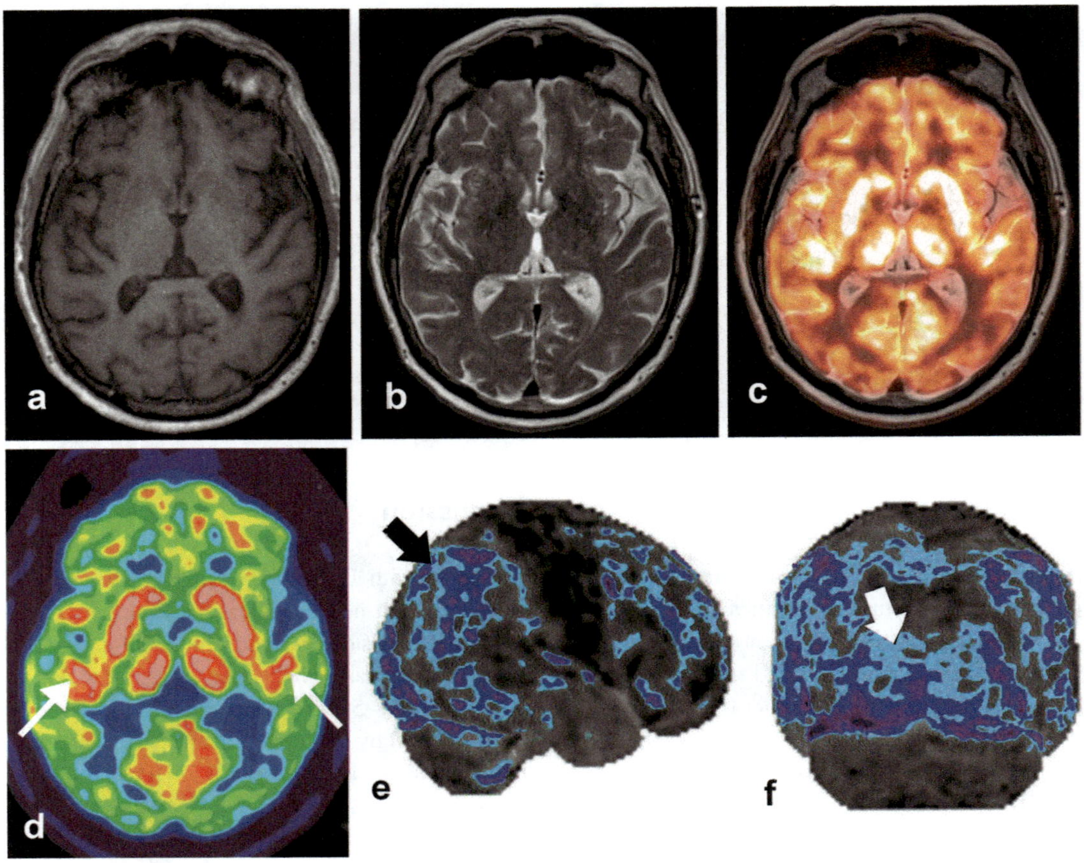

Fig. 129.1 T1 axial (**a**), T2 axial (**b**), PET/MR T2 axial fusion (**c**), PET axial (**d**), PET surface rendering with threshold in right lateral view (**e**), and PET surface rendering with statistical threshold in posterior view (**f**)

regions of atrophy improving diagnostic accuracy. As in Alzheimer's disease, there is decreased FDG uptake in the posterior temporal and parietal lobes with additional involvement of the occipital lobes. Mesial occipital cortex hypometabolism on FDG PET may be the most specific and sensitive imaging finding for DLB, but is not always seen, especially in the absence of visual hallucinations. Alternatively, the loss of vision due to macular degeneration or retinal artery occlusions can also result in decreased FDG uptake in the mesial occipital lobe, but these patients should not have other features of DLB. In cases where PET is equivocal, dopamine transporter imaging showing decreased activity in the putamina and caudate nuclei can be helpful in the diagnosis of DLB.

Suggested Reading

Mak E, Su L, Williams GB, O'Brien JT. Neuroimaging characteristics of dementia with Lewy bodies. Alzheimers Res Ther. 2014;6(2):18.

Mollenhauer B, Förstl H, Deuschl G, Storch A, Oertel W, Trenkwalder C. Lewy body and parkinsonian dementia: common, but often misdiagnosed conditions. Dtsch Arztebl Int. 2011;107(39):684–91.

Taylor JP, O'Brien J. Neuroimaging of dementia with Lewy bodies. Neuroimaging Clin N Am. 2012;22(1):67–81.

Case 130 Cerebral Amyloid Angiopathy with Alzheimer's Disease

Robert Matthews

History

A 76-year-old male with memory loss and micro-hemorrhages seen on outside MRI. Referred for dementia evaluation (Fig. 130.1).

Diagnosis

Cerebral amyloid angiopathy with Alzheimer's disease

Findings

- Mild cortical atrophic changes are noted on T1-weighted images.
- Multiple small hyperintense signals are seen in the white matter and periventricular space on T2 and FLAIR images reflecting small vessel disease (thin arrows).
- SWI shows multiple foci with drop in signal due to siderosis from microhemorrhages related to cerebral amyloid angiography (arrowheads).
- PET fusion and axial images demonstrate severe decreased FDG uptake in the parieto-temporal lobes with moderate decreased uptake in the frontal lobes characteristic of advanced Alzheimer's disease (curved arrows).

Discussion

Cerebral amyloid angiopathy (CAA) is a cerebrovascular disease characterized by the deposition of β-amyloid in the media and adventitia of small and medium size arteries of the cerebral cortex and leptomeninges. This causes a fibrinoid degeneration of the vessel wall between the tunica media and tunica intima with microaneurysm formation, and subsequent microhemorrhage. CAA occurs with advancing age. Although found at autopsy in only 33% of 60–70-year-olds, the prevalence of age-related CAA increases to 75% in those older than 90 years. The combination of multiple intracranial hemorrhages, cerebral volume loss, and leukoencephalopathy may lead to progressive cognitive dysfunction and dementia. CAA-related dementia may progress slowly, similar to patients with Alzheimer disease dementia, with which CAA is frequently associated. In 40% of CAA patients with dementia, Alzheimer pathology is found at autopsy. On the other hand, up to 90% of patients with Alzheimer disease have changes of CAA at autopsy. However, dementia may be present in patients with CAA in the absence of pathologic changes of Alzheimer disease and may in those cases be related to small vessel ischemic changes.

The most common MR findings of CAA are a non-traumatic intracranial hemorrhage that is

R. Gupta et al., *PET/MR Imaging*, https://doi.org/10.1007/978-3-319-65106-4_130

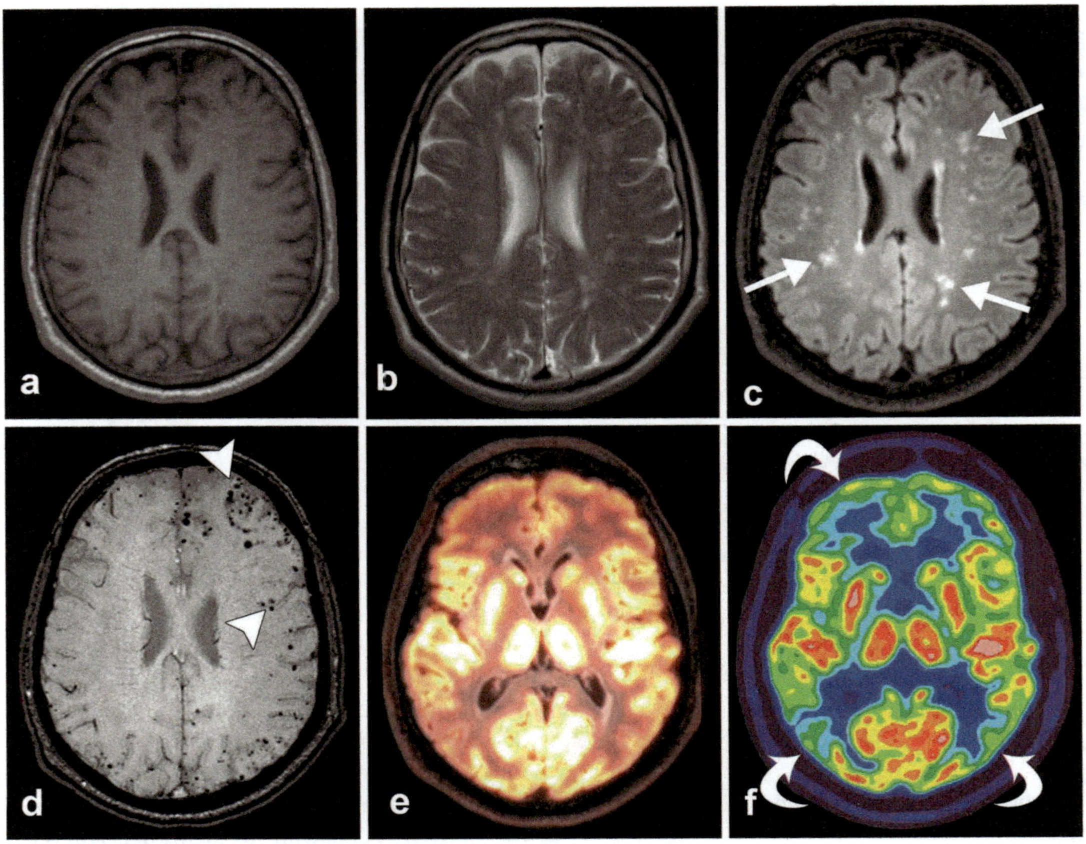

Fig. 130.1 3D T1 axial (**a**), T2 axial (**b**), FLAIR axial (**c**), susceptibility-weighted imaging axial (**d**), PET/MR FLAIR axial fusion, more inferior level (**e**), and PET axial, more inferior level (**f**)

either lobar or rarely cerebellar in location, leukoencephalopathy, and cerebral atrophy. The intracranial hemorrhage involves the cortical-subcortical distribution and generally does not affect the deep white matter, basal ganglia, or brainstem. The bleeding may be subarachnoid, subdural, or intraventricular hemorrhage. Small microhemorrhages less than 5 mm may be difficult to see on traditional T1 and T2 imaging. FLAIR imaging may show high-signal foci, best seen during the acute phase of the microhemorrhage. The best MRI sequences to visualize microhemorrhages are T2 gradient echo or susceptibility-weighted imaging where foci of susceptibility are demonstrated by signal dropout due to siderosis in the cortical-subcortical location. Leukoencephalopathy presents as a high T2 or FLAIR signal of the white matter that is a nonspecific finding seen with chronic microvascular disease, demyelination, vasculitis, sequela of prior infection, or even neoplasm.

Amyloid PET tracer binding has been demonstrated in fibrillar amyloid and perivascular beta-amyloid depositions, the underlying pathology of CAA, as well as in beta-amyloid plaques within the cerebral parenchyma that is the hallmark of Alzheimer's disease. Amyloid PET imaging has been used in CAA with high sensitivity and high negative predictive value to effectively rule out CAA. However, amyloid imaging cannot distinguish between amyloid angiopathy and parenchymal fibrillar plaques, and both are highly prevalent in the elderly, with or without dementia. In patients with dementia, FDG PET imaging is useful to differentiate neurodegenerative diseases based on specific patterns of hypometabolism. In particular, this is important with dementia characterized by positive beta-amyloid load, such as Alzheimer's and dementia with Lewy bodies. In patients with larger size bleeds, one could expect findings of focal areas of hypometabolism in a vascular distribution similar to those found in vascular dementia. PET/MR imaging using FDG is helpful to confirm coexistent CAA and Alzheimer disease by demonstrating multiple hemorrhages, leukoencephalopathy, and cerebral atrophy which are typical findings of CAA on MRI, as well as hypometabolism involving the temporoparietal cortices, posterior cingulate, and precuneus regions, which is a classical pattern for Alzheimer dementia.

Suggested Reading

Baron JC, Farid K, Dolan E, Turc G, Marrapu ST, O'Brien E, et al. Diagnostic utility of amyloid PET in cerebral amyloid angiopathy-related symptomatic intracerebral hemorrhage. J Cereb Blood Flow Metab. 2014;34(5):753–8.

Chao CP, Kotsenas AL, Broderick DF. Cerebral amyloid angiopathy: CT and MR imaging findings. Radiographics. 2006;26(5):1517–31.

Drzezga A, Barthel H, Minoshima S, Sabri O. Potential clinical applications of PET/MR imaging in neurodegenerative diseases. J Nucl Med. 2014;55(Suppl 2):47S–55S.

Case 131
Dural Metastases

Ana M. Franceschi and Robert Matthews

History

A 74-year-old female with breast cancer who developed sudden onset of right-sided blindness (Fig. 131.1).

Diagnosis

Dural metastases

Findings

- Large T1 isointense dural lesions in the bilateral temporal lobes (arrowheads) and frontal lobes (thin arrows) that exert mass effect on the cerebral parenchyma.
- Masses demonstrate enhancement following contrast administration.
- Abnormal FDG uptake on the PET/MR fusion imaging consistent with metastases.

Discussion

Dural or pachymeningeal metastases are a less common form of intracranial metastases as compared to more usual brain metastases. Dural metastases may occur by direct extension from skull metastases, retrograde seeding by the vertebral venous plexus, hematologic spread, and lymphatic seeding. The most common primary origins of dural metastases include breast cancer, prostate cancer, lung cancer, and head and neck cancers. Many patients are asymptomatic until the tumor enlargement causes symptoms such as headache, fatigue, confusion, and focal neurological deficits. The most common type of treatment is radiation therapy. Single solitary lesions may benefit from surgical resection especially if there is a mass effect. Chemotherapy is often employed in combination.

Dural metastases may have a variety of findings on MR imaging. They are typically iso- or hypointense to adjacent cerebral cortex on T1-weighted images and iso- or hyperintense to adjacent cortex on T2-weighted images and demonstrate vivid homogeneous enhancement on the post-contrast T1-weighted sequences. On MR spectroscopy, dural metastases demonstrate elevated choline/creatinine ratio, prominent lipid, and occasionally prominent lactate peaks as well. On neuroimaging with PET/MRI, these lesions will demonstrate increased FDG uptake corresponding to regions with abnormal MRI signal. When solitary, dural metastasis may be indistinguishable from meningioma, which is a very common and most often benign tumor. In such cases PET/MRI offers noninvasive method of differentiating FDG avid metastases from benign dural tumors that do not accumulate FDG.

R. Gupta et al., *PET/MR Imaging*, https://doi.org/10.1007/978-3-319-65106-4_131

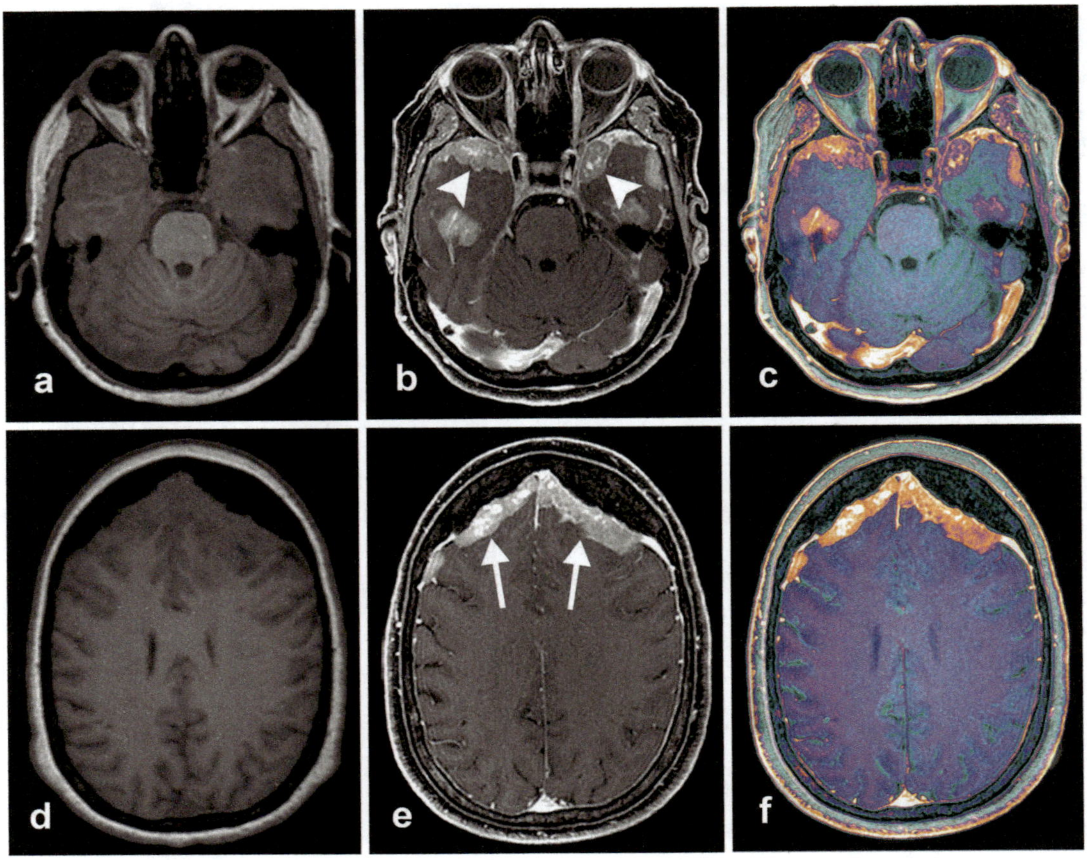

Fig. 131.1 T1 axial (**a**), T1 VIBE post-gadolinium contrast axial (**b**), PET/MR T1 VIBE post-gadolinium contrast axial fusion (**c**), T1 axial, at more superior level (**d**), T1 VIBE post-gadolinium contrast axial, at more superior level (**e**), and PET/MR 3D T1 T1 VIBE post-gadolinium contrast axial fusion, at more superior level (**f**)

Suggested Reading

Barnholtz-Sloan JS, Sloan AE, Davis FG, Vigneau FD, Lai P, Sawaya RE. Incidence proportions of brain metastases in patients diagnosed (1973 to 2001) in the Metropolitan Detroit Cancer Surveillance System. J Clin Oncol. 2004;22(14):2865–72.

Boss A, Bisdas S, Kolb A, Hofmann M, Ernemann U, Claussen CD, et al. Hybrid PET/MRI of intracranial masses: initial experiences and comparison to PET/CT. J Nucl Med. 2010;51(8):1198–205.

Fink KR, Fink JR. Imaging of brain metastases. Surg Neurol Int. 2013;4(Suppl 4):S209–19.

Rohren EM, Provenzale JM, Barboriak DP, Coleman RE. Screening for cerebral metastases with FDG PET in patients undergoing whole-body staging of non-central nervous system malignancy. Radiology. 2003;226(1):181–7.

Case 132
Frontotemporal Dementia

Ana M. Franceschi

History

A 75-year-old female with memory loss and cognitive dysfunction (Fig. 132.1).

Diagnosis

Frontotemporal dementia (FTD)

Findings

- T1 and FLAIR images show cortical atrophy in the bilateral frontal lobes (wide white arrows).
- PET images show severe decreased FDG uptake in the frontal lobes (curved white arrows) and milder decreased uptake in the temporoparietal region (white arrowheads).
- PET surface rendering with statistical threshold images shows areas with the most decreased activity (blue-purple) in the frontal lobes (black thin arrows) and lateral temporal lobes (black arrowheads).

Discussion

Frontotemporal dementia (FTD) is an umbrella term used to describe a group of neurodegenerative disorders characterized by selective atrophy of the frontal and temporal lobes, although other regions of the brain may also be involved including the insula and cingulate gyrus, basal ganglia and thalamus. There is a characteristic clinical presentation, with a predominance of behavioral and psychiatric symptoms including language deficits, while short-term memory loss, typical for Alzheimer's disease, is less pronounced. Up to 20–40% of FTD cases demonstrate an autosomal dominant inheritance pattern. Patients are typically younger than in other forms of dementia, with the average age at presentation being 40–60 years old.

Patients with frontotemporal dementia are further divided into behavioral (frontal lobe predominance) and language (predilection for the left temporal lobe) variants, based on clinical symptomatology and imaging findings. The language variant of FTD is also known as primary progressive aphasia (PPA) and can be additionally subclassified as agrammatic variant primary progressive aphasia (progressive nonfluent aphasia, PNFA), semantic variant primary progressive aphasia (semantic dementia), and logopenic variant primary progressive aphasia.

The classic findings on FDG PET/MR imaging include selective atrophy primarily involving the frontal and temporal lobes, with marked asymmetry between right and left hemispheric involvement, as well as asymmetry in focal involvement of the frontal versus the temporal lobes. Although the frontal and anterior temporal lobes are affected most, the mesial temporal area and subcortical structures may also be affected including the basal

R. Gupta et al., *PET/MR Imaging*, https://doi.org/10.1007/978-3-319-65106-4_132

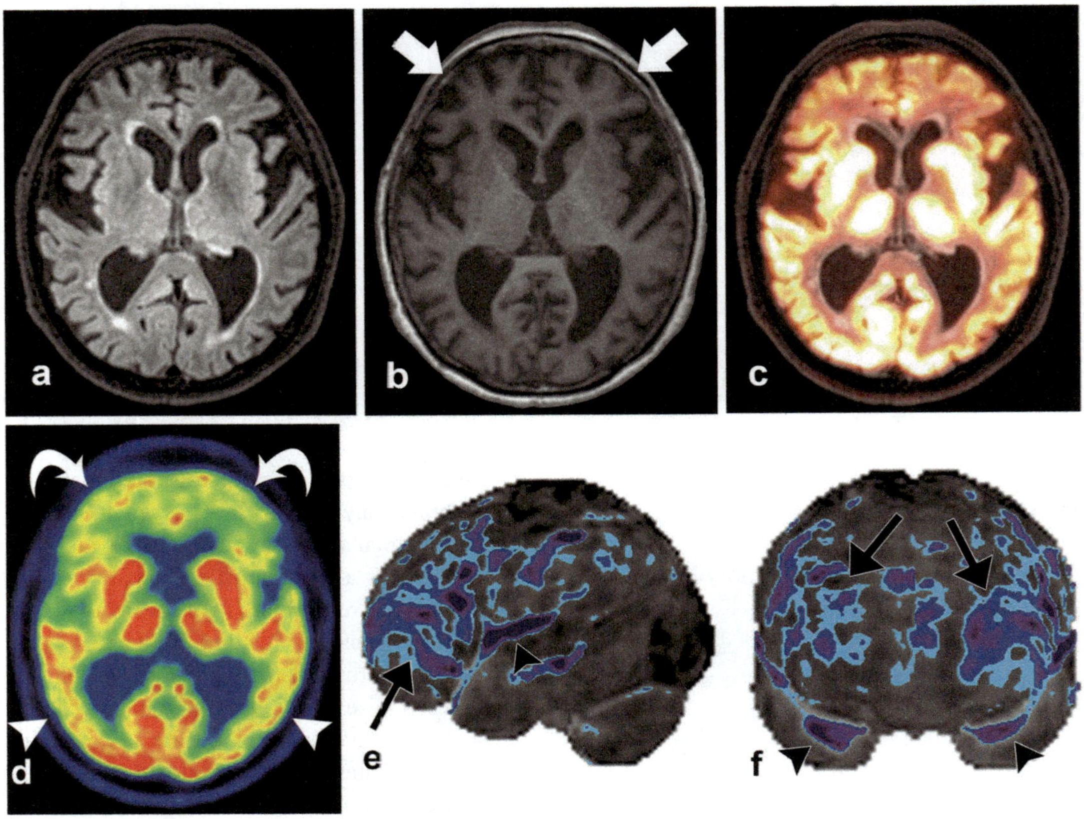

Fig. 132.1 FLAIR axial (**a**), T1 axial (**b**), PET/MR FLAIR axial fusion (**c**), PET axial (**d**), PET surface rendering with statistical threshold in left lateral view (**e**), and PET surface rendering with statistical threshold in anterior view (**f**)

ganglia and thalamus. In the behavioral variant of FTD, prominent frontostriatal pathway dysfunction is also present with a significant reduction in the size of the caudate head in these patients, especially when compared to patients with language variant FTD (primary progressive aphasia). On FDG PET functional images, there is marked hypometabolism corresponding to areas of brain atrophy on MRI structural sequences. As the disease progresses, cerebral volume loss and areas of decreased FDG activity spread in a more diffuse pattern throughout the brain.

Suggested Reading

Agosta F, Galantucci S, Filippi M. Advanced magnetic resonance imaging of neurodegenerative diseases. Neurol Sci. 2017;38(1):41–51.

Gordon E, Rohrer JD, Fox NC. Advances in neuroimaging in frontotemporal dementia. J Neurochem. 2016;138(Suppl 1):193–210.

Kato T, Inui Y, Nakamura A, Ito K. Brain fluorodeoxyglucose (FDG) PET in dementia. Ageing Res Rev. 2016;30:73–84.

Case 133 Neurosarcoidosis

Eric van Staalduinen

History

A 67-year-old male with lesion in the cerebellum that has fluctuated in size over the past couple of years (Fig. 133.1).

Diagnosis

Neurosarcoidosis

Findings

- Axial imaging shows contrast-enhancing lesion in the inferior aspect of the left middle cerebellar peduncle extending to the inferior cerebellar peduncle with increased signal on STIR imaging (thin arrow).
- Abnormal increased FDG uptake in the left cerebellar peduncle lesion.
- Sagittal STIR imaging shows the hyperintense lesion to involve the left middle and inferior cerebellar peduncles (curved arrow).
- PET/MR fusion and MIP images of the chest reveal multiple hypermetabolic mediastinal and hilar lymph nodes proven to be sarcoidosis (arrowheads).

Discussion

Sarcoidosis is a multisystem inflammatory disease of unknown etiology characterized by noncaseating granulomas. Neurosarcoidosis involves the central and peripheral nervous system and is estimated to present symptomatically in approximately 5–16% of sarcoidosis patients. The disease is characterized by granulomatous infiltrates involving the leptomeninges, dura, hypothalamus, pituitary gland, and cranial nerves with a tendency to localize at the base of the brain. Neurosarcoidosis is characterized by its wide range of nonspecific general symptoms including headache, fatigue, dizziness, and fever. Isolated cranial neuropathy, most commonly facial nerve palsy, is the most common symptom, while optic nerve and chiasm involvement are most frequently recognized on imaging. The disease is often indolent, with 67% of patients experiencing a self-limited monophasic illness and the remainder of patients experiencing a chronic remitting-relapsing course. Most patients typically respond rapidly to high-dose steroids. Complications of neurosarcoidosis include hydrocephalus, which is usually associated with a very poor prognosis, vasculitis, and epileptic seizures.

R. Gupta et al., *PET/MR Imaging*, https://doi.org/10.1007/978-3-319-65106-4_133

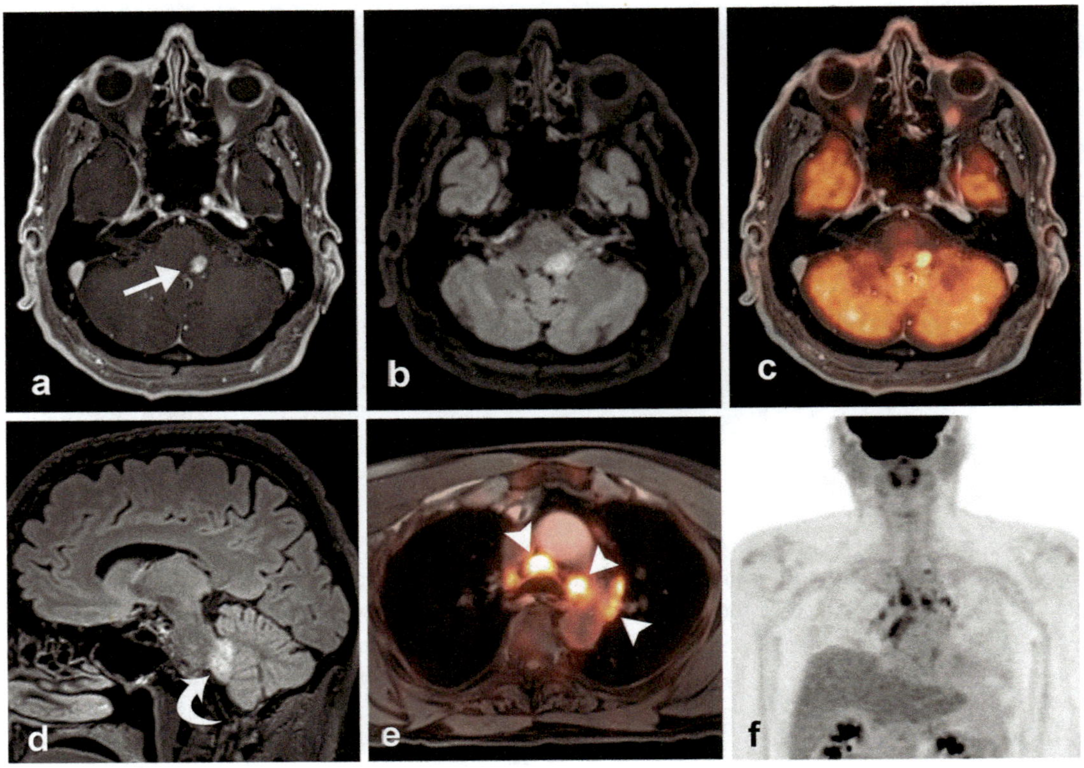

Fig. 133.1 T1 post-gadolinium contrast axial (**a**), FLAIR axial (**b**), PET/MR T1 post-gadolinium contrast axial fusion (**c**), FLAIR sagittal (**d**), PET/MR T1 radial VIBE with fat suppression axial through the chest (**e**), and PET MIP of the chest (**f**)

MRI is considered the most sensitive test in the diagnosis of neurosarcoidosis. The most common finding is basilar leptomeningeal involvement with thickening, and diffuse or nodular enhancement after the administration of intravenous contrast. Neurosarcoidosis can also present with focal masses or diffuse thickening of the dural meninges. MRI signal characteristics are nonspecific with isointense dural lesions on T1-weighted imaging and hypointense dural and intraparenchymal lesions on T2-weighted imaging. Approximately 50% of patients have periventricular T2-hyperintense lesions on FLAIR imaging, while neurosarcoid edema does not exhibit restricted diffusion on diffusion-weighted imaging.

As sarcoidosis is a multisystem inflammatory disease, lesions in the brain also exhibit increased FDG uptake. Since disease activity in sarcoidosis is reflected by the degree of hypermetabolism, FDG uptake has been observed to change in response to treatment. Although increased FDG uptake is not specific for the diagnosis of sarcoidosis, when whole-body FDG PET is performed, the diagnosis of sarcoidosis can be frequently suggested due to its characteristic morphologic pattern of mediastinal and hilar involvement.

Suggested Reading

Dubey N, Miletich RS, Wasay M, Mechtler LL, Bakshi R. Role of fluorodeoxyglucose positron emission tomography in the diagnosis of neurosarcoidosis. J Neurol Sci. 2002;205(1):77–81.

Hebel R, Dubaniewicz-Wybieralska M, Dubaniewicz A. Overview of neurosarcoidosis: recent advances. J Neurol. 2015;262(2):258–67.

Shah R, Roberson GH, Curé JK. Correlation of MR imaging findings and clinical manifestations in neurosarcoidosis. AJNR Am J Neuroradiol. 2009;30(5):953–61.

Smith JK, Matheus MG, Castillo M. Imaging manifestations of neurosarcoidosis. AJR Am J Roentgenol. 2004;182(2):289–95.

Case 134
Tumor Pseudoprogression

Anuj Rajput, Michael Goodman, and Lev Bangiyev

History

A 65-year-old male with history of glioblastoma treated with temozolomide and radiation (Fig. 134.1).

Diagnosis

Tumor pseudoprogression

Findings

- Initial T1 post-gadolinium contrast image shows three nodular-enhancing lesions (thin arrows) within the corpus callosum in this patient who has received chemotherapy and radiation for glioblastoma.
- PET/MRI T1 post-gadolinium contrast fusion image demonstrates no hypermetabolic activity within the enhancing lesions.
- T1 post-gadolinium contrast image performed as follow-up at 6 months demonstrates resolution of previously identified enhancing lesions.

Discussion

Tumor pseudoprogression is a term used to describe an increase in tumor size related to treatment rather than true progression. It is a phenomenon that occurs in patients with high-grade gliomas who recently underwent treatment with radiation, temozolomide chemotherapy, or combination therapy. Pseudoprogression is characterized by the development of new enhancing lesions, which on anatomic imaging may be indistinguishable from true tumor progression. While there is enhancement on T1-weighted images, there is usually a mismatch with low signal intensity on T2-weighted images helping to distinguish them from true tumor with high T2 signal. These lesions do not demonstrate increased metabolic activity on FDG PET imaging, abnormal diffusion restriction, or increased cerebral blood volume. Close imaging follow-up further shows resolution of the suspicious lesions confirming the diagnosis of pseudoprogression.

Correctly identifying pseudoprogression from true progression in treated brain tumors such as glioblastoma is a challenge, particularly in patients receiving combined radiotherapy and an alkylating chemotherapeutic agent such as temozolomide. Pseudoprogression begins as new contrast-enhancing lesions that increase in size or number on follow-up brain imaging. This is followed by a period of stasis and decrease in the size and number of lesions upon further imaging. While the pathophysiology behind tumor pseudoprogression is still poorly understood, postulated mechanisms include radiation injury of oligodendrocytes causing a disruption of myelin synthesis and a temporary increase in the permeability of the blood-brain barrier surrounding the

R. Gupta et al., *PET/MR Imaging*, https://doi.org/10.1007/978-3-319-65106-4_134

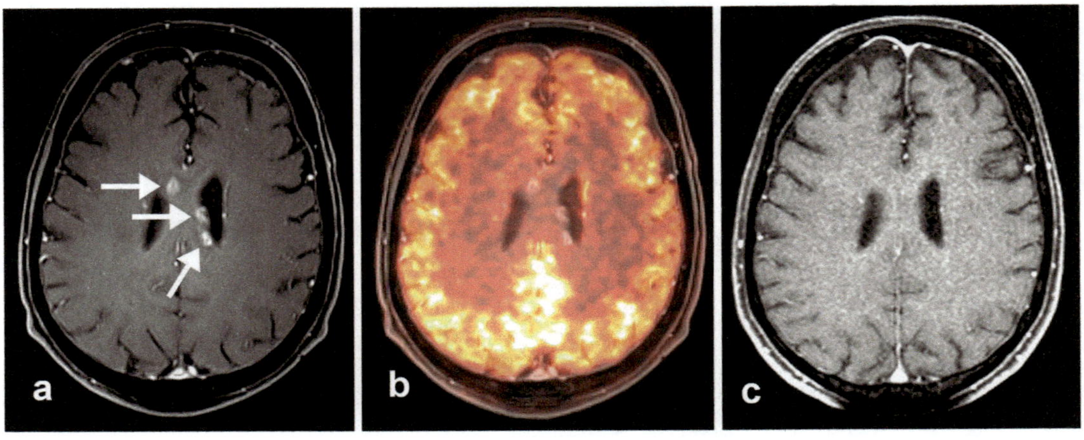

Fig. 134.1 T1 VIBE post-gadolinium contrast axial (**a**), PET/MRI T1 VIBE post-gadolinium contrast axial fusion (**b**), and T1 post-gadolinium contrast axial, follow-up at 6 months (**c**)

tumor. This presents a problem when attempting to employ the Macdonald or RANO criteria, which defines tumor progression as an increase of the contrast-enhancing lesion by at least 25%.

PET imaging is a more effective tool in diagnosing pseudoprogression. Typically, FDG PET/MR imaging demonstrates increased metabolic activity in the case of tumor recurrence while radiation necrosis lesions show no significant FDG uptake. However, high background FDG uptake in the brain parenchyma sometimes makes it challenging to detect low-grade tumor activity. In such patients it is essential to correlate imaging findings with clinical assessment for new symptoms or increased doses of steroids, which would favor true tumor progression. Alternatively, non-FDG radiotracers such as amino acid-based radiotracer have been shown to be more useful in the differentiation of treatment-related changes such as pseudoprogression from true tumor progression.

Suggested Reading

Hygino da Cruz LC Jr, Rodriguez I, Domingues RC, Gasparetto EL, Sorensen AG. Pseudoprogression and pseudoresponse: imaging challenges in the assessment of posttreatment glioma. AJNR Am J Neuroradiol. 2011;32(11):1978–85.

Parvez K, Parvez A, Zadeh G. The diagnosis and treatment of pseudoprogression, radiation necrosis and brain tumor recurrence. Int J Mol Sci. 2014;15: 11832–46.

Case 135
Semantic Dementia

Lev Bangiyev, Michael J. Hoch,
and Timothy M. Shepherd

History

A 66-year-old female presents with progressive language difficulty (Fig. 135.1). She has fluent speech but forgets names of people and things.

Diagnosis

Semantic dementia

Findings

- FLAIR, MPRAGE, and T2 coronal images show severe focal atrophy of the left anterior temporal lobe (large arrow).
- PET fusion and PET coronal image show severe hypometabolic activity in the left anterior temporal lobe (curved arrow).
- PET transaxial image demonstrates mild to moderate global hypometabolic activity. There is preservation of the sensorimotor gyri (thin arrow).

Discussion

Semantic dementia is a variant of primary progressive aphasia and is also categorized as a subtype of frontotemporal lobar degeneration, previously called Pick's disease. The patient initially has difficulty with person and object naming, verbal fluency, dyslexia, and word comprehension. The peak incidence of semantic dementia is approximately 45–65 years old. In the later stage of this condition, patients can become disinhibited and commonly demonstrate dramatic changes in religious or political beliefs.

Neuroimaging with PET/MRI shows characteristic asymmetric focal atrophy involving the temporal lobe, more pronounced anteriorly with relative preservation of the posterior volume. This typically involves the left side first. Parenchymal volume loss or atrophy is evident by prominence of the sulci and enlargement of the CSF spaces. The term "knife blade" describes the most severe cortical atrophy with extreme thinning of the gyri and widening of the sulci. The temporal lobe demonstrates corresponding hypometabolism on FDG PET.

As the disease progresses, eventually volume loss and hypometabolism spread to the contralateral temporal pole and then more diffusely throughout the brain. In the later stages, the process extends to the superior and posterior temporal lobes. The accelerated rate of temporal lobe atrophy distinguishes this disease from Alzheimer's dementia generally affecting the posterior temporal and parietal lobes first.

R. Gupta et al., *PET/MR Imaging*, https://doi.org/10.1007/978-3-319-65106-4_135

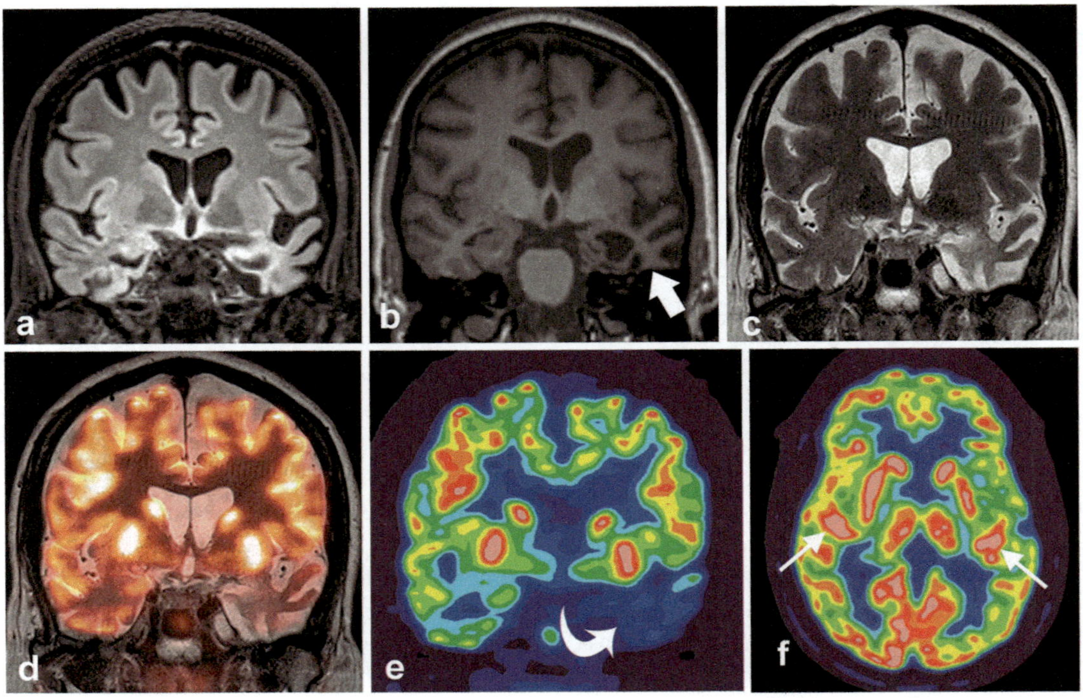

Fig. 135.1 FLAIR coronal (**a**), MPRAGE coronal (**b**), T2 coronal (**c**), PET/MR T2 coronal fusion (**d**), PET coronal (**e**), and PET axial (**f**)

Suggested Reading

Bonner MF, Ash S, Grossman M. The new classification of primary progressive aphasia into semantic, logopenic, or nonfluent/agrammatic variants. Curr Neurol Neurosci Rep. 2010;10(6):484–90.

Diehl J, Grimmer T, Drzezga A, Riemenschneider M, Förstl H, Kurz A. Cerebral metabolic patterns at early stages of frontotemporal dementia and semantic dementia. A PET study. Neurobiol Aging. 2004;25(8):1051–6.

Kruger CE, Dean DL, Rosen HJ, Halabi C, Weiner M, Miller BL, et al. Longitudinal rates of lobar atrophy in frontotemporal dementia, semantic dementia, and Alzheimer's disease. Alzheimer Dis Assoc Disord. 2010;24(1):43–8.

Case 136
Normal Pressure Hydrocephalus

Ana M. Franceschi and Lev Bangiyev

History

A 72-year-old male presents with subacute progression of memory loss, shuffling gait, spasticity, and slightly enlarged ventricles on prior outside MRI (Fig. 136.1). PET/MRI was performed to evaluate for neurodegenerative disease.

Diagnosis

Normal pressure hydrocephalus

Findings

- T1 and T2 axial images show marked dilatation of the lateral cerebral ventricles.
- Congenital cavum septum pellucidum and vergae (thin arrows).
- T1 sagittal demonstrating bowing of the corpus callosum (curved arrow).
- PET fusion axial and sagittal images show preserved cortical radiotracer uptake with dilated ventricles.
- FLAIR fusion image demonstrates incidental small foci of hyperintense signal in the periventricular white matter characteristic of chronic microvascular disease (arrowheads).

Discussion

Normal pressure hydrocephalus (NPH) commonly presents with the typical triad of ataxia, dementia, and urinary incontinence. It is considered as one of the treatable causes of dementia. There are many theories for the etiology of NPH, but none have gained wide acceptance. Likely, there is abnormal resorption of cerebral spinal fluid that ultimately causes the disease. The development of symptoms in a patient with NPH has been explained by two major factors which are mechanical and ischemic. It has been hypothesized that high pulse pressure related to ventricular enlargement and decreased compliance leads to "shear stress."

Imaging plays an important role in confirming the diagnosis. Patients with suspected NPH should be assessed for structural abnormality including aqueductal stenosis or other obstructive lesions. Imaging studies typically show predominant enlargement of the lateral and third ventricles. The assessment of the Evans ratio, which is the maximal ventricular width divided by the largest biparietal distance of the skull extending between the inner tables, can be done on CT or MRI. A ratio greater than 0.3 is consistent with ventriculomegaly. The ventricular dilatation is also out of proportion to the sulcal size. Other

R. Gupta et al., *PET/MR Imaging*, https://doi.org/10.1007/978-3-319-65106-4_136

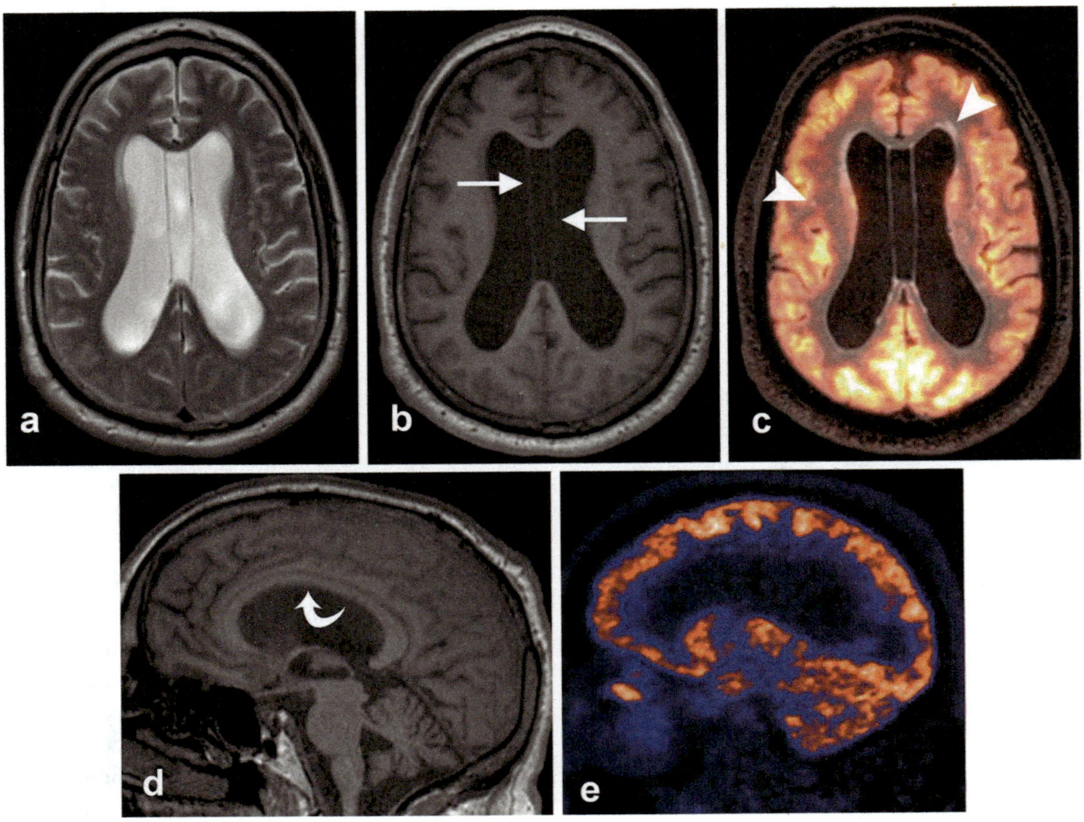

Fig. 136.1 T2 axial (**a**), T1 axial (**b**), PET/MR FLAIR axial fusion (**c**), T1 sagittal midline (**d**), and PET sagittal lateral to midline (**e**)

imaging findings that are suggestive of communicative hydrocephalus include rounding of the temporal horns, bowing of corpus callosum, crowding of the sulci at the vertex, and nonuniform dilatation of the sulci. In these patients, PET/MRI can be used to assess for neurodegenerative disease that may have cofounding or contributing effects on a patients symptoms. Cine phase-contrast MRI has utility in determining an NPH diagnosis. Patients with NPH show increased stroke volume that is suggestive of increased flow that might be the cause of shear stress on the periventricular tissue.

The most common of NPH includes CSF shunting. Prior to placement of a CSF shunt, patients may undergo a trial of CSF removal to predict response to shunting. This can be achieved by either performing a high volume lumbar puncture with removal of >30 ml of CSF or placement of an external lumbar drain. Gait is tested before and after the trial. Patients with predominant gait abnormality and ventriculomegaly show the best response to CSF shunting. Patients with increased white matter burden on MRI have decreased likelihood of improvement after CSF removal trial. Nuclear medicine CSF flow imaging with indium-111 DTPA is an alternative study used less frequently.

Suggested Reading

Bradley WG. Normal pressure hydrocephalus: new concepts on etiology and diagnosis. AJNR Am J Neuroradiol. 2000;21(9):1586–90.

Holodny AI, George AE, de Leon MJ, Golomb J, Kalnin AJ, Cooper PR. Focal dilation and paradoxical collapse of cortical fissures and sulci in patients with normal-pressure hydrocephalus. J Neurosurg. 1998;89(5):742–7.

Shprecher D, Schwalb J, Kurlan R. Normal pressure hydrocephalus: diagnosis and treatment. CurrNeurol Neurosci Rep. 2008;8(5):371–6.

Case 137
Brain Metastases

Anuj Rajput, Michael Goodman, and Lev Bangiyev

History

A 39-year-old female with bilateral breast cancer and suspicious lesions on CT of the brain (Fig. 137.1)

Diagnosis

Brain metastases

Findings

- Peripherally enhancing lesions in the cerebellar hemispheres (curved arrows) that are isointense to brain parenchyma on T1 and mildly hyperintense on T2 sequences. The lesions have central necrotic components characterized by nonenhancing T1 hypointense and T2 hyperintense signal.
- Two contrast-enhancing solid lesions in the cerebellar vermis (arrowhead) are noted.
- PET/MR-fusion image shows increased FDG uptake in the lesions of the cerebellar hemispheres and vertex.
- Additional peripherally enhancing lesion is seen in the right head of caudate nucleus (white arrow) with abnormal FDG uptake in the corresponding lesion that is brighter than the contralateral side caudate nucleus.

Discussion

In adults, metastases are by far the most common brain tumors. Lung cancer is the most common primary malignancy metastasizing to the brain, followed by breast cancer. Other malignancies that commonly metastasize to the brain include the skin, colon, pancreas, testes, ovary, cervix, renal cell carcinoma, and melanoma. The vast majority of patients with brain metastases are asymptomatic and detected by routine imaging during initial staging or follow-up imaging. The development of new neurologic symptoms in a patient with known malignancy can be a sign of brain metastases and should be further evaluated with neuroimaging. Symptoms may include headache, seizure, syncope, focal neurological deficit, or papilledema. Newly diagnosed asymptomatic or symptomatic brain metastases often alter the staging of certain malignancies, thereby changing treatment strategy.

MRI with and without contrast material is the imaging of choice for detection of brain metastases, offering high sensitivity and specificity. Brain metastases can be solitary in approximately 50% of the patients. The typical MRI characteristics of metastases include iso- to hypointense signal on T1-weighted images and hyperintense on T2-weighted images with enhancement follow-

R. Gupta et al., *PET/MR Imaging*, https://doi.org/10.1007/978-3-319-65106-4_137

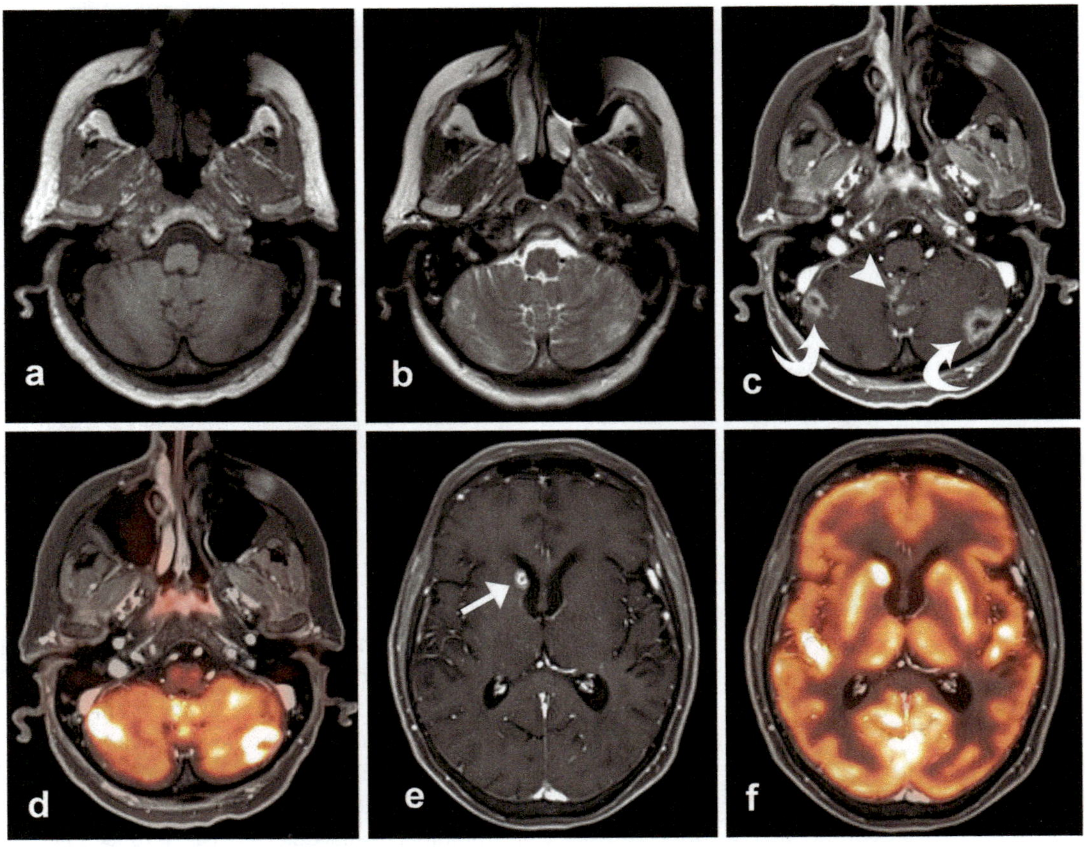

Fig. 137.1 T1 axial through the cerebellum (**a**), T2 axial through the cerebellum (**b**), T1 radial VIBE with fat suppression post-gadolinium contrast axial through the cerebellum (**c**), PET/MR T1 radial VIBE with fat suppression post-gadolinium contrast axial fusion through the cerebellum (**d**), T1 radial VIBE with fat suppression post-gadolinium contrast axial through the frontal horns (**e**), and PET/MR T1 radial VIBE with fat suppression post-gadolinium contrast axial fusion through the frontal horns (**f**)

ing contrast. There is often T2 hyperintense signal in the adjacent white matter consistent with surrounding edema. Metastatic lesions tend to arise at the gray-white matter junction.

PET/MR imaging is increasingly utilized, as a tool in the staging of cancers. FDG PET alone has been found to have lower sensitivity than MRI in detection of brain metastases due to normal high FDG uptake by cerebral cortex. Furthermore, metastases may have FDG uptake similar to the normal brain and have very low contrast or completely blend in with adjacent gray matter. In addition, FDG PET lacks sensitivity in demonstrating small lesions, with 40% probability that a 1 cm metastatic lesion will be detected and an increase to 90% only when the lesion is at least 1.8 cm. When combined with MRI, FDG PET whole-body imaging of cancer patients may include the entire head in the field of view instead of the standard PET/CT whole-body protocol from the base of the skull to the midthigh. Therefore, more effective cancer imaging including evaluation of the brain could be obtained with PET providing metabolic information and MRI allowing for superior tissue delineation and characterization of the findings.

Suggested Reading

Boss A, Bisdas S, Kolb A, Hofmann M, Ernemann U, Claussen CD, et al. Hybrid PET/MRI of intracranial masses: initial experiences and comparison to PET/CT. J Nucl Med. 2010;51(8):1198–205.

Fink KR, Fink JR. Imaging of brain metastases. Surg Neurol Int. 2013;4(Suppl 4):S209–19.

Partovi S, Kohan A, Rubbert C, Vercher-Conejero JL, Gaeta C, Yuh R, et al. Clinical oncologic applications of PET/MRI: a new horizon. Am J Nucl Med Mol Imaging. 2014;4(2):202–12.

Index

R. Gupta et al., *PET/MR Imaging*, https://doi.org/10.1007/978-3-319-65106-4